Practical Neurology Visual Review

SECOND EDITION

José Biller, MD, FACP, FAAN, FAHA
Professor and Chairman
Department of Neurology
Loyola University Chicago
Stritch School of Medicine
Maywood, Illinois

Alberto J. Espay, MD, MSc, FAAN
Associate Professor
Department of Neurology
University of Cincinnati
UC Neuroscience Institute
Cincinnati, Ohio

 Wolters Kluwer | Lippincott Williams & Wilkins
Health

Philadelphia • Baltimore • New York • London
Buenos Aires • Hong Kong • Sydney • Tokyo

Acquisitions Editor: Julie Goolsby
Product Manager: Tom Gibbons
Production Manager: David Saltzberg
Senior Manufacturing Manager: Benjamin Rivera
Marketing Manager: Alexander Burns
Design Coordinator: Holly McLaughlin
Production Service: SPi Global

Printed in China

Library of Congress Cataloging-in-Publication Data
Available upon request

ISBN 978-1-4511-8269-9

To purchase additional copies of this book, call our customer service department at (800) 638-3030 or
fax orders to (301) 223-2320. International customers should call (301) 223-2300.

Visit Lippincott Williams & Wilkins on the Internet: at LWW.com. Lippincott Williams & Wilkins
customer service representatives are available from 8:30 am to 6 pm, EST.

10 9 8 7 6 5 4 3 2 1

RRS1301

PREFACE

"We see what we look for."
"You can observe a lot by watching."—Yogi Berra

Neurologic problems are common in general medical practice and often are a heavy burden for patients and their families. Practitioners, residents/fellows in training, and medical students encounter these disorders with increasing frequency because of the growing size of the aging population.

Current assessment formats for residents/fellows and medical students' education underemphasize bedside teaching. Faculty members strained by the pressures of many competing demands may not be in a position to observe trainees performing physical examinations during their training.

The educational material offered in this second edition of *Practical Neurology Visual Review* provides new venues for teaching and learning the essentials of neurology by utilizing an interactive patient based (real-world situation) audiovisual electronic format (incorporating key semiological, neuroimaging, or other ancillary data when appropriate). One hundred thirty-one carefully edited video clips of patients with an array of commonly and unusually encountered neurological problems are used to teach the following fundamental principles of bedside neurology: (1) description and localization of findings, (2) differential diagnosis, (3) evaluation, (4) management, and (5) counseling. The first two items are considered essential aspects of knowledge, while the last three represent more advanced knowledge and skills. The cases range from the very easy to the very challenging in order to meet the needs of all segments of the intended audience. Each clinical vignette is accompanied by a balanced, practical, and succinct written discussion that includes basic learning objectives, an executive summary, and recommended reading material. As an added feature, most of the videos are also available via the QR codes printed in the book, which should work with most devices.

This audiovisual electronic teaching format may be somewhat unorthodox. However, it is actually more effective in its approach because the technology lends itself to displaying the skills necessary for a physician to form a patient's neurological diagnosis, which is largely based on an effective history, interpersonal communication, and visual information. It is important to acknowledge that the material contained here is not meant to represent an encyclopedic audiovisual electronic clinical neurology library. It is an interactive tool for learning and teaching relevant and practical neurology problems, narrated and demonstrated by real patients—not by actors or "simulated patients," as is the trend in current medical education.

To enhance the educational value, this visual review also includes 373 multiple-choice questions, with cross-references to the video clips and to the second edition of *Practical Neurology*.

On completion of this program, users will be able to recognize an improvement in their core knowledge of

- Neurologic examination and techniques
- Clinical reasoning

- Abstract problem solving
- Attentiveness
- Critical curiosity
- Evidence-based neurology

We hope that by stimulating interest and attention to the process of rational, systematic thinking, this educational material will bring the highest quality neurologic care to as many patients as possible and encourage medical students, residents, and fellows to elect careers in neurology.

José Biller, MD, FACP, FAAN, FAHA
Alberto J. Espay, MD, MSc, FAAN

ACKNOWLEDGMENT

We are forever indebted to each of our patients for enthusiastically agreeing to participate in this project. The editing and final production were the result of the efforts of a dedicated and highly talented and professional team. We especially thank Rocky Rothrock, for the countless hours of passionate video editing; Denise Mehner, from the Office of Visual Media at Indiana University School of Medicine; Tom Gibbons from Lippincott Williams & Wilkins, for his commitment to this product and constant encouragement Linda Turner, from Loyola University, for her extraordinary patience in the organization of the material and for her outstanding secretarial and administrative support; and to our colleagues at Indiana University, Loyola University, and University of Cincinnati.

We are especially grateful to our families for their unwavering support and selfless acceptance of the many hours the creation of this book took us away from their company:

My children, Sofia, Gabriel, and Rebecca; my stepchildren Adam and Emily; my wife Rhonda; and in particular my grandchildren Selim and Ira—JB

My children Isabelle, Samuel, and Elena; my stepchildren Landen and Caid; my lovely wife Kristy; and her nurturing parents Rick and Sue McClarnon—AE

CONTENTS

PREFACE   v

ACKNOWLEDGMENT   vii

SECTION **1** NEUROMUSCULAR   1

CASE 1   Bilateral Carpal Tunnel in Pregnancy   1

CASE 2   Ulnar Neuropathy at the Elbow   3

CASE 3   Combined Median and Ulnar Neuropathy   5

CASE 4   Peripheral Facial Nerve Palsy   7

CASE 5   Hypoglossal Nerve Palsy   9

CASE 6   Brachial Plexopathy (Parsonage-Turner Syndrome)   10

CASE 7   Polyneuropathy/Sensory Neuronopathy   12

CASE 8   L5 Radiculopathy (Disc Herniation)   14

CASE 9   Femoral Neuropathy   16

CASE 10   Foot Drop: History of Arthroscopic Surgery   19

CASE 11   Motor Neuron Disease   21

CASE 12   Myasthenia Gravis   23

CASE 13   Myotonic Dystrophy   25

SECTION **2** SPINAL CORD   27

CASE 14   Posttraumatic Cervical Syringomyelia   27

CASE 15   Lumbar Myelomeningocele/Spina Bifida   29

CASE 16   Cervical Myelopathy (Sarcoidosis)   31

CASE 17   Autoimmune Myelopathy (Stiff Person Syndrome)   33

CASE 18   Ischemic Myelopathy (Antiphospholipid Antibody Syndrome)   36

CASE 19   Paraparesis After Nitrous Oxide Anesthesia   39

SECTION **3** BEHAVIORAL NEUROLOGY   41

CASE 20 Nonfluent Aphasia Secondary to Left Frontal Infarction   41

CASE 21 Nonfluent Aphasia Secondary to LICA Occlusion   44

CASE 22 Fluent Aphasia Secondary to Left Posterior Temporal Infarction   46

CASE 23 Wernicke Aphasia Secondary to Left MCA Infarction   48

CASE 24 Primary Progressive Aphasia   50

CASE 25 Frontotemporal Dementia   52

CASE 26 Alien Hand Syndrome Secondary to Left Frontal/ Callosal Infarction   54

CASE 27 Alexia Without Agraphia   55

CASE 28 Gerstmann Plus Syndrome   56

CASE 29 Anterior Opercular Syndrome (Foix-Chavany-Marie)   58

CASE 30 Amnesia (PCA Infarct)   60

CASE 31 Dementia (Early Alzheimer Disease)   62

CASE 32 Dementia (Late Alzheimer Disease)   64

CASE 33 Dementia with Lewy Bodies   66

SECTION **4** CEREBROVASCULAR   70

CASE 34 Asymptomatic Carotid Artery Stenosis   70

CASE 35 Vertebrobasilar TIAs: Basilar Artery Stenosis   72

CASE 36 Dysphagia/Imbalance: Vertebral Artery Stenosis   74

CASE 37 Pure Motor Hemiparesis Due to Capsular Lacunar Infarction   76

CASE 38 Ataxic Hemiparesis Due to Pontine Infarction   77

CASE 39 Left Internal Carotid Artery Dissection   79

CASE 40 Wallenberg Syndrome Secondary to Vertebral Artery Dissection   81

CASE 41 Multiple Cerebral Infarctions Due to Antiphospholipid Antibody Syndrome   82

CASE 42 Pseudobulbar Palsy (Multiple Strokes)   83

CASE 43 Watershed Infarcts   84

CASE 44 Moyamoya Syndrome Associated with Down Syndrome   86

CASE 45 Takayasu Arteritis   87

CASE 46 Recurrent Facial Palsies (VZV) Followed by Cerebral Infarction   89

CASE 47 Multiple Lobar Hemorrhages Due to Cerebral Amyloid Angiopathy   90

CASE 48 Pure Sensory Stroke Due to Thalamic Hemorrhage   92

CASE 49 Lacunar Hemichoreoathetosis   94

CASE 50 Alexia Without Agraphia Due to Biopsy-Negative Primary CNS Angiitis   96

CASE 51 Superior Sagittal Sinus Thrombosis   99

SECTION 5 MOVEMENT DISORDERS   102

CASE 52 Resting Tremor (and a "Stroke of Luck")   102

CASE 53 Essential Tremor   103

CASE 54 Dystonic Tremor   105

CASE 55 Parkinson Disease   108

CASE 56 Multiple System Atrophy, Parkinsonian Type   111

CASE 57 Corticobasal Syndrome (Corticobasal Degeneration)   113

CASE 58 Progressive Supranuclear Palsy   115

CASE 59 Cervical Dystonia   118

CASE 60 Cerebral Palsy/Dystonia   121

CASE 61 Palatal Tremor Due to Medullary Infarction   122

CASE 62 Hemichorea–Hemiballism   124

CASE 63 Paraneoplastic Chorea/Sensory Neuronopathy   127

CASE 64 Hemifacial Spasm   128

CASE 65 Tic Disorder   130

CASE 66 Hemidystonia (Sarcoidosis)   132

CASE 67 Acute Dystonic Reaction   133

SECTION 6 CEREBELLAR DISORDERS   136

CASE 68 Ataxia Due to Bilateral PICA Infarctions   136

CASE 69 Friedreich Ataxia   138

CASE 70   Cerebellar Ataxia   141

CASE 71   Hereditary Ataxia   143

CASE 72   Spinocerebellar Ataxia Type 3   145

CASE 73   Multiple System Atrophy, Cerebellar Type   147

CASE 74   Lipid Storage Ataxia: Niemann-Pick Type C   149

SECTION **7** DEMYELINATING DISORDERS   151

CASE 75   Bilateral Internuclear Ophthalmoplegia Secondary
to Multiple Sclerosis   151

CASE 76   Nystagmus/Ataxia Secondary to Relapsing–Remitting
Multiple Sclerosis   153

CASE 77   Multiple Sclerosis (Pontine Lesion)   155

CASE 78   Spastic Gait/Dysarthria due to Primary Progressive
Multiple Sclerosis   157

SECTION **8** NEURO-OPHTHALMOLOGY   159

CASE 79   Horner Syndrome in Patient with Wallenberg
Syndrome   159

CASE 80   Adie Tonic Pupil/Ross Syndrome   161

CASE 81   Nonarteritic Anterior Ischemic Optic Neuropathy   163

CASE 82   Postoperative Acute Left CN III Palsy   164

CASE 83   Progressive Left CN III Palsy Secondary to Cavernous
Sinus Mass Lesion   167

CASE 84   Abducens Palsy   168

CASE 85   Chronic Progressive External Ophthalmoplegia   170

CASE 86   Right Homonymous Hemianopsia Due
to PCA Infarct   172

CASE 87   Upbeat Nystagmus: Wernicke Encephalopathy   174

SECTION **9** NEUROINFECTIOUS DISEASES   177

CASE 88   Herpes Zoster (Postherpetic Neuralgia)   177

CASE 89   Recurrent Aseptic Meningitis   178

CASE 90   Postencephalitic Parkinsonism   180

CASE 91   Creutzfeldt-Jakob Disease   182

SECTION **10** NEUROOTOLOGY   185

CASE 92   Vertigo/Imbalance Secondary to Isolated Vermian Infarction   185

CASE 93   Deafness/Tinnitus Secondary to Vestibular (Acoustic) Schwannoma   187

CASE 94   Vertiginous Dizziness   189

CASE 95   Benign Paroxysmal Positional Vertigo   191

SECTION **11** NUTRITIONAL/METABOLIC   194

CASE 96   Wernicke Encephalopathy Secondary to Hyperemesis Gravidarum   194

CASE 97   Cerebrotendinous Xanthomatosis   196

SECTION **12** HEADACHES/PAIN   198

CASE 98   Migraine Headaches/Pregnancy   198

CASE 99   Cluster Headaches   199

CASE 100   CSF Hypotension Syndrome   201

CASE 101   Idiopathic Intracranial Hypertension   203

CASE 102   Trigeminal Neuralgia   205

CASE 103   Atypical Facial Pain   206

SECTION **13** EPILEPSY AND SPELLS   209

CASE 104   Partial Complex Seizures   209

CASE 105   Partial Seizures with Elementary Symptomatology   211

CASE 106   Tuberous Sclerosis Complex   213

CASE 107   Epilepsia Partialis Continua   215

CASE 108   Frontal Lobe Epilepsy   217

CASE 109   Cough Syncope   219

SECTION **14** SLEEP MEDICINE   221

CASE 110   Obstructive Sleep Apnea   221

SECTION **15** GAIT   224

CASE 111   Lower-Body Parkinsonism (Gait Apraxia)   224

CASE 112   Vascular Parkinsonism and Normal Pressure Hydrocephalus   226

CASE 113   Hemiplegic Gait/Spasticity   230

CASE 114   Hemiparkinsonian Gait   232

CASE 115   Adult-Onset Dystonic Gait   234

CASE 116   Psychogenic Gait   236

SECTION **16** NEURO-ONCOLOGY   238

CASE 117   Leptomeningeal Malignancy (Lymphoma)   238

CASE 118   Paraneoplastic Chorea   240

SECTION **17** NEUROLOGIC EMERGENCIES/URGENCIES   243

CASE 119   Acute Cerebellar Infarction (PICA) with Early Hydrocephalus   243

CASE 120   Iatrogenic Emergencies   245

SECTION **18** BORDERLAND BETWEEN NEUROLOGY AND PSYCHIATRY   247

CASE 121   Conversion Disorder (Psychogenic Gait)   247

CASE 122   Somatization Disorder (Psychogenic Stuttering)   248

CASE 123   Psychogenic Tremor   250

SECTION **19** BORDERLAND BETWEEN NEUROLOGY AND MEDICINE   253

CASE 124   Post–Cardiac Arrest Syndrome   253

CASE 125   Tetany in Electrolytic Derangement   256

CASE 126   Acquired Neuromyotonia in Rheumatologic Disease   257

SECTION **20** CLINICOPATHOLOGIC CORRELATIONS   260

CASE 127   Primary CNS Angiitis   260

CASE 128   Cerebrotendinous Xanthomatosis   262

CASE 129   Polymyositis/Myasthenia Gravis   264

CASE 130   Multiple System Atrophy, Cerebellar Type   266

CASE 131   Neoplastic Brachial Plexopathy   269

REVIEW QUESTIONS AND ANSWERS   272

INDEX   323

SECTION 1

NEUROMUSCULAR

CASE 1

BILATERAL CARPAL TUNNEL IN PREGNANCY

OBJECTIVES

- To name the nerve affected in carpal tunnel syndrome.
- To name the most common symptoms of carpal tunnel syndrome.
- To name the most useful diagnostic tests to confirm carpal tunnel syndrome.
- To name the most common treatments for carpal tunnel syndrome.

VIGNETTE

A 32-year-old woman, G1, P0, 38-week gestation, complained of bilateral hand numbness and pain for the last 2 weeks.

CASE SUMMARY

Hand numbness or paresthesias are the most common presenting symptoms of median neuropathy at the wrist (carpal tunnel syndrome). At an incidence of 3.4% in the United States, this is the most common entrapment mononeuropathy. The median nerve is entrapped at the carpal tunnel of the wrist, a narrow fibroosseous tunnel made up on the sides and floor by carpal bones and on the roof by the transverse carpal ligament. The most common symptoms are wrist, hand, and arm pain associated with hand paresthesias. The pain typically is worse at night, disturbing sleep. The paresthesias are most frequently present in the thumb, index finger, middle finger, and radial half of the ring finger. Nocturnal symptoms are often improved by shaking of the hand. Symptoms may be noted with such activities as driving, typing, or holding a phone. Carpal tunnel syndrome is also a common condition in pregnancy (as in our patient), particularly in the last 3 months of pregnancy.

1

The incidence of preeclampsia in pregnant women with carpal tunnel syndrome ranges between 9% and 20%.

Paresthesias may be elicited by gentle tapping over the median nerve (Tinel sign: 50% sensitivity and 77% specificity) or by having the patient hold the wrist in a flexed position (Phalen maneuver: 68% sensitivity and 73% specificity). Weakness of the median inner-vated muscles, especially the abductor pollicis brevis (APB), may be present. Atrophy of the thenar eminence may be noted in more severe cases. Nerve conduction studies and electromyography (EMG) are the most useful tests to confirm the diagnosis. The most common treatments include removal of provoking factors, nonsteroidal anti-inflamma-tory drugs (NSAIDs), and wrist splinting at night in a neutral position. Corticosteroid injections may offer temporary relief. If conservative treatment is unsuccessful or signs of thenar muscle atrophy and weakness develop, surgical decompression (open or endo-scopic) is recommended.

The median entrapment at the wrist by definition spares the anterior interosseous nerve, a branch of the median nerve just 4 cm distal to the medial epicondyle, which supplies the flexor pollicis longus and flexor digitorum profundus to the index and mid-dle fingers, and allows the flexion of these fingers' distal interphalangeal joints. Hence, patients with carpal tunnel syndrome should retain the ability to make an "OK" sign against resistance by the examiner. A lesion involving the anterior interosseous nerve results in an alternative grip pattern when patients are asked to pinch a sheet of paper between the thumb and index fingers using only the fingertips. In this case, the distal finger joints remain uselessly extended while the effort of pinching is transferred to the proximal thumb, whose intact ulnar-supplied adducting power (adductor pollicis) allows it to press the sheet of paper against the intact ulnar-supplied abducting power of the index finger (dorsal interosseous). This pattern of weakness due to anterior interosseous neuropathy is known as the Kiloh-Nevin syndrome (Fig. 1.1).

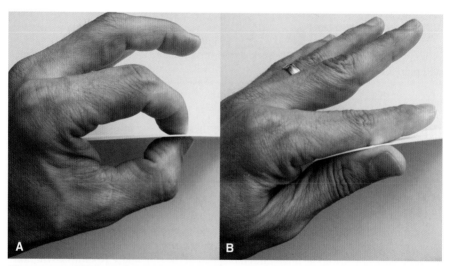

Figure 1.1   Kiloh-Nevin Syndrome. The fingertips suffice to pinch a sheet of paper between the first two fingers, assuming an intact anterior interosseous nerve **(A)**. An alterna-tive, compensatory grip pattern emerges when the distal finger flexors of the first two fingers are weak due to anterior interosseous neuropathy **(B)**.

SELECTED REFERENCES

Biller J, ed. *Practical neurology*, 4th ed. Philadelphia: Lippincott Williams & Wilkins, Wolters Kluwer Health, 2012:Chapter 24.

Espay AJ, Biller J. *Concise neurology*. Philadelphia: Lippincott Williams & Wilkins, Wolters Kluwer Health, 2011:Chapter 9.

Katz JN, Simmons BP. Carpal tunnel syndrome. *N Engl J Med* 2002;346:1807–1812.

MacDermid JC, Wessel J. Clinical diagnosis of carpal tunnel syndrome: a systematic review. *J Hand Ther* 2004;17(2):309–319.

SEE QUESTIONS: 3, 16, 17, 57, 79

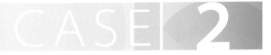

ULNAR NEUROPATHY AT THE ELBOW

OBJECTIVES

- To name the most common symptoms of an ulnar neuropathy.
- To name the most useful diagnostic test to confirm an ulnar neuropathy.
- To name the most common site of compression or irritation of the ulnar nerve.
- To name the most common treatments for ulnar neuropathy.

VIGNETTE

Following a bilateral hernia operation, this 70-year-old man complained of paresthesias on the fourth and fifth digits of his left hand. He also noticed some decrease in grip strength of that hand.

CASE SUMMARY

Ulnar neuropathy is the second most common entrapment neuropathy. The ulnar nerve can be compressed at a variety of sites along its course from the brachial plexus to the hand. By far the most common site of compression is at the elbow where the nerve passes through a fibroosseous canal called the cubital tunnel. The most common sensory symptoms are numbness and paresthesias of the medial forearm, medial hand, fifth digit, and ulnar half of the fourth digit. An early manifestation of ulnar neuropathy is characterized by the inability of the small finger to fully adduct and touch the ring finger (Wartenberg sign). Motor symptoms such as decreased hand dexterity or impaired typing or playing a musical instrument most commonly result from weakness of intrinsic hand muscles. Atrophy of the hypothenar eminence or first dorsal interosseous muscle may be noted (Fig. 2.1). In chronic ulnar neuropathy, paresis of interossei and ulnar lumbricals causes a "claw hand" deformity (Fig. 2.1A). Weakness of the adductor pollicis muscle results in the Froment's prehensile thumb sign, as patients increase pinch grip by relying on the distal flexion of

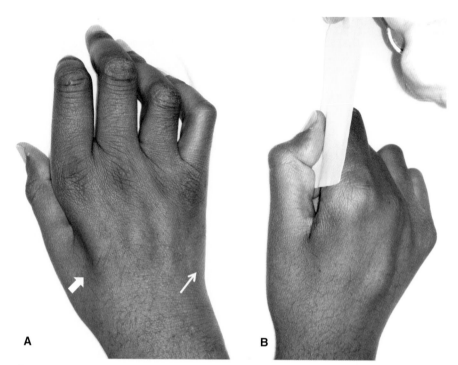

Figure 2.1   Ulnar Neuropathy. Atrophy of intrinsic hand muscles with characteristic "claw hand" deformity **(A)**, particularly marked in the first dorsal interosseous (*thick arrow*) and abductor digiti minimi in the hypothenar eminence (*thin arrow*). The Froment's prehensile thumb sign **(B)** is elicited by asking patients to pinch a sheet of paper between the proximal thumb and index finger. The patient with a weak ulnar-innervated adductor pollicis muscle increases the grip by distally flexing the thumb through the power of an intact anterior interosseous-supplied flexor pollicis longus ("reverse" Kiloh-Nevin syndrome).

the thumb ("reverse" Kiloh-Nevin syndrome), innervated by the anterior interosseous nerve (Fig. 2.1B). This pattern of weakness is different from that of median neuropathy at the wrist (Fig. 2.2). Proximal ulnar nerve lesions result in weakness of ulnar wrist flexion and terminal phalanges of the fourth and fifth fingers. Sensory deficits beyond 2 cm above the wrist localize the lesion to the T1 root, the medial cord, or the medial cutaneous nerve of arm and forearm. Electromyography (EMG) and nerve conduction studies are the most useful tests to confirm the diagnosis.

Conservative treatments such as avoidance of repetitive elbow flexion and extension or direct pressure on the elbow, perhaps adding padded elbow protectors and nonsteroidal anti-inflammatory drugs (NSAIDs), are used first. Surgical options can be explored if conservative measures fail. As in our patient, ulnar neuropathies have been associated with surgical procedures and general anesthesia. Diabetes is a frequent predisposing factor. Controversy exists as to the importance of patient positioning during surgery as a cause of perioperative ulnar neuropathy.

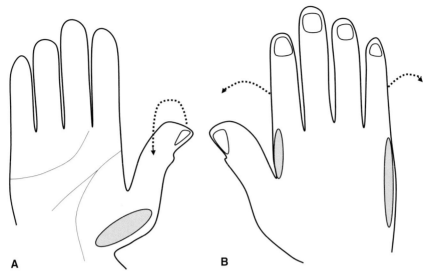

Figure 2.2 **Location of Key Muscles in the Assessment of Hand Weakness.** Median entrapment at the wrist **(A)** most commonly causes weakness in the abductor pollicis brevis (APB). Associated weakness in the deep flexor of the index (flexor digitorum profundus I) and thumb (flexor pollicis longus) indicates a lesion at the elbow, affecting the anterior interosseous nerve. Ulnar neuropathy **(B)** most often causes weakness and atrophy in the first dorsal interosseous (FDI) and abductor digiti minimi (ADM). Associated weakness of the deep flexor of the little finger (flexor digitorum profundus IV) and ulnar wrist (flexor carpi ulnaris), with loss of sensation in medial hand, indicates a lesion at the elbow, affecting the proximal ulnar nerve. (Adapted with permission from Espay AJ, Biller J. *Concise neurology.* Philadelphia: Lippincott Williams & Wilkins, Wolters Kluwer Health, 2011:Chapter 9.)

SELECTED REFERENCES

Biller J, ed. *Practical neurology*, 4th ed. Philadelphia: Lippincott Williams & Wilkins, Wolters Kluwer Health, 2012:Chapter 24.

Goldman SB. A review of clinical tests and signs for the assessment of ulnar neuropathy. *J Hand Ther* 2009;22(3):209–220.

SEE QUESTIONS: 3, 4, 16, 57, 80, 81, 261, 262

CASE **3**

COMBINED MEDIAN AND ULNAR NEUROPATHY

OBJECTIVES

- To identify localizing features when dual neuropathy is present.
- To name the most useful clinical tests that distinguish ulnar from median neuropathy.
- To emphasize the importance of a thorough examination in patients with hand weakness.

After a traumatic injury several years ago, complicated with multiple fractures in the left arm, this 36-year-old man presented with chronic hand weakness (Fig. 3.1). The posture at rest (A–C) showed thenar and hypothenar atrophy with flexion of the third through fifth fingers, associated with contractures (mechanical restriction of the interphalangeal joints to passive extension, C). Forced flexion is only preserved for the distal phalanges of the first (flexor pollicis longus) as well as second through fifth fingers (flexor digitorum

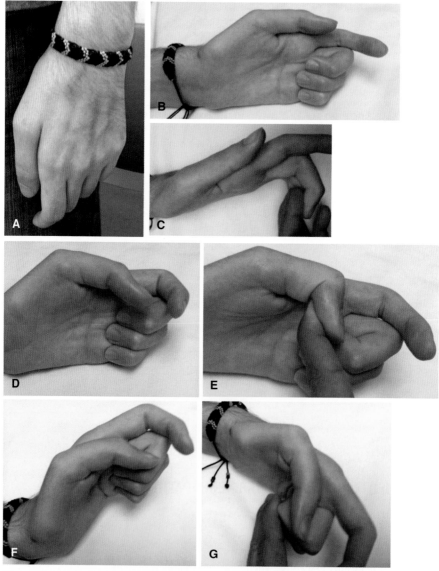

Figure 3.1   Findings in a Case of Chronic Hand Weakness. The examination showed thenar and hypothenar atrophy, wrist flexion weakness, and flexion contractures of third through fifth fingers, with preservation of distal finger flexion and wrist extension.

profundus) (D, E). Wrist extension is normal (F), but wrist flexion is compromised as only minimal resistance overcomes the flexion effort (G). There is some ulnar deviation when wrist flexion is attempted. There was hypesthesia to light touch and temperature in the ulnar aspect of the palm but not above the wrist, in the distal forearm.

CASE SUMMARY

The overall pattern of weakness suggests a partial proximal median nerve injury (with preservation of the anterior interosseous nerve) and distal ulnar nerve injury. The flexor digitorum superficialis (proximal median nerve) is compromised, but the flexor digitorum profundus (anterior interosseous nerve) is not. All thenar muscles (first two lumbricals, opponens pollicis, abductor pollicis brevis, and flexor pollicis brevis) are affected.

The atrophy of interossei and ulnar lumbricals yields a "claw hand," fully expressed in ulnar neuropathy. The preservation of ulnar deviation on wrist flexion (flexor carpi ulnaris) and flexion of the fourth and fifth fingers (flexor digitorum profundus III and IV) suggests preservation of the proximal ulnar nerve. If sensory deficits were to have extended 2 cm above the wrist, the lesion would have been localized to the T1 root, the medial cord, or the medial cutaneous nerve of the arm and forearm.

The adductor pollicis brevis is also weak, and the patient compensates by flexing the distal phalanx of the thumb. Weakness of adductor pollicis results in the Froment's prehensile thumb sign, whereby distal flexion of the thumb is used to increase pinch grip ("reverse" Kiloh-Nevin syndrome). Adductor pollicis and deep head of flexor pollicis brevis are the only thenar muscles regularly supplied by the ulnar nerve.

SELECTED REFERENCES

Biller J, ed. *Practical neurology*, 4th ed. Philadelphia: Lippincott Williams and Wilkins, Wolters Kluwer Health, 2012:Chapter 24.

Espay AJ, Biller J. *Concise neurology*. Philadelphia: Lippincott Williams & Wilkins, Wolters Kluwer Health, 2011:Chapter 9.

SEE QUESTIONS: 3, 4, 16, 57, 80, 81, 261, 262

CASE 4

PERIPHERAL FACIAL NERVE PALSY

OBJECTIVES

- To name the most common symptoms of facial nerve palsy.
- To name the distinguishing characteristics of an upper motor neuron and a lower motor neuron facial weakness.
- To emphasize the importance of a thorough otoneurologic examination in patients suspected of having Bell palsy.
- To name the most common treatments for Bell palsy.

VIGNETTE

A 65-year-old man with a history of carcinoid tumor had new onset of left facial weakness.

CASE SUMMARY

The facial nerve is a mixed motor-sensory and parasympathetic nerve supplying the muscles of facial expression, mucous membranes of the oral and nasal cavities, and salivary and lacrimal glands. It also conveys taste sensation from the anterior two-thirds of the tongue via the lingual nerve and chorda tympani. Sudden facial weakness over the course of a few hours is the most common symptom of a peripheral facial nerve palsy. Pain around the ear or mastoid region may be present. Patients may also complain of numbness or an unusual sensation of the face, but sensory testing should be normal. Depending upon the site of the lesion, there may be associated impairment of taste, lacrimation, or hyperacusis. Taste may be impaired if the lesion is proximal to the chorda tympani. Patients may complain of a metallic taste of the mouth. Sounds may be exaggerated (hyperacusis) if a lesion is proximal to the nerve branch supplying the stapedius muscle, which typically helps dampen loud sounds. Not uncommonly, patients may also have variable degrees of eye dryness.

Our patient had idiopathic peripheral facial paralysis or Bell palsy. Bell palsy is the most common cause of acute facial paralysis. Bell palsy is more common in adults, in patients with diabetes mellitus, and among pregnant women. Herpes simplex virus activation has been suspected as an inciting factor. Atypical facial palsy (longer latency to peak severity and facial hypesthesia) may not be idiopathic but instead result from other causes, such as infections, tumors, or granulomatous diseases (Table 4.1). Early treatment with prednisolone improves the chances of complete recovery, but there is no evidence supporting the use of acyclovir alone or in combination with prednisolone. Artificial tears during the day and lubricating ophthalmic ointment at night are recommended to prevent the complications of corneal exposure. Synkinetic movements may emerge as late complications of Bell palsy.

TABLE 4.1   SECONDARY CAUSES OF FACIAL PALSY

Category	Etiologies
Infections	HSV, HZV
	Lyme disease
	Leprosy
Tumors	Facial nerve neuromas
	Other tumors causing facial nerve compression
Granulomatous diseases	Sarcoidosis
	Melkersson-Rosenthal syndrome

HSV, herpes simplex virus; HZV, herpes zoster virus

SELECTED REFERENCES

Biller J, ed. *Practical neurology*, 4th ed. Philadelphia: Lippincott Williams & Wilkins, Wolters Kluwer Health, 2012:Chapter 15.

Sullivan FM, Swan IRC, Donnan PT, et al. Early treatment with prednisolone or acyclovir in Bell's palsy. *N Engl J Med* 2007;357:1598–1607.

SEE QUESTIONS: 84, 152, 153, 173, 190, 235, 250

CASE **5**

HYPOGLOSSAL NERVE PALSY

- To name the location of the hypoglossal nucleus.
- To name the most common signs and symptoms of hypoglossal nerve palsy.
- To name the most common causes of hypoglossal nerve palsy.

Hypoglossal nerve dysfunction may be supranuclear, nuclear, or infranuclear. A 60-year-old woman developed new-onset vertex headache radiating to the left orbital region, left auricular region, left retromandibular area, and left posterior neck. She also had trouble chewing, swallowing, and controlling her tongue. Her tongue was atrophic on the left.

The hypoglossal nerve (CN XII) provides motor innervation to the intrinsic and extrinsic muscles of the tongue. The hypoglossal nucleus is located in the dorsomedial medulla. The hypoglossal fibers exit the medulla in the preolivary sulcus. The hypoglossal nerve exits the skull through the hypoglossal canal located just above the foramen magnum. Its course is divided into the following segments: medullary, cisternal, skull base, nasopharyngeal/oropharyngeal carotid space, and sublingual segments.

CN XII palsy is uncommon. A unilateral lesion, as in our patient, often leads to difficulty controlling the tongue when chewing, speaking, or sometimes swallowing. Unilateral lesions cause deviation of the tongue to the affected side as contralateral tongue protrusion is weakly opposed or unopposed. Examination of the tongue demonstrates ipsilateral tongue atrophy and fasciculations.

Supranuclear CN XII lesions result in paralysis of the tongue contralateral to the side of the lesion and do not result in denervation atrophy of the tongue musculature as seen in our patient, which resulted from a solitary fibrous tumor. Tumors, predominantly malignant, are the most common cause of unilateral hypoglossal nerve palsy. CN XII palsy may also occur in multiple sclerosis, Guillain-Barré syndrome, trauma, stroke, carotid artery dissections, aneurysms, basilar artery ectasia, surgery, nasopharyngeal carcinoma, metastases, rheumatoid arthritis, and infections.

SELECTED REFERENCES

Keane JR. Twelfth nerve palsy. Analysis of 100 cases. *Arch Neurol* 1996;53:561–566.

Thompson EO, Smoker WRK. Hypoglossal nerve palsy: a segmental approach. *Radiographics* 1994;14: 939–958.

SEE QUESTIONS: 84, 235

CASE 6

BRACHIAL PLEXOPATHY (PARSONAGE-TURNER SYNDROME)

OBJECTIVES

- To review pertinent applied anatomy of the brachial plexus.
- To analyze most common etiologies of brachial plexopathies.
- To review current ancillary evaluation techniques of brachial plexus lesions.
- To briefly discuss the clinical presentation and prognosis of idiopathic brachial plexitis (Parsonage-Turner syndrome).

VIGNETTE

A 53-year-old man complained of right arm weakness.

CASE SUMMARY

Evaluation and management of brachial plexopathies require a thorough knowledge of neuroanatomy. The brachial plexus is formed from the ventral primary rami (spinal nerves or roots) of C5 through T1. A prefixed plexus (when C4 contributes a branch to the brachial plexus) is seen in approximately two-thirds of cases. The brachial plexus is divided into five major components: (a) roots, (b) trunks (upper, middle, and lower), (c) divisions (anterior and posterior), (d) cords (lateral, posterior, and medial), and (e) branches. Typically, the brachial plexus is composed of five roots, three trunks, six divisions (two for each trunk), and three cords (see Fig. 131.1).

Brachial plexus injuries may be complete or incomplete. Injuries may be preganglionic (proximal to the spinal ganglion) or postganglionic. Plexus injuries can result in muscle weakness, neck and shoulder pain, paresthesias or dysesthesias, absent muscle stretch reflexes, and sensory loss. Despite some clinical variations, application of full pressure sensation to the thumb evaluates the corresponding C6 spinal nerve, median nerve, and lateral cord; application of deep pressure to the middle finger evaluates the corresponding C7 spinal nerve, median nerve, and lateral cord; and application of deep pressure to the little finger evaluates the corresponding C8 spinal nerve, ulnar nerve, and the medial cord.

Motor signs are often more prominent than sensory changes. Clinically relevant motor function to be tested should include shoulder abduction (C5); elbow flexion, forearm pronation and supination (C6); extensors of the forearm, hand, and fingers (C7); finger extensors, finger flexors, and wrist flexors (C8); and hand intrinsics (T1).

In our patient, motor signs involved predominantly the deltoid, biceps, brachioradialis, supraspinatus, and infraspinatus and were consistent with an upper plexus lesion. Sensation was intact. The biceps and brachioradialis reflexes were depressed on the involved side.

High-energy trauma to the upper extremity and neck can cause a variety of lesions of the brachial plexus. Upper trunk brachial plexopathies (Erb-Duchenne type, C5-6) may result from traumatic fall onto the side of the head and shoulder with avulsion of the superior aspect of the brachial plexus, or even separation of the head and shoulder

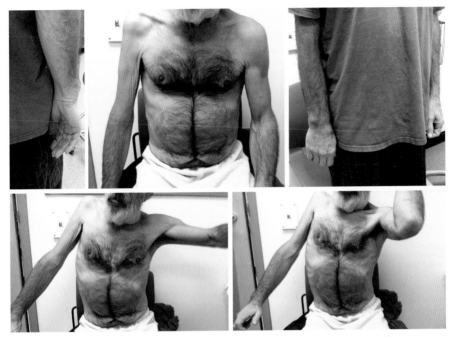

Figure 6.1   Findings in a Case of Right Arm Weakness Due to Traumatic Upper Trunk Brachial Plexopathy. This 52-year-old man became unable to abduct the right arm and flex the elbow after a fall injury 2 years prior to this evaluation. His examination showed severe weakness of arm abduction and elbow flexion in the right arm with wasting of the deltoid and biceps muscles. Biceps and brachioradialis reflexes were absent; supra- and infraspinatus were also involved. There was no wasting or weakness of the hands. Sensation was normal. The right arm was held internally rotated and adducted relative to the left, giving it a "porter's tip" position, classical of upper plexopathy (Erb-Duchenne palsy).

(Fig. 6.1). Birth injury may be a more common presentation, but no cause can be found in cases of idiopathic brachial plexitis (also known as neuralgic amyotrophy or Parsonage-Turner syndrome), as in the vignette patient.

Parsonage-Turner syndrome is an idiopathic brachial plexopathy most commonly seen in young adults and characterized by intense, usually unilateral neck and shoulder pain, with shoulder girdle and proximal arm weakness and atrophy. Involvement of the phrenic nerve may also be seen. Most cases are sporadic and thought to be an immune-mediated inflammatory process. An unusual familial form occurs as an autosomal dominant variety linked to mutations in the *SEPT9* gene on chromosome 17q.

The prognosis of patients with Parsonage-Turner syndrome is generally good, with a slow but progressive recovery over 6 to 18 months. Diagnosis can be substantiated by electrophysiologic testing and magnetic resonance imaging (MRI) of the brachial plexus.

MRI is a useful tool for the diagnosis of postganglionic brachial plexus lesions. MR imaging findings are normal in cases of Parsonage-Turner syndrome. Treatment is largely symptomatic; corticosteroids may be effective with pain control. Lower brachial plexopathies (Dejerine-Klumpke, C8 and T1) often result from trauma, especially arm traction in the abducted position, or malignancies (Pancoast tumor). Lower trunk or medial cord involvement is among the most common peripheral nervous system complications of coronary artery bypass graft surgery.

SELECTED REFERENCES

Bilbey JH, Lamond RG, Mattrey RT. MR imaging of disorders of the brachial plexus. *J Magn Reson Imaging* 1994;4(1):13–18.

Kuhlenbäumer G, Hannibal MC, Nelis E, et al. Mutations in SEPT9 cause hereditary neuralgic amyotrophy. *Nat Genet* 2005;37(10):1044–1046.

Van Eijk JJ, Van Alfen N, Berrevoets M, et al. Evaluation of prednisone treatment in the acute phase of neuralgic amyotrophy: an observational study. *J Neurol Neurosurg Psychiatry* 2009;80:1120–1124.

SEE QUESTIONS: 4, 16, 79, 81, 82, 91

CASE 7

POLYNEUROPATHY/SENSORY NEURONOPATHY

OBJECTIVES

- To review the differential diagnosis of progressive sensory neuronopathy.
- To list empirical treatment options for immune-mediated peripheral neuropathy.
- To summarize treatment options for chronic neuropathic pain.

VIGNETTE

A 37-year-old woman had problems with numbness, tingling, and weakness on her feet. Symptoms gradually progressed to the point where she became wheelchair bound. She also lost about 60 to 70 pounds.

CASE SUMMARY

This 37-year-old woman had a 1-year history of progressive painful numbness and tingling, initially in the feet and legs and subsequently spreading into the hands and face. She had symmetrical distal sensory loss including profound deficits of position and vibratory sense. Muscle stretch reflexes were absent. She had a severe sensory ataxia with a positive Romberg sign. Sural nerve biopsy demonstrated demyelination but no inflammation.

Causes of sensory ataxia include posterior-column myelopathies, sensory ganglionopathies (non–length-dependent proprioceptive and vibratory sensory deprivation), and demyelinating autoimmune polyneuropathies (Table 7.1). Sensory ataxias are not an early manifestation of axonal distal peripheral neuropathies. A considerable number of patients have no identifiable explanation. In our patient, there was a past history of psychiatric disease as well as dramatic weight loss prior to the onset of symptoms. The psychiatric history should raise concerns of a possible toxic exposure, as well as the possibility for an underlying connective tissue disease such as systemic lupus erythematosus (SLE). Our patient had been screened for these conditions with Anti-Hu serology, Anti-Ro

TABLE 7.1 **CAUSES OF SENSORY ATAXIAS**

Localization	Classification	Etiologies
Posterior column	Myelopathies	**Friedreich ataxia** **Metabolic** (Vitamin B_{12} deficiency,[a] folate deficiency,[a] vitamin E deficiency,[a] copper deficiency,[a] POLG1 mutation) **Toxic** (Nitrous oxide myeloneuropathy,[a] clioquinol [antiprotozoal hydroxyquinoline], cassava ingestion) **Infectious** (human immunodeficiency virus [HIV] and human T-cell lymphotropic virus [HTLV] myelopathies, tabes dorsalis) Compressive/vascular myelopathy
Sensory ganglia	Sensory neuronopathies or ganglionopathies	**Metabolic** (thiamine [B_1] deficiency[b]) **Paraneoplastic** (Subacute sensory neuronopathy due to anti-Hu and anti-CV2/CRMP5 antibodies) **Autoimmune** (Sjögren syndrome, Miller-Fisher syndrome; and Bickerstaff brainstem encephalitis) **Drugs** (cisplatin, pyridoxine [B_6] intoxication) **Inherited** disorders with degeneration of dorsal root ganglion cells.
Peripheral nerves	Immune-mediated *demyelinating* neuropathies or polyradiculopathies	Ataxic variant of Guillain-Barré syndrome: Miller Fisher syndrome (Anti-GQ1b) Sensory ataxic neuropathy (Anti-GD1b) Anti-MAG neuropathy

[a]Vitamin B_{12}, E, folate, and copper deficiencies as well as nitrous oxide intoxication may present with a picture reflecting myeloneuropathy or subacute combined degeneration of the spinal cord (pyramidal, cerebellar, and neuropathic signs). Folate supplementation alone improves the anemia and peripheral neuropathy of B_{12} deficiency but not any CNS manifestations. Vitamin E deficiency is similar to Friedreich ataxia plus retinopathy.

[b]CNS manifestations of thiamine deficiency include Wernicke encephalopathy and optic neuropathy. Other manifestations include axonal peripheral neuropathy (*dry beriberi*), in severe cases mimicking the axonal type of Guillain-Barré syndrome, and high-output heart failure (wet beriberi).

MAG, myelin-associated glycoprotein.

Adapted with permission from Espay AJ, Lang AE. *Common movement disorders pitfalls: case-based teaching*. New York: Cambridge University Press, 2012.

(SSA) cytoplasmic antibodies and Anti-La (SSB) antibodies, cerebrospinal fluid (CSF) for elevated protein (as would be seen with a chronic immune-mediated or inflammatory process), and serum B_{12} studies, along with blood work and scans searching for occult systemic disease including malignancy. Even though a malignancy was not detected, the patient's history of cigarette smoking and the lack of objective evidence for inflammation prompted us to remain vigilant with regard to the possibility of malignancy. Spinal cord magnetic resonance imaging (MRI) showed no evidence of T2-high signal abnormalities in the dorsal columns. A positron emission tomography (PET) scan was normal. The patient's predominantly sensory, symmetric demyelinating polyneuropathy fits best with the distal acquired demyelinating symmetric (DADS) neuropathy variant of chronic inflammatory demyelinating polyneuropathy. Patients often, but not always, demonstrate an IgM monoclonal gammopathy with anti-MAG (myelin-associated glycoprotein) antibodies. Presence of these IgM M-proteins is associated with steroid failure.

The patient's course had progressed such that she had constant intense neuropathic pain and was wheelchair bound due to severe sensory ataxia. Therefore, she received empirical treatment for an immune-mediated neuropathy with prednisone and azathioprine with marginal clinical response. Plasma exchange and intravenous immunoglobin (IVIG) would also be additional reasonable treatment options, given the severity of the patient's symptoms.

Treatment of neuropathic pain is a major challenge in this patient. For chronic burning tingling dysesthesias (as experienced by our patient), tricyclic antidepressants remain first-line therapy. Amitriptyline or nortriptyline beginning at 25 mg qhs and gradually increasing as tolerated to 2 mg per kg qhs will provide significant benefit in at least half of patients. Second-line therapy centers on anticonvulsant drugs; carbamazepine, gabapentin, and pregabalin are the most often used. When other measures fail, a trial of mexiletine is worth considering, although the patient must be carefully evaluated for underlying cardiac disease given the drug's tendency to produce cardiac arrhythmia.

SELECTED REFERENCES

Barohn RJ. Approach to peripheral neuropathy and neuronopathy. *Semin Neurol* 1998;18:7–18.

Biller J, ed. *Practical neurology*, 4th ed. Philadelphia: Lippincott Williams & Wilkins, Wolters Kluwer Health, 2012:Chapter 46.

Camdessanché J-P, Jousserand G, Ferraud K, et al. The pattern and diagnostic criteria of sensory neuronopathy: a case-control study. *Brain* 2009;132:1723–1733.

Espay AJ, Biller J. *Concise neurology*. Philadelphia: Lippincott Williams & Wilkins, Wolters Kluwer Health, 2011:Chapter 9.

Espay AJ, Lang AE. *Common movement disorders pitfalls: case-based teaching.* New York: Cambridge University Press, 2012:Chapter 5.

SEE QUESTIONS: 73, 74, 75, 172, 173, 186, 214, 215, 228, 230, 241

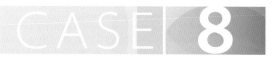

CASE 8

L5 RADICULOPATHY (DISC HERNIATION)

▐ OBJECTIVES ▐

- ■ To review risk factors for lumbar disc herniations.
- ■ To review the clinical presentation of lumbar radiculopathies.
- ■ To discuss the most common etiologies of lumbar radiculopathy.
- ■ To review the management of lumbar disc disease with sciatica.

▐ VIGNETTE ▐

A 31-year-old man developed left buttock and low back pain approximately 1 month earlier. The patient noted that at times the pain was severe and limited his walking and his ability to sit. He had no numbness or weakness; however, he had limitation of movement of his left leg secondary to his pain. He described the pain as a tight feeling on his left buttock shooting down his leg and sometimes up his back when standing or when sitting for prolonged periods. Alleviating factors were sitting with his hip flexed and internally rotated. He also noted relief with Percocet that lasted approximately 3 to 4 hours but did not completely alleviate the pain. He had no loss of bowel or bladder function. He has taken naproxen and cyclobenzaprine in the past with no benefit. He also received acupuncture over the past month with no benefit.

CASE SUMMARY

Low back pain is extremely common, but only a fraction of patients experiencing low back pain during their lifetime have lumbar radiculopathy or sciatica as a consequence of root irritation or compression. Herniation of a lumbar intervertebral disc is one of the most common causes of root compression. The avascular (in adults) biconcave intervertebral discs are located between adjacent vertebral bodies. The intervertebral disc consists of three components: an outer multilaminated annulus fibrosus, the inner gelatinous nucleus pulposus, and the superior and inferior end plates. Most lumbar disc herniations occur between the fourth and fifth lumbar or the fifth lumbar and first sacral interspaces. The spinal nerves exit the spinal canal through the foramina at each level. A disc herniation most frequently irritates the displaced nerve root. Most discs rupture in a posterolateral direction. The incidence of disc rupture is the same among men and women.

The distribution of the leg pain is dependent on the level of nerve root irritation or compression. Radicular or root pain results from inflammation of the nerve root, which has a characteristic burning or lancinating quality. The pain is generally accompanied by dermatomal sensory loss, paresthesias, or dysesthesias. A pain drawing can be very helpful in assessing the dermatomal distribution. Compression of a motor nerve results in weakness, and compression of a sensory nerve results in numbness. Often, accompanying numbness or tingling occurs with a distribution similar to the pain. Nerve root tension signs are used in the evaluation of these patients. A positive straight leg raising sign, also known as Lasègue sign, is almost always present. However, a crossed straight leg raising sign may be even more predictive of a lumbar disc herniation. In this test, straight leg raising of the contralateral limb elicits more specific but less severe pain on the affected side. The back may appear scoliotic. Gait is often abnormal. Muscle weakness may be revealed, particularly when walking on heels and toes.

Our patient had a classic presentation of a lesion affecting the L5 root, including the complaint of lower back, buttock, lateral thigh, and anterolateral calf pain, with associated objective neurological findings of weakness of great toe and foot dorsiflexion (tibialis anterior and extensor hallucis longus) and dermatomal numbness of the lateral leg, dorsomedial foot, and great toe. With L5 root lesions, both the patellar and ankle reflexes are spared.

With lesions affecting the S1 root, the pain generally involves the posterolateral thigh and calf, extending into the heel and lateral toes, and the sensory disturbances generally involve the posterior calf and lateral foot. S1 radiculopathies may cause weakness affecting the gastrocnemius and toe flexors, and the Achilles reflex is depressed (Table 8.1).

Magnetic resonance imaging (MRI) is very sensitive in delineating lumbar disc herniations. There are commonly four stages of a disc herniation: disc degeneration, disc prolapse, extrusion, and disc sequestration (sequestered disc). Computed tomography (CT) myelography may be required in certain instances. Imaging studies must be reserved for cases in which positive findings have been documented. Electromyography (EMG) may be a useful adjunct in selective cases. Most patients with herniated discs respond favorably to conservative therapy. Almost all patients with sciatica and disk herniations deserve a trial of medical therapy with bed rest, anti-inflammatory agents, analgesics, and muscle relaxants. Once the patient has recovered from the worst radicular pain, physical therapy can be instituted. Surgery must be considered among patients with severe and disabling sciatica, those with poor response to at least 6 weeks of conservative therapy, or patients with neurologic deficits such as a foot drop, cauda equina syndrome, or bladder or bowel disturbances.

TABLE 8.1 **ASSESSMENT OF STRENGTH IN FEET AND RELEVANT ROOT LEVELS, MUSCLES, AND NERVES**

Movement	Root Level	Main Muscles	Supplied by...	Which Is Also Key for...
Main plantar flexors	S1-2	Gastrocnemius Soleus	Tibial	Achilles reflex
Main plantar flexors and invertors	L4-5 L5-S2 S1-2	Tibialis posterior Flexor digitorum longus Flexor hallucis longus	Tibial	Sensation to sole Sensation to dorsolateral leg
Main dorsiflexors and toe extensors	L4-5 L5 L5	Tibialis anterior Extensor digitorum longus Extensor hallucis longus	Deep peroneal (tibialis anterior)	Sensation to skin between first and second toes
Plantar evertors	L5 L5	Peroneus longus Peroneus brevis	Superficial peroneal	Sensation to skin in lateral leg and dorsum of feet/toes

The tibial and peroneal nerves form as the anterior and dorsal terminal branches of the sciatic nerve (L4-S2), after it supplies the hamstrings, semitendinosus, semimembranosus, and biceps femoris. See also Table 8.1 for the clinical elements distinguishing the two common causes of foot drop, peroneal neuropathy and L5 radiculopathy.

SELECTED REFERENCES

Biller J, ed. *Practical neurology*, 4th ed. Philadelphia: Lippincott Williams & Wilkins, Wolters Kluwer Health, 2012:Chapter 23.

Brazis PW, Masdeu JC, Biller J. *Localization in clinical neurology*, 6th ed. Philadelphia: Lippincott Williams & Wilkins, Wolters Kluwer Health, 2011.

Pfirmann CW, Metzford A, Zanetti M, et al. Magnetic resonance classification of lumbar intervertebral disc degeneration. *Spine* 2001;26:1873–1878.

Weinstein JN, Tosteson TD, Lurie JD, et al. Surgical vs. nonoperative treatment for lumbar disk herniation. The Spine Patient Outcomes Research Trial (SPORT): a randomized trial. *JAMA* 2006;296(20):2441–2450.

SEE QUESTIONS: 5, 56, 83, 264

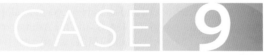

CASE 9

FEMORAL NEUROPATHY

OBJECTIVES

- To describe the normal anatomy of the femoral nerve.
- To list pathological conditions causing femoral neuropathy.
- To describe an unusual cause of femoral neuropathy.

Following thoracolumbar scoliosis surgery, this 48-year-old man presented with pain on the right thigh and around the right hip. He had weakness of right hip flexion and leg extension, sensory impairment over the anteromedial thigh and leg, and an absent right patellar reflex. There was no adductor weakness. There was no Tinel sign over the right inguinal ligament. The video obtained weeks after surgery also showed wasting and atrophy of the distal right quadriceps.

CASE SUMMARY

The femoral nerve, the largest branch of the lumbar plexus, is a mixed sensory and motor nerve. The femoral nerve arises from the posterior division of the ventral rami of L2, L3, and L4 within the psoas muscle and courses onward laterally, reaching the inguinal ligament (Poupart ligament) lateral to the femoral artery. Under the inguinal ligament, the femoral nerve divides into anterior and posterior division. Branches within the pelvis supply the iliacus and psoas muscles. The anterior division supplies motor innervation to the pectineus and sartorius muscles and cutaneous innervation to the anteromedial thigh. The posterior division provides motor innervation to the quadriceps femoris and cutaneous innervation to the medial aspect of the leg and foot.

Our patient had thoracolumbar scoliosis with coronal and sagittal deformity. He was placed in the left lateral decubitus position, and underwent a transthoracic approach with osteotomies of T5-6, T6-7, T7-8, T8-9, with excision of a calcified and partially ossified anterior longitudinal ligament and loosing of the patient's coronal deformity. An inferior vena cava (IVC) filter was placed. Following this, the patient was returned to the full prone position and underwent a posterior thoracolumbar decompression.

Our patient had a postoperative painful right femoral neuropathy proximal to the origin of the branches to the iliacus and psoas muscles. Electromyography (EMG) showed electrodiagnostic findings consistent with a right femoral neuropathy, with decreased recruitment of slightly large amplitude motor unit action potentials (MUAPs) in the right vastus lateralis and vastus medialis. Needle EMG of lumbar paraspinals was normal. Computed tomography (CT) of the pelvis showed asymmetric enlargement of the right iliacus and distal iliopsoas muscle consistent with an intramuscular hemorrhage. Magnetic resonance imaging/magnetic resonance angiography (MRI/MRA) of the pelvis showed muscle edema of the right iliacus, distal iliopsoas, and proximal sartorius (Fig. 9.1). There was no evidence of pseudoaneurysm, dissection, or arterial or venous thrombosis. A follow-up study showed improving soft tissue edema abnormalities of the right iliacus, psoas, and sartorius.

The femoral nerve is subject to a variety of disorders that may affect the nerve anywhere from the nerve roots to the distal branches. Femoral mononeuropathy is uncommon. Femoral neuropathy is usually iatrogenic and caused by trauma from surgery (gynecological, urological, vascular, and abdominal). The neuropathy may be unilateral or less commonly bilateral. Femoral neuropathy may be transient as seen in cases of ilioinguinal blockade for inguinal herniorrhaphy. Self-retaining abdominal retractors exerting constant pressure on the femoral nerve are most frequently implicated. Prolonged lithotomy position (flexion, abduction, and external rotation of the hips) mainly used in vaginal hysterectomy, laparoscopy, or normal delivery may cause a femoral neuropathy by pressing on the stretched inguinal ligament. Other causes include bleeding into the iliac and psoas muscles in patients treated with anticoagulants and thrombolytics, pelvic malignancies, pelvic lymphadenopathy, pelvic irradiation, pelvic fractures, nerve infarctions,

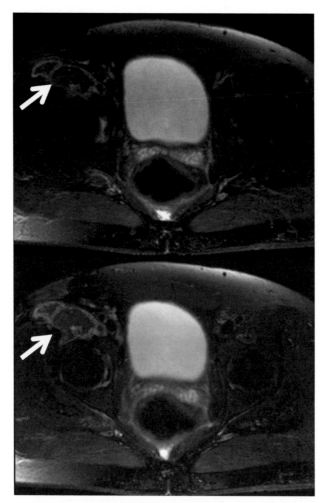

Figure 9.1   Femoral Neuropathy. Postcontrast MRI/MRA of the pelvis showing peripheral rim enhancement of the right iliacus, distal iliopsoas, and proximal sartorius muscle (*arrows*), which suggests evolving intramuscular hematoma.

diabetes mellitus, neurofibromas, schwannomas, yoga, gunshot and stab wounds. Femoral neuropathy may also follow arterial or venous catheterizations. A femoral neuropathy was reported in 0.21% of 9,585 cardiac catheterizations that were due to local hematoma or pseudoaneurysm. Femoral neuropathy may also follow renal transplantation. Severe combined bilateral femoral and sciatic neuropathies have also been observed in the context of alcohol intoxication (*hanging leg syndrome*). Isolated vastus lateralis and vastus medialis atrophy, and localized hypertrophy with onion bulblike formations have been reported.

A femoral neuropathy may be clinically confused with an L4 radiculopathy or lumbar plexopathy. Assessment of hip adduction is key in distinguishing these neuropathic disorders (Table 9.1). Treatment depends on the etiology of the lesion.

TABLE 9.1 **ASSESSMENT OF THE LUMBAR PLEXUS: DISTINGUISHING FEMORAL NEUROPATHY FROM L4 RADICULOPATHY**

Movement	Root Level	Main Muscles	Supplied by...	Which Is Also Key for...
Hip flexion	L1-3	Iliopsoas	Femoral	Sensation to medial thigh and medial lower leg (saphenous)
Leg extension	L2-4	Quadriceps femoris	Femoral	Patellar reflex
Thigh flexor and evertor	L2-4	Sartorius Pectineus	Femoral	
Thigh adduction	L2-4	Adductor longus Adductor magnus	Obturator nerve	Sensation to skin in medial thigh
Internal rotation and knee flexion	L2-4	Gracilis	Obturator nerve	

Femoral neuropathies cause weakness of hip flexion (iliopsoas) and leg extension (quadriceps femoris), absent patellar reflex, **normal** hip adduction, and hypesthesia of the anteromedial thigh and leg. Lesions at or below the inguinal ligament level spare thigh flexion as the femoral branches to the iliopsoas are preserved. **L2-4 radiculopathy or plexopathy** causes weakness of iliopsoas, quadriceps, **and** hip adductors.

SELECTED REFERENCES

al Hakim M, Katirji B. Femoral mononeuropathy induced by the lithotomy position: a report of 5 cases with a review of the literature. *Muscle Nerve* 1993;16(9):891–895.

Brazis PW, Masdeu JC, Biller J. *Localization in clinical neurology*, 6th ed. Philadelphia: Lippincott Williams & Wilkins, Wolters Kluwer Health, 2011.

Petchprapa CN, Rosenberg ZS, Sconpienza LM, et al. MR imaging of entrapment neuropathies of the lower extremity. Part 1. The pelvis and hip. *Radiographics* 2010;30:983–1000.

Scherer K, Skeen M, Strine S, et al. Hanging leg syndrome: combined bilateral femoral and sciatic neuropathies. *Neurology* 2006;66:1124–1125.

SEE QUESTIONS: 5, 56, 83, 263

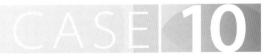

CASE 10

FOOT DROP: HISTORY OF ARTHROSCOPIC SURGERY

OBJECTIVES

- To review the clinical presentation of a lower motor neuron type of foot drop.
- To discuss the most common etiologies of foot drop.

VIGNETTE

A 61-year-old woman had a 2-week history of painless weakness of her right foot.

CASE SUMMARY

 A peroneal neuropathy is the most common isolated mononeuropathy of the lower extremities. The common peroneal nerve descends into the leg as the lateral division of the sciatic nerve. After rounding the head of the fibula, the common peroneal nerve splits into two branches: the deep peroneal nerve and the superficial peroneal nerve. Patients presenting with a foot drop often have either a peroneal neuropathy or an L5 radiculopathy (Table 10.1). Central nervous system (CNS) causes are rare.

Neuropathy of the common peroneal nerve is a frequent clinical condition, generally caused by compression at the fibular head. Chronic compression from habitual leg crossing is a common mechanism. Peroneal entrapment neuropathy has also been reported from sitting in a cross-legged position (yoga foot drop), tibial fracture, short casts or braces, arthroscopic knee surgery, excessive climbing, repetitive kicking, nerve infarcts, Baker cysts, hematoma, tumor, or leprosy. Peroneal nerve entrapment at the fibular head has also been reported in patients with hemiparetic strokes.

Dancers are susceptible to a number of entrapment neuropathies, including superficial and deep peroneal nerve entrapments. Prolonged crash dieting and exertional compartment syndrome may also result in peroneal neuropathy and foot drop. Compression of the peroneal nerve by an intraneural ganglion cyst or other masses (e.g., neurofibroma) may result in a painful foot drop. Bilateral foot drop may result from thiamine deficiency. Foot drop may also occur among pregnant patients who had a prolonged and difficult labor from compression of the lumbosacral trunk by a fetal head. Caustic effects on the sciatic nerve from certain drugs injected intramuscularly in the buttock, particularly among children, may result in a paralytic foot drop. Rarely, intermittent pneumatic compression devices to prevent deep venous thrombosis may cause bilateral peroneal neuropathies. Pressure palsy of the peroneal nerve at the fibular head results in foot drop and loss of sensation over the lateral calf, dorsal malleolus, and dorsum of the foot. Sensory loss is much more apparent with lesions of the superficial division of the peroneal nerve. With lesions of the deep division of the peroneal nerve, the sensory loss is often confined to a small area between the first and second toes. The weakness of ankle dorsiflexion, ankle eversion, and toe extension (dorsiflexion) is accompanied by an excessive foot slapping of the forefoot against the floor.

TABLE 10.1	**ASSESSMENT OF COMMON CAUSES OF FOOT DROP**	
	Common Peroneal	**L5 Radiculopathy**
Impaired action	Weakness of ankle/toe dorsiflexion and *eversion*	Weakness of ankle dorsiflexion and *inversion*
Distinctively weak muscles	Extensor hallucis longus	Flexor digitorum longus (non-peroneal L5)
Hypesthesia	Lateral leg and dorsum of the foot, but spares fifth toe	Lateral leg, dorsomedial foot, and large toe

Palpation along the fibular head may elicit signs of tenderness or discover a mass. As demonstrated by our patient, with lesions at the fibular head, the deep branch of the peroneal nerve is affected more commonly than the whole nerve. Electrophysiological testing—nerve conduction velocities (NCVs) and electromyography (EMG)—are very helpful in the evaluation of these patients. EMG sampling of the short head of the biceps femoris is the preferred above-the-knee muscle to test for localization purposes in cases of foot drop. Since the peroneal division of the sciatic nerve proximal to the fibular head supplies this muscle, abnormalities at the biceps femoris muscle localizes the deficit to the sciatic nerve rather than the peroneal nerve. Magnetic resonance imaging (MRI) of the lower thigh is also highly accurate in the evaluation of unusual causes of peroneal neuropathy. Ankle foot orthosis prevents tripping due to foot drop. Surgery is seldom indicated in most cases of peroneal neuropathies.

SELECTED REFERENCES

Biller J, ed. *Practical neurology*, 4th ed. Philadelphia: Lippincott Williams & Wilkins, Wolters Kluwer Health, 2012:Chapter 25.

Brazis PW, Masdeu JC, Biller J. *Localization in clinical neurology*, 6th ed. Philadelphia: Lippincott Williams & Wilkins, Wolters Kluwer Health, 2011.

Kennedy JG, Baxter DE. Nerve disorders in dancers. *Clin Sports Med* 2008;27(2):329–334.

Vastamaki M. Decompression for peroneal nerve entrapment. *Acta Orthop Scand* 1986;57:551–554.

SEE QUESTIONS: 5, 56, 83, 264

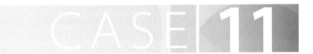

MOTOR NEURON DISEASE

OBJECTIVES

■ To review the differential diagnosis of slowly progressive asymmetric lower extremity weakness.

■ To list the basic diagnostic workup for patients with suspected motor neuron disease.

■ To outline treatment strategies for patients with motor neuron disease.

VIGNETTE

A 34-year-old woman had a year-long history of right lower extremity weakness. Her problems were dated to a fall several months prior to this assessment, followed by subsequent falls and difficulties lifting her right foot when walking. She had no speech or swallowing difficulties, urinary or bowel complaints, numbness, or upper extremity complaints.

CASE SUMMARY

Our patient was a 34-year-old woman with gradually progressive painless muscle weakness and atrophy, initially affecting her right leg and then spreading to the left. She had no sensory loss or bladder or bowel disturbances. Examination demonstrated a lower motor neuron pattern of asymmetric lower extremity weakness without any upper motor neuron signs. Imaging of the spine, cerebrospinal fluid (CSF) analysis, and routine laboratory studies were normal.

The electrophysiologic studies indicated relatively normal motor nerve conduction velocities. The needle examination showed chronic and active neurogenic changes in multiple muscles. Together, these findings indicated a lower motor neuron syndrome that could be due to anterior horn cell disease, lumbosacral polyradiculopathy, or multifocal motor neuropathy.

Variants of motor neuron disease include amyotrophic lateral sclerosis (ALS), primary lateral sclerosis, progressive muscular atrophy (PMA), and progressive bulbar palsy (Table 11.1). ALS is the most common degenerative motor neuron disease of adulthood. It is recognized by the presence of both upper motor neuron (UMN) and lower motor neuron (LMN) signs in multiple spinal segments. Among patients with findings restricted to the LMN, PMA is in general a slower form of motor neuron disease associated with abnormalities of the survivor motor neuron gene. Patients with pure LMN syndromes with predominant bulbar weakness may also have X-linked bulbospinal neuropathy (Kennedy disease) or multifocal motor neuropathy (MMN). Patients with MMN have asymmetric focal weakness of the distal limbs and have marked conduction block on nerve conduction studies, and approximately half of them demonstrate elevated levels of anti-GM1 antibodies. Patients with pure LMN syndrome should also be screened for a possible monoclonal gammopathy. As with any focal LMN disorder, particularly involving paraparesis, meticulous imaging of the spine is mandatory to exclude structural lesions (tumor, spinal vascular malformation, syrinx, etc.). Inflammatory disorders of the roots, such as an immune-mediated polyradiculopathies or infectious polyradiculopathies, should be

TABLE 11.1   DIFFERENTIAL DIAGNOSIS AND VARIANTS OF MOTOR NEURON DISEASE

	Main Disorders
Restricted to UMN	HTLV-1 myelopathy
	Multiple sclerosis
	Stiff person syndrome (SPS)[a]
	Adrenomyeloneuropathy
	Primary lateral sclerosis
	Hereditary spastic paraparesis
	Lathyrism
Restricted to LMN	Progressive muscular atrophy
	Multifocal motor neuropathy
	Kennedy's X-linked bulbospinal neuronopathy
	Monomelic amyotrophy
	Adult-onset spinal muscular atrophy type IV
	Postpolio muscular atrophy

HTLV, human T-cell lymphotropic virus-1.
[a]Hyperreflexia is the only UMN sign allowed in the diagnostic criteria for SPS.

considered and evaluated with CSF studies. Infiltrating processes such as sarcoidosis or fungal or carcinomatous meningitis might also affect multiple motor nerve roots and lead to a progressive clinical course.

In our patient, following a thorough laboratory evaluation, the diagnosis was motor neuron disease. Therapy of motor neuron disease generally involves rehabilitation measures, including in this patient's case splinting for foot drop and assessment of ambulation and mobility with equipment and safety devices. Muscle cramps may be treated with quinine. Patients with substantial spasticity are treated with antispasticity drugs. Patients developing upper extremity involvement require experienced occupational therapy, including equipment, to facilitate their activities of daily living (ADL) function.

Assessment of forced vital capacity (FVC) looking for diaphragmatic involvement is indicated; when the FVC falls below 60% of predicted, patients should be treated with bilevel positive airway pressure (BIPAP). As patients develop bulbar dysfunction with dysphagia and speech difficulty, symptomatic management with equipment for speech and percutaneous endoscopic gastrostomy (PEG) for dysphagia are indicated. In general, patients are best managed in multidisciplinary clinics. At the present time, the only drug that has been proven in double-blind randomized clinical trials to affect the progression of motor neuron disease is the antiglutamatergic agent riluzole.

SELECTED REFERENCES

Biller J, ed. *Practical neurology*, 4th ed. Philadelphia: Lippincott Williams & Wilkins, Wolters Kluwer Health, 2012:Chapter 45.

Espay AJ, Biller J. *Concise neurology*. Philadelphia: Lippincott Williams & Wilkins, Wolters Kluwer Health, 2011:Chapter 9.

Pascuzzi RM. ALS, motor neuron disease, and related disorders: a personal approach to diagnosis and management. *Semin Neurol* 2002;22:75–87.

SEE QUESTIONS: 1, 5, 11, 15, 18, 77, 173, 186, 214

CASE **12**

MYASTHENIA GRAVIS

OBJECTIVES

- To review the differential diagnosis for fluctuating proximal weakness.
- To summarize the diagnostic workup for myasthenia gravis (MG) and the Lambert-Eaton myasthenic syndrome (LEMS).
- To illustrate the evaluation and management of patients with seronegative MG.
- To review treatment options for patients with autoimmune MG.

VIGNETTE

A 43-year-old man, previously healthy, had progressive muscle weakness and fatigability.

The patient is a 43-year-old man who presents with several months of fatigable and fluctuating limb muscle weakness, relatively worse in the later hours of the day. The patient has no cranial symptoms. Examination confirms the presence of proximal limb muscle weakness. The history suggests and the examination confirms the presence of fluctuating and fatigable muscle weakness.

Although MG presents with fluctuating or fatigable weakness, the majority of patients have some degree of cranial/bulbar involvement. Twenty-five percent of patients present with diplopia, 25% with eyelid ptosis, and by 1 month 80% have some degree of ocular involvement. Ten percent of myasthenics present with bulbar symptoms, 10% with lower extremity weakness, and 10% with generalized weakness, whereas respiratory failure is the presenting symptom in 1%.

LEMS is far less common than MG and is associated with proximal limb muscle weakness, particularly in the lower extremities, with a relative paucity of cranial weakness. The absence of dry mouth (and other antimuscarinic, anticholinergic symptoms), as well as the preservation of muscle stretch reflexes, would be against the diagnosis of LEMS in our patient. An acquired myopathy such as polymyositis, dermatomyositis, inclusion body myositis, or thyroid disease are also in the differential, but far less likely to cause the degree of fluctuation in strength described and shown by this patient. Metabolic or genetic disorders such as adult-onset acid maltase deficiency and Desmond myopathy are additional myopathies in the differential.

In our patient, serologic studies showed no detectable acetylcholine receptor (AChR) antibodies (about 80% sensitive for MG). In addition, there were no detectable voltage-gated P/Q calcium channel antibodies (typically seen in LEMS). Of patients with suspected autoimmune MG who are seronegative for AChR antibodies, about 50% are estimated to have antibodies to muscle-specific tyrosinase kinase (MuSK). Our patient was seronegative for MuSK antibodies. Pharmacological testing demonstrated a positive response to cholinesterase inhibitors, supporting the diagnosis of a neuromuscular junction transmission disorder.

Neurophysiologic studies demonstrated normal compound muscle action potential (CMAP) amplitudes, normal nerve conduction velocities, and the presence of a decremental response to low rates of repetitive stimulation. The electromyography (EMG) needle examination was normal. The decremental response with normal baseline CMAP amplitudes favored the diagnosis of MG. In LEMS, the baseline motor amplitudes are uniformly low (Table 12.1). Therefore, the clinical presentation, response to cholinesterase inhibitors, and neurophysiologic studies lead to a diagnosis of myasthenia gravis.

Management of MG includes the use of immunotherapy and pyridostigmine and performance of a thymectomy in patients with suspected thymoma or those AChR antibody positive patients younger than 60 years with generalized MG. Our patient's residual deficits despite benefits to cholinesterase inhibitors led to the performance of a thymectomy with histological findings of thymic hyperplasia. The response to thymectomy tends to be delayed one or more years following the procedure. Our patient was therefore treated with immunosuppressive therapy, in this case mycophenolate mofetil, with improvement in strength 1 to 2 months after initiating therapy. In addition to thymoma, alert clinicians must be mindful that MG patients have an increased risk of developing other autoimmune disorders such as rheumatoid arthritis, SLE, and pernicious anemia. Finally, patients should avoid drugs that impair acetylcholine release and may worsen MG, such as quinidine/quinine, procainamide, P-type calcium channel blockers, most antibiotics, and drugs causing hypermagnesemia (largely, laxatives and antacids).

TABLE 12.1	KEY CLINICAL FEATURES TO DISTINGUISH DISORDERS MIMICKING MYASTHENIA GRAVIS
MG-Like Disorders	**Key Clinical Findings and Tests**
Lambert-Eaton myasthenic syndrome	Dry mouth, CMAP amplitude increase >100% with high-frequency repetitive stimulation (50 Hz)
Botulism	Dry mouth, fixed dilated pupils, descending paralysis, CMAP amplitude decrement with postexercise or tetanic facilitation
Hypermagnesemia	Administration of magnesium from antacids and laxatives, or given during the treatment of eclampsia
Miller-Fisher variant of Guillain-Barré syndrome	Areflexia, descending weakness, GQ1b autoantibodies
Tick paralysis	Descending weakness, examination of skin and scalp for ticks
Diphtheric neuropathy	Tonsillar exudates

SELECTED REFERENCES

Burns TM, Royden Jones H Jr. Myasthenia gravis. In: Royden H, Jones JR, Srinivasan J, et al. *Netter's neurology*, 2nd ed. Philadelphia: Elsevier Saunders, 2012:Chapter 73.

Pascuzzi RM. Pearls and pitfalls in the diagnosis and management of neuromuscular junction disorders. *Semin Neurol* 2001;21:425–440.

Sanders DB, El-Salem K, Massey JM, et al. Clinical aspects of MuSK antibody positive seronegative MG. *Neurology* 2003;60:1978–1980.

SEE QUESTIONS: 1, 2, 11, 12, 13, 18, 73, 74

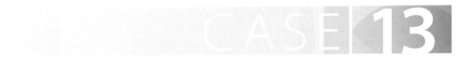

MYOTONIC DYSTROPHY

OBJECTIVES

- To recognize the importance of examining the mother in evaluating a floppy or weak newborn.
- To recognize the classical facies of myotonic dystrophy and illustrate the clinical phenomena of grip myotonia and percussion myotonia.
- To emphasize the systemic complications of myotonic dystrophy.
- To list the differential diagnosis of myotonic dystrophy including current subtypes.

VIGNETTE

A 31-year-old woman gave birth to a hypotonic baby.

CASE SUMMARY

This 31-year-old woman gave birth to a floppy baby 2 weeks earlier. Although the mother has no past neurological or neuromuscular history of symptoms, simple observation demonstrates classic features of myotonic dystrophy with a myopathic lugubrious facies and mild eyelid ptosis. In addition, the patient demonstrates a classic grip and percussion myotonia. In men, the diagnosis can be even more obvious given the presence of frontal balding. Ninety percent of patients have posterior subcapsular cataracts. Myotonic dystrophy typically produces substantial distal extensor muscle weakness, often more pronounced than in proximal muscle groups.

The diagnosis is usually obvious from the examination and family history, but mild or atypical cases may require laboratory investigation. Myotonic dystrophy type 1 is associated with an abnormal CTG trinucleotide repeat on chromosome 19. Myotonic dystrophy is associated with electromyography (EMG) changes of myotonic discharges and small myopathic voluntary motor units.

The importance of making a diagnosis is twofold. Myotonic dystrophy patients acquire numerous systemic complications. Cardiac conduction abnormalities can be life threatening, but preventable. Obstructive and central sleep apnea, endocrinopathies (testicular atrophy and impotence in men), dysphagia, gallbladder disease, hypersomnolence, apathy, and learning disabilities are examples of relatively common associated disorders. Pregnant women have increased risk of fetal loss. The second important aspect of establishing the diagnosis in this autosomal dominant condition is the fact that many patients are unaware that they have the disease. Therefore, examination of relatives is indicated.

Treatment remains symptomatic, including equipment to help with activities of daily livings (ADLs) such as ankle-foot orthosis. Screening and management of cardiac disease, respiratory insufficiency, and gastrointestinal involvement should be included in the long-term evaluation and management plan. Myotonia in such patients is usually not so disabling as to require membrane stabilizing medication. As the patients age, their myotonia becomes less pronounced.

The differential diagnosis includes proximal myotonic myopathy (PROMM) DM2, similar in clinical appearance to myotonic dystrophy except that patients tend not to have distal weakness (instead, weakness is proximal). PROMM patients tend to have more symptomatic muscle stiffness from myotonia. Myotonic dystrophy type 2 is clinically similar to type 1 other than a tendency to have combined proximal and distal muscle weakness; also, type 2 is associated with a different expansion than that of myotonic dystrophy type 1.

Congenital myotonic dystrophy should be considered in any floppy baby or weak newborn. It is the most severe form of the disease and typically inherited from the mother. The best diagnostic test is a brief evaluation of the infant's mother (as in the presented video). Myotonia congenita is a benign autosomal dominant condition involving more severe muscle stiffness and myotonia but without systemic complications or progressive weakness. These patients often have bulky muscles as opposed to atrophy and may require membrane stabilizing medications.

SELECTED REFERENCES

Biller J, ed. *Practical neurology*, 4th ed. Philadelphia: Lippincott Williams & Wilkins, Wolters Kluwer Health, 2012:Chapter 47.

Srinivasan J, Segarceanu M, Ho D, et al. Hereditary myopathies. Chapter 75. In: Royden Jones H Jr, Srinivasan J, Allam GJ, et al. *Netter's neurology*, 2nd ed. Philadelphia: Elsevier Saunders, 2012.

Thornton C. The myotonic dystrophies. *Semin Neurol* 1999;19:25–33.

SEE QUESTIONS: 1, 58, 77, 202

SECTION 2

SPINAL CORD

CASE 14

POSTTRAUMATIC CERVICAL SYRINGOMYELIA

OBJECTIVES

- To describe a patient with posttraumatic cervical spinal cord dysfunction.
- To review the classification of syringomyelia and different conditions associated with this entity.

VIGNETTE

In 1960, this 65-year-old woman became instantly paralyzed from the neck down after a diving accident when she hit the bottom of a pool. Two days later, she had an emergency cervical laminectomy. She was then placed on tongs and gradually improved her sensation and movements, more in the arms than in her legs. However, she subsequently developed a motor deficit on the right side of her body and a sensory deficit on the left side of her body, particularly to pain and temperature.

CASE SUMMARY

Several years after sustaining a serious high cervical spinal cord injury that initially rendered her quadriplegic, and following a very satisfactory recovery after emergency cervical laminectomy, our patient developed a progressive neurologic syndrome characterized by decreased mobility on the right side of her body, particularly affecting the intrinsic muscles of her right hand. She also lost the sensation of pain, heat, and cold on the left side.

Examination was remarkable for contractures, impaired dexterity, and muscular atrophy of her right hand causing a clawhand (*main en griffe*) appearance, right-sided long-tract signs, and loss of pain and temperature appreciation on the left side (not shown on

TABLE 14.1	**SENSORY DISSOCIATION SYNDROME: INTRINSIC SPINAL CORD LESIONS**
Tumors	• Ependymoma (most common in adults) • Astrocytoma (most common in children) • Hemangioblastoma
Vascular	• Arteriovenous malformations • Cavernous malformations • Hematoma • Infarcts (aortic surgery among diabetics)
Other	• Syringomyelia • Hydromyelia • Abscess (myelitis) • Demyelination

Wasting of the hand and a dissociated sensory loss (hypesthesia to pain and temperature with preservation of proprioception), especially if in a halfcape distribution, suggest an intrinsic lesion of the cervical and upper thoracic cord.

the tape) without a classical cape or hemicape distribution. There was no right-sided segmental anesthesia, facial analgesia, or thermal hypesthesia. She had preservation of light-touch sensation, position sense, and vibration sense. There was no Horner syndrome, brainstem findings, scoliosis, digital ulcerations, or Charcot joints.

Our patient had cervical spinal cord dysfunction due to a central cord syndrome associated with a characteristic sensory dissociation syndrome manifested by loss of pain and heat and cold sensations, with sparing of touch, vibration, and position sense (syringomyelic dissociation) (Table 14.1). In addition to the cervical postlaminectomy changes, magnetic resonance imaging (MRI) showed a tubular cystic cavitation of the spinal cord extending from C3 through C7, consistent with the diagnosis of syringohydromyelia. There was no Chiari malformation or other extrinsic lesion at the level of the foramen magnum. The syrinx did not communicate with the fourth ventricle. There was no evidence of intramedullary mass lesion nor MRI changes suggestive of adhesive spinal arachnoiditis. There was no evidence of basilar impression or platybasia. A final diagnosis of posttraumatic noncommunicating syringohydromyelia was reached.

Syringomyelia may at times present with confusing unilateral symptoms such as segmental limb hypertrophy rather than segmental amyotrophy, which is a common feature from extension of the syrinx into the anterior horn cells. A neuropathic shoulder arthropathy may be a feature of syringomyelia. Scoliosis in childhood may develop secondary to syringomyelia. Syringomyelic deformities tend to be kyphoscoliotic. An isolated Horner syndrome may be a presenting feature. Isolated segmental myoclonus and periodic limb movements have been described. Respiratory failure, postural tachycardia, and gastrointestinal dysfunction may be associated with syringomyelia.

A central cord syndrome is seen in syringomyelia (syringohydromyelia) and trauma. Syringomyelia is a chronic cavitating disorder of the spinal cord, usually located at the lower cervical or upper thoracic spinal cord level, causing a progressive myelopathy. Idiopathic (nontraumatic) syringomyelia has been associated with hindbrain malformations (Chiari I malformation without hydrocephalus and Chiari II malformation with hydrocephalus), spinal cord tumors (particularly intramedullary cervical spinal cord tumors), chronic adhesive spinal arachnoiditis (postoperative, postinfectious, and postsubarachnoid hemorrhage), and trauma. Terminal syringomyelia has been associated with the tethered cord syndrome. The term *idiopathic syringomyelia* is applied when no cause is found; idiopathic syringomyelia is very rare.

Classically, syringomyelia has been classified into the following varieties: (a) communicating, (b) posttraumatic, (c) tumor related, (d) arachnoiditis related, and (e) idiopathic. Posttraumatic syringomyelia may develop months to years after a traumatic spinal cord injury. Approximately 3% to 4% of persons with traumatic spinal cord injury develop symptomatic posttraumatic syringomyelia (also referred to as cystic myelopathy). Enlarging posttraumatic syringomyelia results in a progressive neurologic deficit extending some distance beyond the initial site of injury. When syringomyelia or other intramedullary process is suspected, MRI is the diagnostic imaging procedure of choice. MRI is also useful for the postoperative evaluation of these patients. Computed tomography (CT) myelography may be useful in demonstrating the extent of obstruction to cerebrospinal fluid (CSF) flow. Treatment of syringomyelia involves a variety of surgical options, depending on the neuroimaging features of the syrinx and its pathogenesis.

SELECTED REFERENCES

Asano M, Fujiwara K, Yonenobu K, et al. Post-traumatic syringomyelia. *Spine* 1996;21:1446–1453.
Barnett HJM, Foster JB, Hudgson D. *Syringomyelia.* London: WB Saunders, 1973.
Olivero WC. Pathogenesis of syringomyelia. *Am J Neuroradiol* 1999;20:2024–2025.
Schurch B, Wichmann W, Rossier AB. Post-traumatic syringomyelia (cystic myelopathy): a prospective study of 449 patients with spinal cord injury. *J Neurol Neurosurg Psychiatry* 1996;60(1):61–67.
Schwartz ED, Falcone SF, Quencer RM, et al. Post-traumatic syringomyelia: pathogenesis, imaging, and treatment. *AJR Am J Roentgenol* 1999;173:487–492.

SEE QUESTIONS: 14, 15, 35, 39, 58, 212, 265

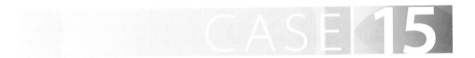

LUMBAR MYELOMENINGOCELE/SPINA BIFIDA

OBJECTIVES

- To present an adult patient with sequelae of a surgically corrected lumbosacral myelomeningocele.
- To review the different entities associated with spinal dysraphism or myelodysplasia.
- To emphasize the urologic morbidity associated with myelodysplasia.

VIGNETTE

A 50-year-old woman was evaluated because of gait difficulties.

CASE SUMMARY

 Our patient had a history of a lumbosacral myelomeningocele (L5-S1) repaired at the age of 3 months, with subsequent neurogenic bladder and recurrent urinary tract infections and pyelonephritis. She also had a history of syringomyelia and Chiari malformation. The patient currently voided spontaneously with the Crede maneuver and catheterized herself intermittently. Several postvoid residuals were in the range of 100 to 200 mL. She also had some degree of rectal incontinence.

There was a history of left club foot repair at the age of 3 years and a right fifth toe partial amputation secondary to osteomyelitis. She had required numerous tendon transfers. Examination demonstrated residual lower extremity paresis, variable loss of sensation in an L5-S1 distribution, decreased sensation over sacral dermatomes (S3-4 distribution, not shown), and foot deformities. Achilles tendon reflexes were absent bilaterally. Magnetic resonance imaging (MRI) showed postoperative changes, but no evidence of tethering of the cord.

Our patient has myelodysplasia or spinal dysraphism. Spinal dysraphism includes a group of developmental disorders resulting from defects in neural tube closure. Closure of the spinal canal begins at the cephalad end approximately 20 days after fertilization, proceeds caudally, and is complete at approximately day 28. The causes of spinal dysraphism are largely unknown; genetic and environmental influences have been implicated. Its incidence appears to be increased among the offspring of mothers who had folic acid deficiency and/or received treatment with valproic acid or carbamazepine during pregnancy.

Most caudal neural tube closure defects occur in the lumbar region. Involvement above L3, in general, precludes ambulation. Involvement below S1 allows for unaided ambulation. Patients with lesions between L3 and S1 require assisting devices for ambulation. Patients with myelodysplasia have considerable urologic morbidity. Children with myelodysplasia often have disturbances of bowel function as well.

Lesions of myelodysplasia may include spina bifida occulta, meningocele, myelomeningocele, or lipomyelomeningocele. Spina bifida occulta refers to congenital defects of spinal column formation without involvement of the spinal cord or meninges. In many of these patients a cutaneous abnormality (i.e., tuft of hair, cutaneous angioma or lipoma, or dermal sinus tract) may overlie the lower spine. A meningocele occurs when the meningeal sac extends beyond the confines of the vertebral canal but does not contain neural elements. A myelomeningocele occurs when neural tissue (spinal cord tissue, nerve roots, or both) is included in the sac. A lipomyelomeningocele is defined by the presence of fatty tissue and neural elements within the sac.

Myelomeningoceles account for most of the dysraphic states. The incidence ranges from 1 case per 1,000 live births in the United States to almost 9 per 1,000 in Ireland. The incidence is lower in Asian countries. Virtually all affected neonates have abnormal bladder function. Most children with a myelomeningocele have an associated Chiari II malformation.

SELECTED REFERENCES

Bruner JP, Tulipan N, Paschall RL, et al. Fetal surgery for myelomeningocele and the incidence of shunt-dependent hydrocephalus. *JAMA* 1999;282:1819–1825.

Elwood JH, Nevin NC. Factors associated with anencephalus and spina bifida in Belfast. *Br Prev Med* 1973;27:73–86.

McLone DG. Results of treatment of children born with a myelomeningocele. *Clin Neurosurg* 1983;30: 407–412.

Sutherland RS, Mevorach RA, Baskin LS, et al. Spinal dysraphism in children: an overview and an approach to prevent complications. *Urology* 1995;46(3):294–304.

SEE QUESTIONS: 85, 192, 226, 238, 266

CASE 16

CERVICAL MYELOPATHY (SARCOIDOSIS)

OBJECTIVES

- To emphasize the rarity of sarcoidosis exclusively manifested by myelopathy.
- To discuss the differential diagnosis of an expanding intramedullary mass.
- To highlight the importance of careful systemic examination in patients with unexplained myelopathy.
- To review current treatment for sarcoid myelopathy.

VIGNETTE

A 44-year-old woman had a history of progressive hand numbness and pain. Four years earlier, she experienced a tingling sensation in the medial aspect of her left hand. The tingling had progressed to involve her entire left hand and the fourth and fifth fingers of her right hand. She also complained of electric shocklike pains down the medial aspect of both arms. She noted that when taking hot showers, her symptoms were worse. She had difficulties in writing and holding objects, and could no longer exercise.

The pain came in waves lasting approximately 15 minutes. The pain was worse when she was hugged. She has not experienced any visual changes or double vision, weakness, dysarthria, vertigo, or sphincteric difficulties.

CASE SUMMARY

Our patient had a subacute cervical myelopathy. Magnetic resonance imaging (MRI) of the spinal cord showed an intramedullary enhancing mass accompanied by expansile surrounding edema from the C3 to C7 level. A spinal cord tumor was initially suspected by the referring physician. Radiological differential diagnosis included ependymoma, demyelinating disease, multiple sclerosis, metastasis, or transverse myelitis. MRI of the brain showed no intracranial mass, abnormal parenchymal or leptomeningeal enhancement, or other focal abnormalities. The cerebellar tonsils were borderline low. Chest radiograph showed bilateral hilar and right paratracheal lymphadenopathy. Pathological findings of the skin biopsy were consistent with those of sarcoidosis (Fig. 16.1).

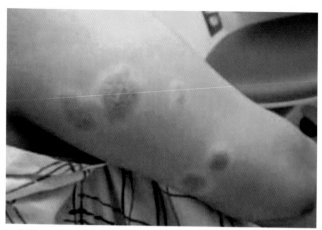

Figure 16.1   Multiple chronic, indurated plaques of sarcoidosis in the arm. These lesions typically do not cause pruritus or pain.

Sarcoidosis is a chronic multisystem granulomatous disease characterized by noncaseating granulomatous reaction of unknown origin. Sarcoidosis most frequently involves the lymph nodes and lungs, but any organ can be compromised. Nervous system involvement represents 5% to 15% of cases. Neurological involvement in the form of myelopathy is one of the rarest manifestations of the disease, affecting less than 0.5% of patients with sarcoidosis. Granulomatous inflammation of the spinal cord and meninges may produce isolated mass lesions or multiple patchy lesions and meningitis. Previous or concurrent skin lesions and eye involvement (i.e., iritis and uveitis) should assist with the diagnosis.

Past history of unexplained cranial neuropathies, aseptic meningitis, or hypothalamic/pituitary dysfunction should raise suspicion (Table 16.1). Differential diagnosis of sarcoidosis includes indolent malignancies such as lymphoma, tuberculosis, fungal infections, and other smoldering granulomatous conditions. Thus, whenever possible, tissue should be obtained in an effort to secure the diagnosis. The importance of searching other locations that are easier and safer to biopsy than the spinal cord itself must be stressed. If there is no readily accessible biopsy site, a blind biopsy of skeletal muscle may be positive in approximately half of the patients.

It has also been suggested that in patients suspected of spinal cord sarcoidosis from MRI findings, a transbronchial lung biopsy be attempted, even if chest roentgenograms or chest computed tomography (CT) are normal. Laboratory data supporting the diagnosis of sarcoidosis include elevation of blood and cerebrospinal fluid (CSF) angiotensin-converting enzyme (ACE) levels and the presence of hilar lymphadenopathy on chest imaging. Elevation of CSF globulin or gamma globulin has been reported in cases of progressive myelopathy due to sarcoidosis.

The clinical course of sarcoid myelopathy is highly variable, including exacerbations and spontaneous remissions. Mainstay of treatment is with corticosteroids. In general, patients with spinal cord involvement have an impressive and relative rapid improvement of clinical and radiographic manifestations when treated with corticosteroids.

TABLE 16.1   **CLINICAL CLUES IN NEUROSARCOIDOSIS**

Cranial nerves	Peripheral facial palsy, often bilateral
	Progressive monocular visual loss (compressive optic neuropathy)
	Subacute monocular visual loss (inflammatory optic neuritis)
	Relapsing painful ophthalmoplegia (similar to Ramsay Hunt syndrome)
	Other cranial neuropathies (vertigo, sensorineural deafness, facial numbness, dysphagia, dysphonia, and ageusia or anosmia)
Sensorimotor assessment	Painful peripheral neuropathies (including as mononeuritis multiplex)
	Other focal motor or sensory findings (important MS mimicker)
	Ascending paralysis with areflexia (Guillain-Barré syndrome; CSF pleocytosis instead of albuminocytologic dissociation)
Other clinical manifestations	Encephalopathy with hyperreflexia (diabetes insipidus)
	Proximal weakness and hyperreflexia (hypercalcemia)
	Erythema nodosum and other skin lesions
	Uveitis and parotiditis (Heerfordt syndrome)
Other paraclinical manifestations	CSF: Lymphocytic pleocytosis with low glucose (aseptic meningitis)
	Serum: High ACE, calcium, and alkaline phosphatase; low gonadotropin, TSH, and ACTH (hypopituitarism)
	Chest x-ray: lymph node enlargement

CSF, cerebrospinal fluid; ACE, angiotensin-converting enzyme.

SELECTED REFERENCES

Delaney P. Neurologic manifestations of sarcoidosis. Review of the literature with a report of 23 cases. *Ann Intern Med* 1977;87:336–346.

Morimoto T, Takeuchi K, Morikawa T, et al. Spinal cord sarcoidosis without abnormal shadows on chest radiography or chest CT diagnosed by transbronchial lung biopsy. *Nihon Kokyuki Gakkai Zasshi* 2001;39:871–876.

Pierre-Kahn V, Capelle L, Sbai A, et al. Intramedullary spinal cord sarcoidosis. Case report and review of the literature. *Neurochirurgie* 2001;47:439–441.

Stern BJ, Krumholz A, Johns C, et al. Sarcoidosis and its neurological manifestations. *Arch Neurol* 1985;42:909–917.

SEE QUESTIONS: 10, 12, 17, 39, 58, 190, 240

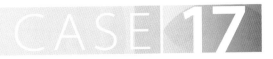

AUTOIMMUNE MYELOPATHY (STIFF PERSON SYNDROME)

OBJECTIVES

- To discuss the main clinical features of stiff person syndrome (SPS).
- To summarize the different red flags guiding the practitioner to conditions mimicking SPS.
- To elaborate an appropriate diagnostic and treatment plan for patients with suspected SPS.

VIGNETTE

A 57-year-old woman with an 8-month history of generalized stiffness with episodic muscle spasms. The spasms began in both lower legs and spread onto the arms over a few months. Each of these lasted for about 30 minutes, with increasing frequency of up to 10 episodes per day. Between episodes, she is feeling stiffer and, as a result, slower. She has come to rely on a cane for ambulation given her fear of falls.

CASE SUMMARY

This middle-aged woman insidiously developed muscle rigidity and superimposed episodic spasms over several months. Examination showed markedly slowed movements due to the presence of rigidity with hyperreflexia without other upper motor neuron signs. She exhibited a cautious gait and exaggeration of normal lumbar lordosis. These features led to the suspicion of stiff person syndrome (SPS), which was confirmed by the identification of high titers of anti–glutamic acid decarboxylase (anti-GAD) antibodies. Clonazepam, increased to a dose of 1 mg four times a day, decreased the excessive rigidity, greatly reduced the frequency of the spasms, and improved her gait velocity and postural reflexes, as shown in the second video.

SPS is characterized by progressive muscular stiffness and gait difficulty with stimulus-sensitive superimposed painful muscle spasms leading to exaggerated lumbar lordosis and impaired ambulation, which progresses to becoming deliberate and slow, in part due to fear of falling (Fig. 17.1A–C). As shown in the video, the spasms may be spontaneous or stimulus sensitive and typically begin with an abrupt jerk, followed by tonic activity that slowly subsides over seconds to, less commonly, minutes. This is

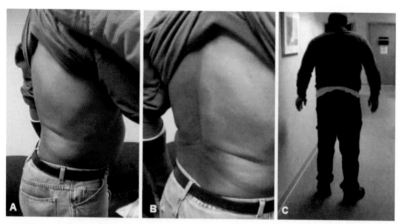

Figure 17.1 Enhanced lumbar lordosis. **A, B:** Note the cast on the left arm was due to a fracture sustained during a recent fall. Patients have increased fear of falling, which may partly explain the boardlike posture with arms extended seen during walking **(C)**. As a clinical paradox, the excessive slowness, which may suggest parkinsonism at a superficial glance, is due to a hyperkinetic disorder, excessive rigidity. (From Espay AJ, Chen R. Rigidity and spasms from autoimmune encephalomyelopathies: stiff-person syndrome. *Muscle Nerve* 2006;34(6):677–690, with permission from Wiley Periodicals, Inc.)

TABLE 17.1   DISORDERS TO CONSIDER IN SPS-LIKE PRESENTATIONS

Disorder	Diagnostic Findings
Tetanus	Laceration or open wound
Strychnine poisoning	Exposure to rat pesticide
Neuromyotonia	Neuromyotonic discharges on EMG
	VGKC antibodies
Cramp–fasciculation syndrome	AChR antibodies
Hyperekplexia	*GLAR1* gene mutation
Primary generalized dystonia	*DYT1* gene mutation
Encephalomyelitis lethargica	Lymphocytic pleocytosis
Neuroborreliosis	*Borrelia burgdorferi* titers

VGKC, voltage-gated potassium channel; AChR, acetylcholine receptor; GLAR1, gene encoding the *a*1 subunit of the glycine receptor.

in contrast with the much faster exaggerated startle reaction of hyperekplexia, where brainstem hypersensitivity results from deficiency of glycine-mediated fast inhibitory postsynaptic potentials (IPSP) unlike the slow gamma aminobutyric acid (GABA)-mediated IPSP of SPS.

Highly specific anti-GAD antibodies are present in most patients, in whom other autoimmune diseases, such as diabetes, hyperthyroidism, hypothyroidism, pernicious anemia, and vitiligo, may co-occur. Anti-GAD antibodies have 99% specificity for the diagnosis of SPS, now most commonly measured by radioimmunoassay or enzyme-linked immunosorbent assay. The diagnosis is also supported by electromyography (EMG), which shows a typical pattern of continuous low-frequency firing of normal motor units in agonist and antagonist muscles of the affected region and at least in one axial muscle. Importantly, for the diagnosis to be suspected pyramidal (except for exaggerated muscle stretch reflexes and loss of abdominal cutaneous reflexes), extrapyramidal, lower motor signs, and sphincter and sensory disturbances must be absent. Presence of these features should suggest an alternative diagnosis. The closest mimickers are tetanus and peripheral nerve hyperexcitability syndromes, such as neuromyotonia (Table 17.1).

The management of SPS rests on removing the pathogenic antibodies and enhancing GABA neurotransmission. Immunosuppressants, plasmapheresis, and intravenous immunoglobulin (IVIG) have been reported as potentially beneficial. High-dose benzodiazepines (diazepam and clonazepam, especially) may decrease the rigidity and abolish the excessive motor unit activity on EMG. For our patient, response to both of these therapies can be appreciated in the second video. Of note, tricyclic antidepressants may worsen SPS symptoms and abrupt withdrawal of pharmacotherapy can be life threatening.

SELECTED REFERENCES

Biller J, ed. *Practical neurology*, 4th ed. Philadelphia: Lippincott Williams & Wilkins, Wolters Kluwer Health, 2012:Chapter 24.

Espay AJ, Chen R. Rigidity and spasms from autoimmune encephalomyelopathies: stiff-person syndrome. *Muscle Nerve* 2006;34(6):677–690.

Espay AJ, Biller J. *Concise neurology*. Philadelphia: Lippincott Williams & Wilkins, Wolters Kluwer Health, 2011:Chapter 53.

SEE QUESTIONS: 267, 268, 269

CASE 18

ISCHEMIC MYELOPATHY (ANTIPHOSPHOLIPID ANTIBODY SYNDROME)

OBJECTIVES

- To review the arterial blood supply of the spinal cord.
- To discuss the main clinical features of spinal cord infarction in the distribution of the anterior spinal artery.
- To summarize the main etiologies of arterial spinal cord infarction.
- To remind clinicians of unusual coagulopathies as the etiology of arterial spinal cord infarction.

VIGNETTE

A 48-year-old woman was evaluated because of weakness and flexion spasms of both legs. During the daytime, she needed to catheterize herself every 2 hours.

CASE SUMMARY

Our patient had a spinal cord infarction (SCI). SCI is an uncommon but often devastating vascular disorder, accounting for approximately 1.2% of all strokes. A variety of causes are described (Tables 18.1 and 18.2). Initial investigations were geared to exclude the most common causes of a rapidly producing partial transverse spinal cord lesion, such as spinal cord compression, spinal cord trauma, acute parainfectious or demyelinating myelopathies, and central cord syndromes caused by tumors or hemorrhages. Arterial SCI can occur when the blood supply to the spinal cord is interrupted anywhere from the aorta to the intramedullary vasculature by a thrombotic or embolic vessel occlusion, inadequate systemic perfusion pressure, or a combination of both mechanisms.

Three basic vascular systems supply the spinal cord: (i) three spinal arteries (a single anterior spinal artery and paired posterior spinal arteries), (ii) radicular arteries, and (iii) terminal extramedullary and intramedullary arteries. The anterior spinal artery descends in the anterior sulcus of the spinal cord, supplying the anterior two-thirds of the spinal cord including the anterior horns, corticospinal tracts, and lateral spinothalamic tracts. The two posterior spinal arteries descend along the posterior surface of the spinal cord as an anastomotic network and supply the posterior one-third of the spinal cord including the dorsal columns. The anterior and posterior spinal arteries join in an anastomotic loop at the conus medullaris. Only a few radicular arteries supply the spinal cord. Among those, the arteria radicularis magna or artery of Adamkiewicz supplies the lower anterior thoracic and lumbosacral spinal cord. The artery of Adamkiewicz arises from the aorta and generally enters the spinal canal typically on the left side (T9-T12). The extramedullary and intramedullary systems are the terminal branches supplying the spinal cord; they are made up of the peripheral vasocorona that encircle the spinal cord and the central or sulcal arteries arising from the anterior spinal artery.

The spectrum of spinal cord vascular disease is broad. It covers thrombotic and embolic (arterial or venous) infarctions (Tables 18.1 and 18.2); lacunar infarctions; transient

TABLE 18.1 **CAUSES OF ARTERIAL SPINAL CORD INFARCTION**

- Atherosclerosis
- Severe arterial hypotension or cardiac arrest
- Aortic surgery
- Traumatic laceration of the aorta
- Dissecting aortic aneurysm
- Thrombo-occlusive aortic disease
- Peripheral vascular surgery
- Infection (lues, tuberculosis)
- Vasculitis
- Neoplastic spread to the spinal cord
- Hypertensive small vessel disease
- Subarachnoid hemorrhage
- Sickle cell anemia
- Systemic lupus erythematosus
- Polyarteritis nodosa
- Antiphospholipid antibody syndrome
- Disseminated intravascular coagulation
- Cervical spondylosis
- Spine fracture or dislocation
- Ankylosing spondylitis
- Vertebral artery occlusion or dissection
- Rib resection for sympathectomy
- Lumbar sympathectomy
- Thoracoplasty for tuberculosis
- Thoracotomy
- Intercostal artery ligation
- Esophageal surgery
- Celiac plexus block
- Decompression sickness (Caisson disease)
- Atheromatous emboli
- Cholesterol emboli
- Fibrocartilaginous emboli
- Atrial myxoma
- Aortic or spinal cord angiography
- Intraaortic balloon pump
- Lumbar artery compression
- Supine hyperlordosis (OR), cervical flexion myelopathy after valproic acid overdose

Cheshire WP, Santos CC, Massey EW, Howard JF Jr. Spinal cord infarction: etiology and outcome. *Neurology* 1996;47:321–330; Williams LS, Bruno A, Biller J. Spinal cord infarction. *Top Stroke Rehabil* 1996;3(Jan):41–53.

ischemic attacks (TIAs, embolic or hemodynamic); hematomyelia; epidural, subdural, and subarachnoid hemorrhage; and spinal cord vascular malformations.

SCI remains a diagnostic challenge. Manifestations are protean and are often associated with striking clinical variability due to the greater vulnerability of the gray matter to ischemia, variations in the number and caliber of the radicular arteries and the availability of collateral vessels. SCI may present as with a classic anterior spinal artery distribution infarct with bilateral motor and sensory deficits, or as an anterior spinal artery unilateral

TABLE 18.2 CAUSES OF VENOUS SPINAL CORD INFARCTION

- Thrombophlebitis
- Chronic meningitis
- Caisson disease
- Acute myelogenous leukemia
- Spinal cord glioma
- Polycythemia rubra vera
- Esophageal vein sclerotherapy
- Liver abscess (embolization of venous material)
- Fibrocartilaginous emboli
- Spinal cord DAVF

DAVF, dural arteriovenous fistula
Adapted from Williams LS, Bruno A, Biller J. Spinal cord infarction. *Top Stroke Rehabil* 1996;3(Jan):41–53.

infarct, a posterior spinal artery unilateral infarct, a central infarct, bilateral spinal artery infarct, or a transverse SCI. The anterior spinal artery infarct typically is associated with back or neck pain of sudden onset, paralysis, and loss of pain and temperature sensation below the level of the infarction with sparing of position, vibration, and light touch. Bladder and bowel function are impaired. Onset and evolution of symptoms may be more gradual as in cases of hypoxic myelopathy and spinal cord claudication. The anterior spinal artery syndrome most commonly occurs in watershed or boundary zones where distal branches of major arterial systems of the spinal cord anastomose, between the T1 and T4 segments and at the L1 segment. Magnetic resonance imaging of the spinal cord is the procedure of choice to exclude a compressive lesion masquerading as spinal cord ischemia. If not available or contraindicated, spinal CT myelography should be performed. Once spinal cord compression has been ruled out, a lumbar puncture can be performed to exclude inflammatory, infectious, or neoplastic processes.

After extensive evaluation, our patient was found to have persistent elevations of antiphospholipid antibodies titer. Her SCI was attributed to a prothrombotic state due to a primary antiphospholipid antibody syndrome (APAS). Reported neurologic involvement associated with antiphospholipid antibodies includes ischemic strokes, TIAs, ocular ischemia, migrainous-like events, cerebral venous thrombosis, vascular dementia (with or without Sneddon syndrome), acute ischemic encephalopathy, transient global amnesia, seizures, chorea, Guillain-Barré syndrome, and transverse myelopathy. It is generally accepted that oral anticoagulation with warfarin is the preferred treatment for the prevention of thromboembolic events in patients with APAS. Our patient received warfarin titrated to a moderate-intensity international normalized ratio (INR) range (INR 2.0 to 3.0).

SELECTED REFERENCES

Cheshire WP, Santos CC, Massey EW, Howard JF Jr. Spinal cord infarction: etiology and outcome. *Neurology* 1996;47:321–330.

Cuadrado MJ, Hughes GRV. Antiphospholipid (Hughes) syndrome. *Rheum Dis Clin North Am* 2001;27:507–524.

Novy J, Carruzzo A, Maeder P, Bogousslavsky J. Spinal cord ischemia. Clinical and imaging patterns, pathogenesis, and outcomes in 27 patients. *Arch Neurol* 2006;63:113–1120.

Williams LS, Bruno A, Biller J. Spinal cord infarction. *Top Stroke Rehabil* 1996;3(Jan):41–53.

SEE QUESTIONS: 10, 12, 14, 18

CASE 19

PARAPARESIS AFTER NITROUS OXIDE ANESTHESIA

OBJECTIVES

- To emphasize a rare neurological complication of nitrous oxide exposure.
- To discuss the differential diagnosis of cobalamin (B_{12}) deficiency.
- To remind the practitioner that nitrous oxide can cause cobalamin (B_{12}) deficiency.
- To highlight the importance of careful assessment of vitamin B_{12} levels prior to any exposure to nitrous oxide.

VIGNETTE

A 46-year-old previously healthy man with abdominal pain and diarrhea was hospitalized and found to have an increased white blood count (WBC). He had a sigmoid colon resection with a colostomy under epidural anesthesia; he also received general anesthesia with nitrous oxide.

Following surgery, he complained of weakness in both lower extremities, numbness on both feet, lack of bilateral bladder control, and impaired erections.

CASE SUMMARY

A nonvegan man with possible subclinical cobalamin (vitamin B_{12}) deficiency developed lower extremity weakness and numbness, loss of bladder control, and impaired erections after exposure to nitrous oxide anesthesia. He also had received epidural anesthesia. Examination demonstrated predominantly distal lower extremity paresis, patellar hyperreflexia, Achilles areflexia, and sensory changes on L5-S1 distribution. He also had bilateral extensor plantar responses (not shown on the tape). Magnetic resonance imaging (MRI) of the thoracic and lumbosacral spine showed minimal posterior epidural fluid collection at the T12-L1 level, probably representing a resolving discrete epidural hematoma.

Electromyography (EMG) findings were consistent with an acute bilateral lumbosacral radiculopathy involving the L5-S1 nerve roots. Urodynamic studies showed a hypotonic neurogenic bladder with intact sensation. He was found to have low serum vitamin B_{12}. We interpreted his clinical and laboratory findings as strong evidence of a myeloneuropathy due to exposure to nitrous oxide in an individual who had subclinical vitamin B_{12} deficiency. We felt the small epidural hematoma noted on MRI was not clinically significant.

The most common cause of cobalamin deficiency is pernicious anemia due to autoimmune parietal cell dysfunction, associated with defective gastric secretion and absence of intrinsic factor. Cobalamin deficiency may also be caused by inadequate dietary intake (vegans), atrophy of the gastric mucosa, partial or total gastrectomy, functionally abnormal intrinsic factor, inadequate proteolysis of dietary cobalamin, insufficient pancreatic protease, bacterial overgrowth in the intestine, terminal ileum disease, tropical sprue, genetic enzyme deficiencies (methylmalonic aciduria), tapeworm infection, disorders of plasma transport of cobalamin, dysfunctional uptake and use of cobalamin by cells, drugs such as metformin, and nitrous oxide administration. Classic pernicious anemia produces cobalamin deficiency due to failure of the stomach to secrete intrinsic factor. Pernicious anemia is also associated with other autoimmune diseases, such as Addison disease, Graves disease, and hypoparathyroidism. In pernicious anemia, the neurological manifestations reflect myelin degeneration of the dorsal and lateral columns of the spinal cord, peripheral nerve dysfunction, and cerebral dysfunction. Myelopathy, peripheral neuropathy, and optic neuropathy are common neurologic complications of pernicious anemia.

Patients often present with paresthesias of toes and fingers, weakness, clumsiness, distal loss of proprioception, and unsteady gait. Loss of position sense in the second toe and loss of vibratory sense for a 256-Hz but not a 128-Hz tuning fork are the earliest signs of dorsolateral column involvement. A Lhermitte sign may be present. Confusion, irritability, memory impairment, perversion of taste and smell, diminished visual acuity, optic atrophy, and impaired micturition may occur as well.

Nitrous oxide (N_2O) is widely used in anesthesia and is also used as a propellant in the food industry (e.g., in whipped cream dispensers). Nitrous oxide is a potent oxidant that has multiple deleterious effects on cobalamin metabolism. In humans, the use of nitrous oxide is associated with neurologic and hematologic abnormalities. Patients with unrecognized cobalamin deficiency may be particularly susceptible to brief exposures to nitrous oxide, which inactivates cobalamin-dependent methionine synthase and may cause a myeloneuropathy. In healthy subjects, this side effect on the methionine synthase methylcobalamin complex may be well compensated for by the large vitamin B_{12} stores in the liver and bone marrow. For patients with a preexisting vitamin B_{12} deficiency, even a short course of nitrous oxide anesthesia may deplete the few remaining stores. Furthermore, the inactivation of methionine synthase by nitrous oxide may be more rapid in patients with low concentrations of vitamin B_{12}.

Initial reported clinical features for nitrous oxide toxicity may be acral paresthesias and a "reverse" Lhermitte sign, corresponding with vibration and position sensory loss and hypo- or areflexia in the legs. Later features may include distal leg weakness, hand clumsiness, erectile dysfunction, neurogenic bladder, and encephalopathy, at a time when hyperreflexia and Babinski signs as well as more dense proprioceptive loss may emerge. Nerve conduction studies show an axonal sensorimotor neuropathy.

Clinicians should be aware of this condition when confronted with patients with a myeloneuropathy after surgical or dental procedures. Since vitamin B_{12} levels may be normal or reduced, appropriate screening should include serum homocysteine and methylmalonate levels, which may be elevated before B_{12} is measurably low. The risk may be avoided by promptly administering cobalamin to patients with suspected or confirmed vitamin B_{12} deficiency before surgery involving nitrous oxide anesthesia. Since approximately 14% of the population may have a cobalamin deficiency, awareness of this information is critical. Our patient subsequently received intramuscular injections of vitamin B_{12}, 1,000 μg daily for 5 days and then 1,000 μg every month. He also received folate replacement therapy.

SELECTED REFERENCES

Green R, Kinsella LJ. Current concepts in the diagnosis of cobalamin deficiency. *Neurology* 1995;45:1435–1440.

Marie RM, Le Biez E, Busson P, et al. Nitrous oxide anesthesia-associated myelopathy. *Arch Neurol* 2000;57:380–382.

McMorrow AM, Adams RJ, Rubenstein MN. Combined system disease after nitrous oxide anesthesia: a case report. *Neurology* 1995;45:1224–1225.

Rosener M, Dichgans J. Severe combined degeneration of the spinal cord after nitrous oxide anaesthesia in a vegetarian. *J Neurol Neurosurg Psychiatry* 1996;60:354–356.

Shulman RM, Geraghty TJ, Tadros M. A case of unusual substance causing myeloneuropathy. *Spinal Cord* 2007;45:314–317.

SEE QUESTIONS: 10, 14, 15, 39, 58, 141, 172, 192, 210, 213, 270

SECTION 3

BEHAVIORAL NEUROLOGY

CASE 20

NONFLUENT APHASIA SECONDARY TO LEFT FRONTAL INFARCTION

OBJECTIVES

- To present characteristic features of Broca aphasia.
- To name the most common types of aphasia.
- To review one of the most common etiologies of Broca aphasia.

VIGNETTE

One week after quadruple coronary artery bypass, a 62-year-old man with history of coronary artery disease, hypertension, hyperlipidemia, and prior left hemispheric cortical infarct had sudden onset of language difficulties and right-sided weakness.

CASE SUMMARY

One week following four-vessel coronary artery bypass graft (CABG) surgery, and while on 81 mg of aspirin daily, our patient had sudden onset of language impairment. Upon arising from bed and going to the restroom, he abruptly became unable to speak. His wife immediately called 911. Past medical history was remarkable for arterial hypertension, hyperlipidemia, three myocardial infarctions, and a left parietal ischemic stroke. The patient was treated with intra-arterial tissue plasminogen activator (tPA).

On subsequent evaluation, he had nonfluent verbal output. Speech was poorly articulated, effortful, and dysprosodic. He was able to utter the most meaningful words of a sentence, but often omitted words (telegraphic speech or agrammatism). Repetition was impaired. There was relative preservation of comprehension of spoken language. There was a faciobrachial distribution of his right hemiparesis. Echocardiography showed left

41

ventricular dilatation, reduced global left ventricular systolic function, left atrial dilatation, regional wall motion abnormality, mild mitral regurgitation, and a thickened aortic valve without significant stenosis. A diagnosis of Broca aphasia due to a cardioembolic left frontal infarction involving branches of the superior division of the middle cerebral artery (MCA) was made and warfarin therapy initiated (target INR range, 2.0 to 3.0).

Aphasia refers to loss or impairment of language processing caused by brain damage. When assessing language function, one must note verbal fluency, auditory comprehension, naming, repetition, reading, and writing. Repetition should include sentences with functor words. "No ifs, ands, or buts" is commonly used. The traditional perisylvian aphasias are (i) Broca aphasia, (ii) Wernicke aphasia, (iii) global aphasia, and (iv) conduction aphasia. The other four traditional aphasic syndromes arise from lesions outside the perisylvian region and include anomic aphasia and the three types of transcortical aphasias (transcortical motor, transcortical sensory, and mixed transcortical) (Table 20.1). The perisylvian aphasias are "nonrepetitive" (repetition is impaired), whereas the extraperisylvian aphasias are "repetitive" (repetition is preserved).

Broca aphasia is characterized by nonfluent verbal output, poor repetition, and relatively intact comprehension of spoken language. Prosody is often disturbed. Writing (even with the nonparalyzed left hand) and oral reading abilities are impaired. Patients with Broca aphasia are aware of their language deficits and often become frustrated and depressed. Lesions producing this type of aphasia are typically located in the posterior portion of the inferior frontal gyrus, anterior to the motor strip, of the dominant hemisphere. Usually the lesions extend to the neighboring cortex and underlying white matter. The most common cause of Broca aphasia is arterial occlusion of the superior division of the left middle cerebral artery branches.

Wernicke aphasia is characterized by fluent and effortless speech output (although meaningless or paraphasic), impaired auditory comprehension, and poor repetition. Patients are typically unaware of their errors. Lesions producing this type of aphasia are typically located in the posterior part of the superior temporal gyrus of the dominant hemisphere. Global aphasia is characterized by nonfluent speech, poor auditory comprehension, and poor repetition. Lesions are typically located throughout the perisylvian region of the dominant hemisphere, encompassing at least part of the frontal, temporal, and parietal lobes. Conduction aphasia is characterized by fairly fluent speech, relatively intact auditory comprehension, but poor repetition and some phonemic paraphasias. The arcuate fasciculus connecting Broca and Wernicke areas is often involved, but lesions circumscribed to the supramarginal gyrus, primary auditory cortex, and large posterior

TABLE 20.1   CLASSIFICATION OF APHASIA TYPES BASED ON LANGUAGE FEATURES

Type	Fluency	Comprehension	Repetition
Broca	Nonfluent	Intact (relative)	Impaired
Wernicke	Fluent	Impaired	Impaired
Global	Nonfluent	Impaired	Impaired
Conduction	Fluent	Intact	Impaired
Anomic	Fluent	Intact	Intact
Transcortical motor	Nonfluent	Intact	Intact
Transcortical sensory	Fluent	Impaired	Intact
Mixed transcortical	Impaired	Impaired	Intact

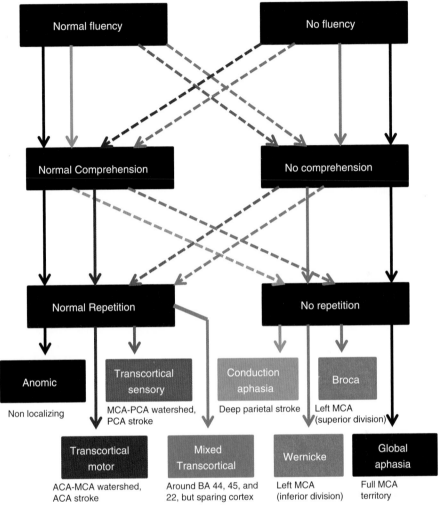

Figure 20.1 This diagram illustrates the classic aphasias and their localizing value in acute settings. The "repetitive" left four are often due to watershed infarcts outside the perisylvian region. The "nonrepetitive" right four result from large vessel occlusions in the perisylvian region and the localizing value of each.

perisylvian lesions also cause conduction aphasia. In most aphasias, reading impairment and writing impairment parallel oral language comprehension and expression deficits. Paraphasic errors and word-finding difficulties can be seen in many types of aphasia. Assessment of the fluency, comprehension, and repetition of language should enable the clinician to determine the type of aphasia and its localizing value (Fig. 20.1).

Clinical presentation of ischemic stroke differs depending on the affected area(s) of the brain. The most common causes are atheromatous disease in large- and medium-sized extracranial and/or intracranial arteries, small vessel disease, and cardiac embolism. Rare causes include border-zone ("watershed") infarcts due to arterial hypotension and poor cerebral perfusion, cervicocephalic arterial dissection, other nonatherosclerotic vasculopathies, and hypercoagulable states.

The MCA territory is most commonly involved in patients with ischemic stroke. Clinical picture of MCA territory infarction varies according to site of occlusion (e.g., stem, superior division, inferior division, and lenticulostriate branches) and available collaterals. Clinical features of MCA territory infarction are extremely varied (e.g., complete MCA territory, deep territory, superficial anterior [superior] territory, and superficial posterior [inferior] territory). Embolism of cardiac origin accounts for approximately 15% to 20% of all ischemic strokes. Stroke occurs after CABG with a frequency ranging between 1% and 5%. Two-thirds of strokes occur by the second postoperative day and predominantly involve the cerebral hemispheres.

SELECTED REFERENCES

Alexander MP, Benson DF. The aphasias and related disturbances. In: Joynt RJ, ed. *Clinical neurology*, Vol 1. Philadelphia: JB Lippincott Co, 1993:1–58.

Biller J, ed. *Practical neurology*, 4th ed. Philadelphia: Lippincott Williams & Wilkins, Wolters Kluwer Health, 2012:Chapter 3.

Mesulam MM. *Principles of behavioral neurology*, 2nd ed. New York: Oxford, 2000.

SEE QUESTIONS: 32, 53, 174, 271, 272

CASE **21**

NONFLUENT APHASIA SECONDARY TO LICA OCCLUSION

OBJECTIVES

- To demonstrate a brief evaluation of a patient with an acute aphasic syndrome.
- To name the perisylvian aphasias.
- To analyze the most common characteristics and evolution of global aphasia.

VIGNETTE

A 69-year-old African-American woman with a history of arterial hypertension and diabetes was evaluated because of sudden onset of speech difficulties.

CASE SUMMARY

Our patient had sudden onset of language difficulties. The video shown was obtained within 24 hours of symptom onset. On initial evaluation, her spontaneous speech was markedly reduced but not to a state of mutism. She was able to utter only a few words (e.g., well, yes, and OK). Naming, repetition, and comprehension of spoken language were compromised. Reading and writing (not shown) were also affected. She had a minimal right central facial paresis, a right-hand pronator drift, and a right Babinski sign.

Despite minimal associated neurologic deficits, her acute aphasia fits best with a nonfluent, nonrepetitive aphasia with impaired comprehension, thus resembling a global aphasia. Further investigations showed an acute left frontal infarction and an occluded cervical left internal carotid artery at its origin.

We suspected intracranial embolism to be the most likely mechanism of her frontal infarction. She was treated with aspirin and received speech therapy. Her aphasia subsequently evolved into a Broca aphasia.

Aphasia refers to loss or impairment of language processing caused by brain damage. When assessing language function, one must note verbal fluency, auditory comprehension, naming, repetition, reading, and writing. The traditional *perisylvian* aphasias are (i) Broca aphasia, (ii) Wernicke aphasia, (iii) global aphasia, and (iv) conduction aphasia. The common element to these aphasias is the universal impairment of repetition.

Figure 20.1 summarizes the essential features of these aphasias. The other four aphasic syndromes include anomic aphasia and the three types of transcortical aphasias (transcortical motor, transcortical sensory, and mixed transcortical). In these *nonperisylvian* aphasias (due to lesions outside the perisylvian region), repetition is preserved.

Broca aphasia is characterized by nonfluent speech, poor repetition, and relatively intact comprehension. Lesions producing this type of aphasia are typically located in the posterior portion of the inferior frontal gyrus of the dominant hemisphere. Wernicke aphasia is characterized by fluent and effortless speech output, impaired auditory comprehension, and poor repetition. Lesions producing this type of aphasia are typically located in the posterior part of the superior temporal gyrus of the dominant hemisphere. Global aphasia is characterized by nonfluent speech, poor auditory comprehension, and poor repetition. Most patients with classical global aphasia have an associated right hemiplegia, right hemisensory abnormalities, and right homonymous visual field loss.

For these classic, nonrepetitive aphasias, the causative lesions are typically located throughout the perisylvian region of the dominant hemisphere, affecting the frontal (Broca), temporal (Wernicke), or parietal lobe (conduction), or a combination of the three (global). Rare cases are reported, however, with global aphasia associated with two discrete lesions in the dominant hemisphere (one frontal and one temporoparietal) but less severe neurologic deficits. The latter situation is usually due to embolic strokes, but may also result from intraparenchymal hemorrhages and cerebral metastases. As with our patient, global aphasia may evolve into a Broca aphasia. Conduction aphasia is characterized by fairly fluent speech, relatively intact auditory comprehension, but poor repetition. The arcuate fasciculus connecting Broca and Wernicke areas is often involved, but lesions circumscribed to the supramarginal gyrus, primary auditory cortex, and large posterior perisylvian lesions also cause conduction aphasia. In most aphasias, reading impairment and writing impairment parallel oral language comprehension and expression deficits. Paraphasic errors and word-finding difficulties can be seen in many types of aphasia.

Occlusion of the internal carotid artery (ICA) can produce symptoms and signs of infarction in either the middle cerebral artery (MCA) or, less commonly, the anterior cerebral artery (ACA) territories, or both. Posterior cerebral artery (PCA) territory infarctions can also be seen with ICA occlusion if a fetal origin (from a large posterior communicating artery) of the PCA is present. The single feature distinguishing the ICA syndrome from a middle cerebral artery syndrome is the presence of amaurosis fugax. The carotid pulse may be absent ipsilaterally. A Horner syndrome may be present due to oculosympathetic involvement along the course of the internal carotid artery.

SELECTED REFERENCES

Benson DF, Ardila A. *Aphasia: a clinical perspective.* New York: Oxford University Press, 1996.

Biller J, ed. *Practical Neurology,* 4th ed. Philadelphia: Lippincott Williams & Wilkins, Wolters Kluwer Health, 2012:Chapter 3.

Legatt AD, Rubin MJ, Kaplan LR, et al. Global aphasia without hemiparesis: multiple etiologies. *Neurology* 1987;37:201–205.

Mesulam MM. *Principles of behavioral neurology,* 2nd ed. New York: Oxford, 2000.

SEE QUESTIONS: 33, 66, 89, 167, 183

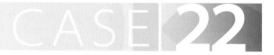

FLUENT APHASIA SECONDARY TO LEFT POSTERIOR TEMPORAL INFARCTION

OBJECTIVES

- To define aphasia.
- To name the most common types of aphasia.
- To name the most common anatomic location for each type of aphasia.

VIGNETTE

A 49-year-old right-handed woman, a high school math teacher, without known vascular risk factors, had sudden onset of speech difficulties and headaches.

CASE SUMMARY

Our patient had a master's degree in math education. She had no prior history of heart disease, arterial hypertension, diabetes, dyslipidemia, or cigarette smoking. She had a history of two previous miscarriages. While skiing, she suddenly became disoriented and could not remember her daughter's friend's name. She was diagnosed with an acute ischemic stroke involving the left posterior temporal region.

She then complained of residual confusion when writing or spelling and often hunting for words particularly with multisyllabic words. She also made mistakes while reading aloud and had difficulty following conversations. She suspected her memory was reasonably clear for recent details, events, and conversations. She doubted having new problems with mathematics, but she did have trouble remembering phone numbers and quickly transcribing them. She was very much concerned about her ability to return to work as a teacher, given the state of her language deficits.

On initial evaluation, our patient's conversational speech was unremarkable for dysarthria. Prosody was normal. Phrase length was long and language was grammatic, but there were occasional phonemic paraphasias. Letter fluency was impaired. Confrontation naming on the Boston naming test was quite impaired with only 32/60 items named spontaneously and without errors. This improved to 47/60 after self-correction and successive approximation. Comprehension of conversatioanl speech was quite good, but comprehension of syntactically complex or subtly worded questions was clearly impaired.

Writing was marked by good letter formation, although spelling was clearly defective for her level of education. Mental arithmetic was average for age and clearly complicated by poor comprehension, and questions had to be restated several times. Written arithmetic was very well preserved and superior for age. Constructional praxis in assembling blocks to match a template and in copying geometric figures from memory was quite good.

Our patient's aphasia fits best into the category of conduction aphasia, a fluent aphasia with overtly normal comprehension, though subtle impairments in more extensive evaluation, but clearly abnormal repetition. Further investigations showed hyperhomocysteinemia and transient elevation of β_2 glycoprotein 1 antibodies. She received treatment with aspirin plus clopidogrel and also a combination of folic acid, pyridoxine (vitamin B_6), and cobalamin (vitamin B_{12}).

Aphasia refers to loss or impairment of language processing caused by brain damage. When assessing language function one must note verbal fluency, auditory comprehension, naming, repetition, reading, and writing. Repetition should include sentences with functor words. "No ifs, ands, or buts" is commonly used. The traditional perisylvian aphasias are (i) Broca aphasia, (ii) Wernicke aphasia, (iii) global aphasia, and (iv) conduction aphasia. Figure 20.1 summarizes the essential features of these aphasias. The other four extra-perisylvian aphasic syndromes include anomic aphasia and the three types of transcortical aphasias (transcortical motor, transcortical sensory, and mixed transcortical) where repetition is preserved.

Broca aphasia is characterized by nonfluent speech, poor repetition, and relatively intact comprehension. Lesions producing this type of aphasia are typically located in the posterior portion of the inferior frontal gyrus of the dominant hemisphere. Wernicke aphasia is characterized by fluent and effortless speech output, impaired auditory comprehension, and poor repetition. Lesions producing this type of aphasia are typically located in the posterior part of the superior temporal gyrus of the dominant hemisphere. Global aphasia is characterized by nonfluent speech, poor auditory comprehension, and poor repetition. Lesions are typically located throughout the perisylvian region of the dominant hemisphere, encompassing at least part of the frontal, temporal, and parietal lobes.

Conduction aphasia is characterized by fairly fluent speech, relatively intact auditory comprehension, but poor repetition. The arcuate fasciculus connecting Broca and Wernicke areas is often involved, but lesions circumscribed to the supramarginal gyrus, primary auditory cortex, and large posterior perisylvian lesions also cause conduction aphasia. In most aphasias, reading impairment and writing impairment parallel oral language comprehension and expression deficits. Paraphasic errors and word-finding difficulties can be seen in many types of aphasia.

Commonly used formal scored tests for evaluation of patients with aphasia include the Boston Diagnostic Aphasia Examination (BDAE), the Western Aphasia Battery (WAB), and the Token Test.

SELECTED REFERENCES

Biller J, ed. *Practical neurology*, 4th ed. Philadelphia: Lippincott Williams & Wilkins, Wolters Kluwer Health, 2012:Chapter 3.

Mesulam MM. *Principles of behavioral neurology*, 2nd ed. New York: Oxford, 2000.

SEE QUESTIONS: 48, 174

CASE 23

WERNICKE APHASIA SECONDARY TO LEFT MCA INFARCTION

OBJECTIVES

- To name the most common types of aphasia.
- To name the most common anatomic location for each type of aphasia.
- To present characteristic language abnormalities in a patient with Wernicke aphasia.

VIGNETTE

A 63-year-old right-handed man, retired construction worker, and part-time professional musician with history of hypertension and hyperlipidemia presented to his local hospital with sudden onset of right-sided weakness and language difficulties. He was treated with intravenous tPA.

CASE SUMMARY

Our patient had a sudden onset of right-sided weakness and language difficulties. At the local emergency room, his blood pressure was 230/120 mm Hg. He received intravenous labetalol, and after a computed tomography (CT) scan was obtained and blood pressure parameters became within appropriate range for thrombolytic therapy, intravenous tPA was administered. His right-sided hemiparesis improved, but his language impairment persisted.

Additional ancillary investigations showed an elevated antinuclear antibody (ANA) (1:2,560) nucleolar pattern, elevated cholesterol, low-density lipoprotein (LDL), and triglycerides. Echocardiography showed left ventricular hypertrophy and aortic valve sclerosis, but no evidence of intracardiac thrombi or right-to-left shunt. Carotid ultrasound showed mild plaque formation of both carotid artery bulbs. Magnetic resonance imaging (MRI) showed a large middle cerebral artery territory infarction. Magnetic resonance angiography (MRA) showed decreased visualization of a few branches of the inferior division of the left middle cerebral artery. He received antiplatelet therapy, antihypertensives, and a statin. He was referred for further evaluation.

On examination, he was at times anxious and agitated. Verbal output was fluent and phrase lengths of up to 23 words observed. Utterances frequently contained neologistic paraphasias. He also had a number of phonemic paraphasias. Naming and repetition were severely impaired. He could not reliably follow any more than one-step command. Comprehension of sentences spoken by others was quite impaired. Comprehension of syntactically complex questions and stories was also clearly defective. Reading out loud and reading comprehension were abnormal. He could not read simple sentences without being paraphasic.

Written expression was accurate for his name but no other autobiographical information. He could not recite automatic sequences (days of the week and months of the year). He could complete simple sentences by selecting the appropriate word, but this quickly became inaccurate with increasing complexity. He attempted to augment the spoken word with spontaneous physical gestures on a number of occasions. He also frequently provided circumlocution/verbal description to help himself in communicating his message. There was right-arm ideomotor apraxia and a residual right superior homonymous quadrantanopia.

In summary, our patient's language impairment was characterized by increased verbal output, impaired repetition, and impaired comprehension of spoken language, characteristic of Wernicke aphasia. He also had frequent semantic and neologistic paraphasias. A literal paraphasia is when a syllable is substituted within a word (phonemic substitution). Words can be substituted only by meaningless words (neologisms). Further ancillary investigations showed persistent elevations of IgG anticardiolipin (aCL) and antiphosphatidylethanolamine (aPE) antibodies. Antiplatelet therapy was discontinued. He was started on warfarin (INR target range, 2.0 to 3.0) and referred for speech therapy.

Aphasia refers to loss or impairment of language processing caused by brain damage. When assessing language function one must note verbal fluency, auditory comprehension, naming, repetition, reading, and writing. The traditional ("nonrepetitive") perisylvian aphasias are (i) Broca aphasia, (ii) Wernicke aphasia, (iii) global aphasia, and (iv) conduction aphasia. Figure 20.1 summarizes the essential features of these aphasias. The extra-perisylvian aphasic syndromes include anomic aphasia and the three types of transcortical aphasias (transcortical motor, transcortical sensory, and mixed transcortical) where repetition is preserved.

Broca aphasia is characterized by nonfluent speech, poor repetition, and relatively intact comprehension. Lesions producing this type of aphasia are typically located in the posterior portion of the inferior frontal gyrus of the dominant hemisphere. Wernicke aphasia is characterized by fluent and effortless speech output, impaired auditory comprehension, and poor repetition. The content of speech is often unintelligible because of frequent errors in phonemes and word choices. Lesions producing this type of aphasia are typically located in the posterior part of the superior temporal gyrus of the dominant hemisphere. Wernicke aphasia most commonly occurs due to infarction in the distribution of the inferior division of the left middle cerebral artery.

Patients with Wernicke aphasia are often misdiagnosed as having a psychiatric disorder, especially as associated hemiparesis and sensory loss may be absent. Recovery in Wernicke aphasia is less favorable than in Broca aphasia. Patients recovering from Wernicke aphasia may develop the profile of a conduction or anomic aphasia. Global aphasia is characterized by nonfluent speech, poor auditory comprehension, and poor repetition. Lesions are typically located throughout the perisylvian region of the dominant hemisphere, encompassing at least part of the frontal, temporal, and parietal lobes. Conduction aphasia is characterized by fairly fluent speech, relatively intact auditory comprehension, but poor repetition. The arcuate fasciculus connecting Broca and Wernicke areas is often involved, but lesions circumscribed to the supramarginal gyrus, primary auditory cortex, and large posterior perisylvian lesions may also cause conduction aphasia. In most aphasias, reading impairment and writing impairment parallel oral language comprehension and expression deficits. Paraphasic errors and word-finding difficulties can be seen in many types of aphasia.

SELECTED REFERENCES

Biller J, ed. *Practical neurology*, 4th ed. Philadelphia: Lippincott Williams & Wilkins, Wolters Kluwer Health, 2012:Chapter 3.

Brazis PW, Masdeu JC, Biller J. *Localization in clinical neurology*, 6th ed. Philadelphia: Lippincott Williams & Wilkins, Wolters Kluwer Health, 2011.

Devinsky O. *Behavioral neurology. 100 maxims in Neurology Series*, Vol 1. London: Edward Arnold, 1992:88–90.

Mesulam MM. *Principles of behavioral neurology*, 2nd ed. New York: Oxford, 2000.

SEE QUESTIONS: 70, 88, 174, 233, 273, 274

CASE **24**

PRIMARY PROGRESSIVE APHASIA

OBJECTIVES

- To present characteristic features of the syndrome of primary progressive aphasia (PPA).
- To describe the diagnostic features of the three PPA phenotypes: progressive nonfluent aphasia, semantic dementia, and logopenic aphasia.
- To name the most common etiologies associated with each of the phenotypes of the PPA syndrome.

VIGNETTE

Nine years earlier, this 72-year-old right-handed man consulted us because of difficulty "coming up with proper words." Since then, he had progressive difficulties with several cognitive functions, most specifically forgetting names and nouns and having impaired reading. Most specific complaints consisted of his inability to name objects even though he could describe their meaning. He also frequently forgot names of relatives and friends.

CASE SUMMARY

 Our patient was a Ph.D. research physiologist whom we followed clinically since 1997. Evaluation at that time indicated an anomic aphasia with normal comprehension, anterograde memory, executive function, and visual perception.

In 2000, he noted worsening ability to read and find words and to comprehend certain nouns. His wife also suspected changes on his recent memory. His judgment had also deteriorated as he engaged in risky ventures. Examination at that time demonstrated well-preserved social graces. Verbal output was largely fluent but showed worsening word-finding difficulties particularly with nouns. Speech was more empty, anomic, and circumlocutory. Occasional semantic paraphasias were also present in conversational speech.

He was able to solve complex and abstract problems nonverbally. There was also mild decline in anterograde visual memory. Constructional praxis remained above average for age but mildly worse than on previous examinations.

In 2001, he felt overall quite good, but unhappy and frustrated. However, he continued to do and enjoy woodworking and mowing the lawn. He nevertheless fell from a ladder when inappropriately standing on the top step and injured his shoulder. His son described this as one of many instances of his apparent lack of judgment. Another example included filling a lawn mower with a lit cigar in his mouth.

Examination showed an alert and awake man whose affect and mood appeared to be euthymic and reactive. Conversational speech was clearly empty and anomic, with a number of literal and semantic paraphasias. Confrontation naming remained severely impaired.

Both reading and written comprehension were clearly impaired, although reading comprehension was significantly worse. Nonverbal problem solving remained quite good on the Wisconsin Card Sorting Test. Nonverbal reasoning with matrices also continued to be well preserved. Visual memory for geometric designs was impaired and worse than in previous evaluations.

In summary, our patient had a slowly progressive language disorder. He maintained normal cognitive abilities early on in the course of his disease process. Based on the distinctive clinical manifestations, neuropsychological findings, and neuroimaging investigations, we concluded he had primary progressive aphasia (PPA), with a semantic dementia phenotype

PPA is a distinctive but unusual clinical syndrome characterized by a slow deterioration of language functions with relative preservation of other cognitive functions for at least the first 2 years from symptom onset. PPA has been divided into three clinical phenotypes: (1) nonfluent progressive aphasia (NFPA), characterized by apraxia of speech and deficits in processing complex syntax, associated with left inferior frontal and insular atrophy; (2) semantic dementia, characterized by fluent speech and semantic memory deficits, associated with left anterior temporal damage; and (3) logopenic aphasia, characterized by slow speech and impaired syntactic comprehension and naming, showed atrophy in the left posterior temporal cortex and inferior parietal lobule. The underlying pathology is most commonly a tauopathy such as corticobasal degeneration or frontotemporal lobar degeneration due to MAPT mutations (FTLD-tau) in cases of PNFA, ubiquitin- and TDP-43-positive proteinopathies associated frontotemporal lobar degeneration with or without progranulin (FTLD-U) in cases of semantic dementia, and Alzheimer disease in the case of logopenic aphasia.

Semantic dementia results in a syntactically fluent but empty speech, with semantic paraphasias and shrinking vocabulary (poor word retrieval). As shown in the video, our patient also exhibited surface dyslexia, a selective reading deficit that affects the print-to-sound translation of irregularly pronounced words, which is a common feature of semantic dementia and, less commonly, other neurodegenerative dementias such as Alzheimer disease. Unlike the behavioral (nonlanguage) variant of frontotemporal lobar degeneration, personality remains well preserved until advanced stages of the disease. Brain MRI is supportive of the clinical diagnosis by demonstrating a focal pattern of atrophy, predominantly affecting the left temporal lobe (Fig. 24.1).

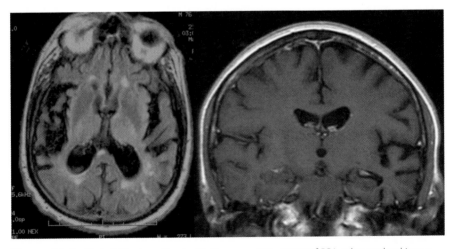

Figure 24.1   Brain MRI of a patient with the semantic variant of PPA, who evolved into a corticobasal syndrome. Focal atrophy in the left temporal lobe is prominent. In this case, postmortem studies confirmed Alzheimer disease.

SELECTED REFERENCES

Kertesz A, Munoz DG. Primary progressive aphasia. *Clin Neurosci* 1997;4(2):95–102.
Mesulam MM. *Principles of behavioral neurology*, 2nd ed. New York: Oxford, 2000.
Mesulam MM. Primary progressive aphasia. *Ann Neurol* 2001;49:421–423.
Sobrido MJ, Abu-Khalil A, Weintraub S, et al. Possible association of the tau H1/H1 genotype with primary progressive aphasia. *Neurology* 2003;60:862–864.

SEE QUESTIONS: 86, 174, 275

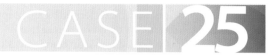

FRONTOTEMPORAL DEMENTIA

OBJECTIVES

- To present characteristic features of the syndrome of frontotemporal dementia (FTD).
- To describe the typical features of the three major FTD phenotypes: behavioral variant, progressive nonfluent aphasia, and semantic dementia.
- To name the most common etiologies associated with each phenotype of the FTD syndrome.

VIGNETTE

Four years earlier, this 58-year-old woman displayed belligerence and foul language, which were unprecedented in her characteristic sophisticated behavior. Several months later, she went on to show difficulties interacting meaningfully with other people. She would occasionally ask what "a fried egg" was, if she had been asked this for breakfast. A year into her illness, she became paranoid, believed her husband was hitting her, and exhibited violent behavioral outbursts. Quetiapine first and risperidone later were given for about 3 months after a hospitalization in the psychiatry ward. With her behavioral outbursts controlled, she became restless and needed to pace about constantly. She also developed stereotypies whereby she would tap her lap or rub her fingers repeatedly. She also exhibited a marked decrease in verbal output with a persistent grin and constant mumbling, occasionally interrupted by echolalia. She needed help to attend all of her personal needs. Her mother is reported to have had Alzheimer disease at the age of 60 years.

CASE SUMMARY

In addition to her progressive global aphasia (beyond that shown by the patient of the prior case) and echolalia, this patient displayed a range of abnormal behaviors hinging around a dramatic change in her personality. Her perseverative behaviors and stereotypies associated with disinhibition and early irritability, in the setting of marked atrophy of the frontal and antero-temporal lobes, were highly suggestive of the behavioral variant of frontotemporal dementia (bvFTD). Akathisia may have emerged as the result of prior neuroleptic exposure but could also have represented underlying motor disinhibition. Given her positive family history, a mutation in tau or progranulin may be the underlying genetic etiology.

The behavioral variant of FTD is suspected in cases where impairments in abstraction, attention, problem solving, and planning occur in the context of personality disorders, echolalia, perseveration, and stereotypical use of words and gestures. Parkinsonism and "sweet tooth" are common. Frontotemporal dementias are becoming the most common cause of presenile dementia and, as a group, may yield the greatest inheritability as up to 40% of patients have a positive family history of dementia. The possible behavioral subgroups within the bvFTD are the "pseudopsychopathic," where disinhibition and irritability result from orbitobasal-predominant atrophy; the mutism and apathy form due to anterior cingulate-predominant atrophy; and the "pseudodepression" type in which psychomotor retardation is associated with dorsolateral prefrontal pattern of atrophy. The motor variants of FTD typically include parkinsonian presentations and include the "classical" presentation of progressive supranuclear palsy (PSP, Steele-Richardson-Olszewski syndrome), corticobasal syndrome, progressive akinesia and freezing of gait, and, as it has been more recently identified, motor neuron disease.

The two more common genetic causes of FTD are progranulin (*PGRN*) and tau (*MAPT*) mutations (Table 25.1), both on chromosome 17 (the preloci nomenclature was that of "frontotemporal dementia with parkinsonism associated with chromosome 17," or FTDP-17). More recently, mutations in *C9orf72* in chromosome 9 have been recognized as the most important cause of those with FTD and motor neuron disease. Treatment for these FTDs remains symptomatic, with little response to levodopa for motor function and sometimes paradoxical worsening of behaviors to acetylcholinesterase inhibitors.

TABLE 25.1   **FTDP-17T/*MAPT* VERSUS FTDP-17U/*PGRN***

	FTDP-17T/*MAPT*	FTDP-17U/*PGRN*
Age	Younger, 40s	Older, >50 y
Predominant clinical phenotype	Parkinsonism and personality change are more common	Language abnormalities, parkinsonism less common (except for CBS)
Most common presenting deficits	Behavioral/personality changes, semantic impairment	Anomia, apathy (or disinhibition), apraxia
Disease duration	Mean: 12 y Range: 3–10 y	Mean: 5 y Range: 1–15 y
Common clinical presentations	bvFTD, CBS, PSPS, AD	PNFA, CBS, AD, PDD/DLB
Distribution of atrophy	Anteromedial temporal lobe and orbitofrontal region; caudate	Inferior frontal, temporal, and inferior parietal lobe
Pattern of atrophy	Symmetric	Asymmetric

FTDP-17T/MAPT, frontotemporal dementia with parkinsonism associated with chromosome 17, due to tau mutations in the MAPT gene; FTDP-17U/PGRN, frontotemporal dementia with parkinsonism associated with chromosome 17, due to PGRN mutations; bvFTD, behavioral variant of frontotemporal dementia; PNFA, progressive nonfluent aphasia; PSPS, progressive supranuclear palsy syndrome; PDD, Parkinson disease dementia; DLB, dementia with Lewy bodies.

SELECTED REFERENCES

Espay AJ, Biller J. *Concise neurology.* Philadelphia: Lippincott Williams & Wilkins, Wolters Kluwer Health, 2011:Chapter 6.

Espay AJ, Litvan I. Parkinsonism and frontotemporal dementia: the clinical overlap. *J Mol Neurosci* 2011;45(3):343–349.

Rohrer JD, Guerreiro R, Vandrovcova J, et al. The heritability and genetics of frontotemporal lobar degeneration. *Neurology* 2009;73(18):1451–1456.

SEE QUESTIONS: 276, 277, 278, 279

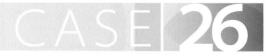

CASE 26

ALIEN HAND SYNDROME SECONDARY TO LEFT FRONTAL/CALLOSAL INFARCTION

OBJECTIVES

■ To recognize the phenomenon of alien hand syndrome.
■ To describe the clinical features of the three types of motor alien hand syndrome.

VIGNETTE

A 67-year-old right-handed woman had a 2-year history of progressive abnormal right grip and uncontrollable fisting attitude of her right hand.

CASE SUMMARY

The most common lesions in the corpus callosum are gliomas, lymphomas, and demyelinating diseases. Our patient had a striking syndrome secondary to an infarction of the midportion of the corpus callosum and medial aspect of left frontal lobe regions supplied by the anterior cerebral artery (ACA). Infarction of the corpus callosum may be more common than previously thought and is often the result of cerebral embolism. Cardiac embolism due to atrial fibrillation was identified as the cause of our patient's ischemic stroke.

Alien hand syndrome is an unusual disorder. The term alien hand syndrome was initially used to describe interhemispheric disconnection phenomena among patients with lesions involving the anterior aspects of the corpus callosum. Three varieties of alien hand syndrome have been reported: lesions involving the corpus callosum plus dominant medial frontal cortex, lesions involving the corpus callosum alone, and lesions involving posterior cortical and subcortical areas.

Based on magnetic resonance imaging (MRI) findings and her history of grasping behavior (despite lacking crural paresis), our patient's diagnosis best fulfills criteria for a *frontal alien hand syndrome.* This syndrome results from damage to the supplementary motor area, anterior cingulate gyrus, medial prefrontal cortex of the dominant hemisphere, and anterior corpus callosum. Symptoms of the frontal alien hand syndrome always occur in the dominant hand with prominent motor phenomena including reflexive grasping, groping, and utilization behavior of the dominant hand (e.g., compulsive manipulation of tools). The second type of alien hand syndrome, the *callosal alien hand syndrome*, requires only a callosal lesion and is characterized by intermanual conflict with manual interference of the nondominant hand. There typically is not associated limb paresis.

The third, *sensory* or *posterior-variant alien hand syndrome* results from lesions in the parietotemporal region and generally involves the nondominant hand, which tends to levitate rather than interfere with the dominant hand. There is also relevant sensory impairment with triple (sensory, visual, and cerebellar) ataxia and hemispatial neglect.

Hence, the alien hand syndrome is associated with acute focal lesions such as stroke or corpus callosum surgery in the case of the frontal and callosal variants, but with neurodegenerative disorders, such as the corticobasal syndrome due to corticobasal degeneration or the posterior variant of Alzheimer disease in the case of the posterior variant.

SELECTED REFERENCES

Giroud M, Dumas R. Clinical and topographical range of callosal infarction: a clinical and radiological correlation study. *J Neurol Neurosurg Psychiatry* 1995;59:238–242.

Marey-Lopez J, Rubio-Nazabal E, Alonso-Magdalena L, et al. Posterior alien hand syndrome after a right thalamic infarct. *J Neurol Neurosurg Psych* 2002;73:447–449.

Suwanwela NC, Lelacheavasit N. Isolated corpus callosal infarction secondary to pericallosal artery disease presenting as alien hand syndrome. *J Neurol Neurosurg Psychiatry* 2002;72:533–536.

SEE QUESTIONS: 253, 280, 281

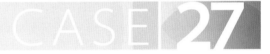

ALEXIA WITHOUT AGRAPHIA

OBJECTIVES

- To review the different types of alexias.
- To demonstrate an example of alexia without agraphia.

VIGNETTE

A 49-year-old man with history of poorly controlled arterial hypertension and cigarette smoking presented to an emergency room 48 hours after the acute onset of chest pain; he was taken to the Cardiac Cath Lab and found to have a right coronary artery occlusion and a left ventricular thrombus. Immediately following cardiac catheterization, he complained of not being able to see. The patient had an emergent catheter cerebral angiogram and received intra-arterial tPA followed by Integrilin.

The video examination was conducted 10 days after the index event.

CASE SUMMARY

Our patient had alexia without agraphia and a right homonymous hemianopia. Three types of alexia are recognized: (i) alexia without agraphia, (ii) alexia with agraphia, and (iii) aphasic alexia (frontal or third alexia). Other rare types of alexia include hemialexias following posterior corpus callosum section, and unilateral paralexias associated with unilateral inattention syndromes.

As in our patient, infarcts in the distribution of the callosal branches of the posterior cerebral artery (PCA) involving the left occipital region and the splenium of the corpus callosum result in alexia without agraphia. Alexia without agraphia, first described by Dejerine in 1892, is an isolated inability to read. With a left occipital cortex stroke, all visual information can only be processed in the normal right occipital cortex. With a second lesion in the splenium of the corpus callosum, the visual information cannot be transferred from the right to the left hemisphere language cortex. Hence, these patients can write correctly and speak and spell normally, but are unable to read words and sentences including their own. Their ability to name letters and numbers may be intact, but there can be inability to name colors, objects, and photographs. Alexia without agraphia has also been reported with infarcts of the left lingual gyrus with or without involvement of the splenium of the corpus callosum. Dejerine postulated a disconnection syndrome between the intact right visual cortex and the left hemisphere language areas, particularly the angular gyrus.

These patients may be unable to name visual stimuli but can name them after tactile exploration or verbal description, a phenomenon termed *optic aphasia*.

SELECTED REFERENCES

Alexander MP, Benson DF. The aphasias and related disturbances. In: Joynt RJ, ed. *Clinical neurology*, Vol 1. Philadelphia: JB Lippincott, 1993:1–58.

Espay AJ, Biller J. *Concise neurology*. Philadelphia: Lippincott Williams & Wilkins, Wolters Kluwer Health, 2011:Chapter 6.

Friedman R, Ween JE, Martin AL. Alexia. In: Heilman KM, Valenstein E, eds. *Clinical neuropsychology*. New York: Oxford University Press, 1993.

Geschwind SH. Disconnection syndromes in animals and man. *Brain* 1965;88:237–294, 585–644.

SEE QUESTIONS: 34, 52, 53, 282

CASE 28

GERSTMANN PLUS SYNDROME

OBJECTIVES

- To illustrate a reversible angiopathic syndrome in the postpartum period.
- To review causes of arterial ischemic strokes associated with pregnancy and puerperium.

Approximately 3 days postpartum, this 38-year-old woman developed headaches in the context of increased blood pressure. She then noticed visual blurring, word-finding difficulties, and right-sided weakness.

CASE SUMMARY

This 38-year-old left-handed woman developed new-onset headaches in the context of increased blood pressure 3 days after delivery of healthy twins from her first pregnancy. She had no seizures and reported no prior history of migraine headaches. No vasoconstrictor drugs had been used, and no medications were given to suppress lactation.

She was initially diagnosed with migraine headaches and released from a local emergency room (ER). She was soon readmitted to an outside hospital with similar complaints and was diagnosed with postpartum preeclampsia. Cerebrospinal fluid (CSF) analysis showed 19 WBCs, 30 RBCs, a protein content of 73, and normal glucose concentration. She was diagnosed with aseptic meningitis and discharged home.

A few days later, she had loss of peripheral vision, word-finding difficulties, and right-arm weakness. She was found to have fluctuating blood pressure, right–left disorientation, finger agnosia, and dyscalculia. Magnetic resonance imaging (MRI) showed diffusion restriction involving the left posterior brain region. Magnetic resonance angiography (MRA) demonstrated multisegmental arterial narrowing of both middle cerebral arteries, both anterior cerebral arteries, and basilar artery. She was then suspected of having a primary central nervous system (CNS) angiitis and was transferred to our institution for further evaluation.

A repeat lumbar puncture was normal. Transthoracic and transesophageal echocardiography were normal. Extensive investigations for hypercoagulability were unremarkable. Follow-up MRI/MRA showed interval evolution of the left posterior parietal–occipital arterial infarct and near-complete resolution of the caliber irregularities of the cerebral vessels seen on prior MRA. She was diagnosed with probable postpartum cerebral angiopathy or reversible cerebral vasoconstriction syndrome (RCVS).

The video, obtained a few months after hospital admission, demonstrated residual right–left disorientation, right inferior homonymous quadrantanopsia, and some difficulties with simple arithmetics. There was right-sided hyperreflexia and a right Babinski sign. There were no obvious naming difficulties, agraphia, or finger agnosia. Blood pressure had normalized.

Stroke in pregnancy and puerperium results from a vast number of etiologies, such as thromboembolism, cardioembolism, primary or secondary hypercoagulable states, non-atherosclerotic arteriopathies, arterial hypotension, preeclampsia/eclampsia, amniotic fluid embolism, migrainous infarction, and cervicocephalic arterial dissections.

The immediate postpartum period is a time of high stroke risk. There was an association between preeclampsia and eclampsia and stroke. Hypertensive disorders of pregnancy (including preeclampsia, eclampsia, and the syndrome of hemolysis, elevated liver enzymes, and low platelets known as HELLP syndrome) represent a comorbid condition in almost half of pregnant patients with ischemic stroke and in two-thirds of patients with hemorrhagic stroke.

Cerebral angiopathy in the postpartum period is unusual. Diagnosis is based on clinical findings and angiography. Postpartum cerebral angiopathy, a form of RCVS, is a reversible clinicoradiologic syndrome characterized by sudden onset of severe headaches, vomiting, seizures, and occasional focal neurologic deficits occurring in the puerperium. CSF is usually normal. A discrete CSF pleocytosis is possible; red blood cells and protein content may be elevated. A vasoconstrictive response to acute severe hypertension is likely to play a major pathogenetic role in this condition. Neurologic deficits at times result from infarction, which often involve the posterior aspects of the cerebral hemispheres. Other complications include intracerebral hemorrhage and localized convexity nonaneurysmal subarachnoid hemorrhage. Some patients have had exposure to ergot derivatives or sympathomimetic agents including bromocriptine, ergonovine, ergometrine maleate, or methylergonovine.

Angiography demonstrates multifocal narrowing of intracranial arteries. As MRA and computed tomography angiography (CTA) provide excellent imaging of the intracerebral circulation noninvasively, catheter cerebral angiography is currently seldom utilized. Transcranial Doppler ultrasound (TCD) examination is useful in detecting changes in mean flow velocity and together with MRA allows for noninvasive evaluation of these patients. Hemorrhagic stroke in postpartum cerebral angiopathy is unusual. Treatment of RCVS includes withdrawal of vasoactive substances. Clinical outcome is usually favorable.

Two years later, our patient delivered a healthy baby girl by cesarean section, induced at the 36th week of gestation. Patients who had a stroke during pregnancy without a specific, identifiable, persistent risk factor for stroke are at relatively low risk of recurrent strokes with subsequent pregnancies. When patients with a prior history of stroke decide to pursue another pregnancy, care is better undertaken by multidisciplinary teams of physicians including neurologists, high-risk obstetricians, as well as cardiologists, hematologists, and internists.

SELECTED REFERENCES

Bogousslavsky J, Despland PA, Regli F, et al. Postpartum cerebral angiopathy: reversible vasoconstriction assessed by transcranial Doppler ultrasounds. *Eur Neurol* 1989;29:102–105.

David EF, Wityk RJ. Cerebrovascular disorders. In: *Cherry and Merkatz's complications of pregnancy.* Philadelphia: Lippincott Williams & Wilkins, 2000:465–485.

Donaldson JO. Eclampsia and postpartum cerebral angiopathy. *J Neurol Sci* 2000;178(1):1.

Kittner SJ, Stern BJ, Feeser BR, et al. Pregnancy and the risk of stroke. *N Engl J Med* 1996;335:768–774.

SEE QUESTIONS: 20, 34, 52, 94

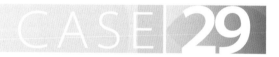

ANTERIOR OPERCULAR SYNDROME (FOIX-CHAVANY-MARIE)

OBJECTIVES

- To review the clinical characteristics of a vasculopathic anterior opercular (Foix-Chavany-Marie) syndrome.
- To describe nonvascular etiologies of the Foix-Chavany-Marie syndrome.

VIGNETTE

A 53-year-old right-handed man with diabetes, hypertension, a history of cigarette smoking, and previous right middle cerebral artery (MCA) infarct with residual left hemiparesis had sudden onset of slurred speech and right-sided weakness. Due to inability handling secretions, he had a tracheostomy and percutaneous endoscopic gastrostomy (PEG) placement at the local hospital. Due to clinical deterioration, he was transferred for further evaluation.

CASE SUMMARY

Our patient had multiple vascular risk factors. He experienced acute onset of right-sided weakness and slurred speech and found to be markedly dysarthric with a decreased gag reflex and severely impaired swallowing. As he became unable to handle his own secretions, he had a tracheostomy and placement of a PEG tube. He was then transferred to our center for further evaluation and management.

Subsequent examination was remarkable for preserved verbal comprehension, a positive snout reflex, bilateral palmomental reflexes, bilateral upper motor neuron facial weakness with preservation of emotional facial movements, and quadriparesis, right hemibody involved to a greater extent than the left hemibody. He was unable to open his mouth or protrude or move his tongue on command. On repeated occasions, he was observed to yawn spontaneously. Due to his tracheostomy, we were unable to assess whether he was anarthric or severely dysarthric. Diffusion-weighted magnetic resonance imaging (MRI) showed signal changes consistent with an acute left anterior opercular infarct and an old right opercular infarct. Magnetic resonance angiography (MRA) showed an occluded left internal carotid artery.

The anterior opercular syndrome (Foix-Chavany-Marie) syndrome, or the syndrome of facio–pharyngo–glosso–masticatory diplegia with automatic–voluntary movement dissociation is a cortico–subcortical type of suprabulbar palsy due to bilateral anterior perisylvian lesions involving the primary cortex and parietal opercula. Patients with this syndrome lack voluntary control of facial, pharyngeal, lingual, masticatory, and sometimes ocular muscles. However, there is preservation of reflexive and automatic functions of these muscles. These patients may blink, laugh, or yawn spontaneously, but cannot open their mouth or close their eyes on command. They do not have emotional lability. The gag reflex is decreased, and swallowing is severely impaired. The anterior opercular syndrome must be distinguished from Broca aphasia, oral–buccal apraxia, pseudobulbar palsy, and bulbar palsy.

The Foix-Chavany-Marie syndrome most often results from bilateral vascular lesions of the opercula or their corticofugal projections. The anterior opercular syndrome has also been associated with developmental bilateral perisylvian cortical polymicrogyria or central macrogyria, meningoencephalitis due to herpes simplex encephalitis, trauma, and neurodegenerative disorders. A reversible form has also been reported in children with epilepsy.

SELECTED REFERENCES

Brazis PW, Masdeu JC, Biller J. *Localization in clinical neurology*, 6th ed. Philadelphia: Lippincott Williams & Wilkins, Wolters Kluwer Health, 2011.

Graff-Radford NR, Bosch EP, Stears JC, et al. Developmental Foix-Chavany-Marie syndrome in identical twins. *Ann Neurol* 1986;20:632–635.

Weller M. Anterior opercular cortex lesions cause dissociated lower cranial nerve palsies and anarthria but no aphasia: Foix-Chavany-Marie syndrome and "automatic voluntary dissociation" revisited. *J Neurol* 1993;240:199–208.

SEE QUESTIONS: 33, 49, 66, 115, 116, 117, 118, 120, 122, 123

CASE 30

AMNESIA (PCA INFARCT)

OBJECTIVES

- To review the anatomic circuits and connecting pathways involved in amnesia.
- To identify disorders associated with acute-onset memory loss.
- To evaluate the leading causes of amnestic syndromes.

VIGNETTE

A 50-year-old right-handed man had sudden difficulties in comprehending written words and remembering the names of family members and associates. He also had right-sided headaches and right-sided visual field impairment. Past medical history was remarkable for hypertension and thrombocytopenia of unknown cause.

CASE SUMMARY

Our patient had acute onset of memory loss, anomia, alexia, and a right superior homonymous quadrantanopia consistent with an infarct in the territory of the left posterior cerebral artery (PCA). T2-weighted magnetic resonance imaging (MRI) of the brain showed hyperintensities involving the inferomedial left PCA. Follow-up brain MRI showed hyperintensities on T2-weighted and fluid-attenuated inversion recovery (FLAIR) images involving the left hippocampus, amygdala, and left occipital lobe (Fig. 30.1). On diffusion-weighted images these areas showed restricted diffusion. Magnetic resonance angiography (MRA) showed focal stenosis of the left PCA at the P1-P2 junction.

Our patient was initially thought to have herpes simplex encephalitis. Herpes simplex encephalitis, the most common cause of sporadic viral encephalitis, often presents with a subacute and progressive course characterized by headache, fever, altered sensorium, seizures, and occasionally focal neurologic deficits. Our patient had no recorded fever. Moreover, the course of his illness was acute and nonprogressive. Indeed, he awoke with his deficits. Although herpes viruses have a predilection for the limbic system, involving one or both mesial temporal lobes, involvement of the diencephalon and occipital cortex is rare.

An amnestic syndrome is a state characterized by selective impairment of learning and memory in an otherwise alert and responsive patient. Strokes may cause a number of behavioral changes including amnesia. The PCAs and their branches supply the mammillary bodies, thalami, and medial and basal temporal lobes including the hippocampi. Infarcts in the anterior distribution of the left PCA result from verbal and visual amnesia, color anomia, homonymous superior quadrantanopia, and alexia without agraphia. Smaller infarcts localized to the anterior, midline, or mediodorsal nuclei of the thalamus may cause an isolated amnestic syndrome or anomia. Alexia without agraphia has also been reported with infarcts involving the left lingual gyrus with or without involvement of the splenium of the corpus callosum.

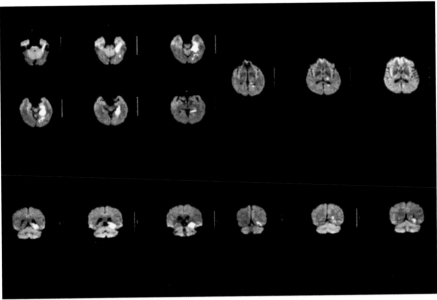

Figure 30.1   Brain MRI of this patient. Areas of hyperintensity correspond with the distribution of the left PCA.

Memories are formed in the frontal lobes, basal forebrain, thalami, and mesial temporal lobes circuitry. Amnesia refers to a pervasive impairment in the ability to recall and recognize unique events and unique stimuli. Retrograde amnesia refers to amnesia for information learned before onset of illness. Anterograde amnesia implies amnesia for information that should have been acquired after onset of illness. Etiologies of amnesia are myriad; amnestic syndromes of sudden onset (Table 30.1) usually show gradual but incomplete recovery.

Some sudden amnestic syndromes are transitory, such as those seen with partial complex seizures, postconcussive states, and transient global amnesia. Amnestic syndromes of subacute onset as seen in patients with Wernicke-Korsakoff syndrome, herpes simplex encephalitis, tuberculosis, and other basilar meningitides are associated with variable degrees of recovery and usually leave important sequelae. Slowly progressive amnestic states may be caused by tumors involving the floor and walls of the third ventricle, Alzheimer disease, or other degenerative dementias.

TABLE 30.1   **AMNESTIC SYNDROMES WITH SUDDEN ONSET**

- Bilateral hippocampal infarction due to atheroembolic occlusive disease of the PCAs or their inferior temporal branches
- Trauma to diencephalic or inferomedial temporal regions
- Spontaneous subarachnoid hemorrhage
- Carbon monoxide and other hypoxic states[a]
- Wernicke encephalopathy[a]

---

[a]These disorders may have a prodromal (subclinical state) but often exhibit a latency between neuronal injury and onset of neurological deficits, which can be sudden.

SELECTED REFERENCES

Benson DF, Marsden CD, Meadows JC. The amnesic syndrome of posterior cerebral artery occlusion. *Acta Neurologica Scandinavica* 1974;50:133–145.

De Renzi E, Zambolin A, Crisi G. The pattern of neuro-psychological impairment associated with left posterior cerebral artery infarcts. *Brain* 1987;110:1099–1116.

Ott BR, Saver JL. Unilateral amnesic stroke. Six new cases and a review of the literature. *Stroke* 1993;24:1033–1042.

Papez JW. A proposed mechanism of emotion. *Arch Neurol Pathol* 1937;38:725–743.

SEE QUESTIONS: 49, 115, 164, 283

CASE 31

DEMENTIA (EARLY ALZHEIMER DISEASE)

OBJECTIVES

- To discuss the diagnosis of dementia.
- To discuss the diagnosis of Alzheimer disease.
- To discuss treatment of Alzheimer disease.

VIGNETTE

A 75-year-old man had a 1-year history of progressive memory problems.

CASE SUMMARY

Our patient had difficulties with short-term memory. His wife noted that her husband had troubles with simple calculations and remembering recent conversations. On one occasion, while staying at an unfamiliar environment, he became confused, unclothed, and attempted to enter the hotel rooms of other guests. Past medical history was notable for pulmonary fibrosis and hyperlipidemia. He had no history of previous stroke, head trauma, or central nervous system (CNS) infection. He did not drink alcohol excessively and was on no medications that could impair cognition. There was no family history of dementia.

On examination, he was oriented to person, place, and time except that he had difficulty naming the month. Immediate recall and attention were unremarkable. He was able to name two of three objects on testing short-term recall. He was not aphasic, was able to follow multistep commands, and had no construction apraxia. He was diagnosed as having early Alzheimer disease and treated with galantamine.

Dementia is defined as a decline in memory and at least one other cognitive domain impairing social or occupational functioning. Dementia results from many causes including degenerative, vascular, infectious, psychiatric, toxic, metabolic, traumatic, and brain structural etiologies. Most nondegenerative causes can be excluded with appropriate history and a thorough general and neurologic examination, neuroimaging, and laboratory evaluation. Neuropsychologic testing further defines the specific cognitive abnormalities. The most common cause of dementia is Alzheimer disease. Hippocampal, mesial temporal lobe, and parietal lobe atrophy may be seen on computed tomography (CT) or magnetic resonance imaging (MRI). Positron emission tomography (PET) may demonstrate bilateral temporoparietal hypometabolism. More recently, the use of biomarkers in the diagnosis of Alzheimer disease has received considerable attention in the literature, including abnormal Aβ metabolism as demonstrated by low amyloid β-42 (with high phosphorylated tau) on cerebrospinal fluid (CSF) and increased uptake on the Pittsburgh compound B (PIB PET) of fibrillar Aβ of senile plaques in neocortical regions.

Other common degenerative dementias include dementia with Lewy bodies, and frontotemporal lobar degeneration. An algorithm for the diagnosis and evaluation for dementia is illustrated in Figure 31.1.

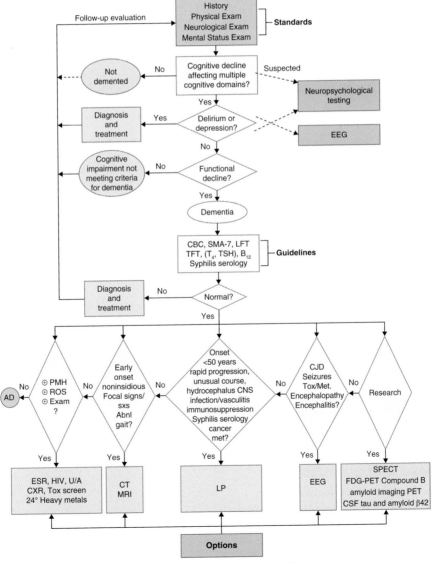

Figure 31.1   Algorithm for the diagnosis and evaluation of dementia.

Definitive Alzheimer disease requires histopathologic confirmation based on brain biopsy or autopsy brain specimens. Alzheimer disease is diagnosed clinically when there is a gradual and progressive decline or impairment of recent memory and at least one other cognitive domain (aphasia, apraxia, agnosia, visuospatial dysfunction, or dysexecutive state). The observed cognitive deficits should not be attributable to other psychiatric, neurologic, or systemic diseases. Moreover, the cognitive deficits should be unrelated to delirium, which precludes the unequivocal diagnosis of dementia among hospitalized patients. Extensive test batteries sensitive to dementia are available. Most popular screening test is the Mini–Mental State Examination (MMSE). A newer screening test more sensitive at detecting mild cognitive impairment and early dementia is the Montreal Cognitive Assessment (MOCA).

Treatment of dementia is directed at the underlying cause, especially if there is a potentially reversible cause. Symptomatic treatment with acetylcholinesterase inhibitor medications (donepezil, rivastigmine, and galantamine) may slow the decline in patients with Alzheimer disease. The *N*-methyl-D-aspartate receptor antagonist (NMDA) memantine can also used for the treatment of moderate-to-severe Alzheimer disease singly or in combination with any of the acetylcholinesterase inhibitors.

SELECTED REFERENCES

American Psychiatric Association. *Diagnostic and statistical manual of mental disorders*, 4th ed. Washington: American Psychiatric Association, 1994.

Biller J, ed. *Practical neurology*, 4th ed. Philadelphia: Lippincott Williams & Wilkins, Wolters Kluwer Health, 2012.

Biller J, Gruener G, Brazis P. *DeMyer's the neurologic examination. A programmed text*, 6th ed. New York: McGraw-Hill Medical, 2011.

Chui H, Zhang Q. Evaluation of dementia: a systematic study of the usefulness of the American Academy of Neurology's Practice Parameters. *Neurology* 1997;49:925–935.

Knopman DS, DeKosky ST, Cummings JL, et al. Practice parameter: diagnosis of dementia (an evidence-based review). Report of the Quality Standards Subcommittee of the American Academy of Neurology. *Neurology* 2001;56:1143–1153.

SEE QUESTIONS: 86, 106, 107, 109, 110

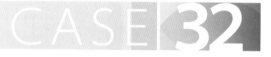

DEMENTIA (LATE ALZHEIMER DISEASE)

OBJECTIVES

- To discuss diagnosis of dementia.
- To discuss treatment of Alzheimer disease.
- To discuss treatment of the behavioral manifestations of Alzheimer disease.

An 85-year-old man had a 3-year history of gradually progressive memory loss.

█ **CASE SUMMARY** ▶

This 85-year-old man had progressive memory loss. His wife had troubles caring for him and became concerned that her husband started wandering out of the house. He also had a history of a right frontal lobe infarct associated with a right internal carotid artery occlusion and bilateral postural hand tremors. He initially received donepezil, but it was subsequently discontinued as his wife felt it was ineffective. He also received low-dose levetiracetam for probable multifocal myoclonus. For mild depression he was given mirtazapine and later escitalopram.

Examination showed him to be disoriented to time and place, with poor immediate and short-term recall, impaired simple calculation abilities, difficulty following multistep commands, and troubles with writing sentences and copying figures. His answers were noted to be hesitant and at times he perseverated. A neuropsychological examination showed significant problems with orientation and very poor short-term recall and recall of recent events. His recognition memory was notably impaired as was his semantic fluency and confrontation naming. He scored 13/30 on the Mini–Mental State Exam (MMSE). He had marked subjective depression on the Geriatric Depression Inventory. It was thought he had a generalized dementia of moderate severity that was greater than expected for his previous stroke.

Dementia is defined as a decline in memory and at least one other cognitive domain (aphasia, apraxia, agnosia, and decline in executive function) impairing social or occupational functioning. Dementia results from many causes including degenerative, vascular, infectious, psychiatric, toxic, metabolic, traumatic, and brain structural etiologies. Most of the nondegenerative causes can be excluded with appropriate history, general and neurologic examination, head imaging study, and laboratory evaluation. Neuropsychologic testing is done to define the specific cognitive abnormalities, which often follow a pattern consistent with a specific diagnosis.

Alzheimer disease is the most common neurodegenerative dementia and progresses from anomia to agnosia to aphasia to apraxia. As demonstrated by his wife's concern for his safety, caring for patients with Alzheimer disease can be quite demanding. Often, patients with advanced stages of the disease, may be agitated, anxious, depressed, and have sleep disorders. Hallucinations (more often visual than auditory), and delusions that family members or caregivers are impostors, as well as bizarre or violent behavior may occur. Impaired judgment and wandering are especially challenging because of safety issues.

Symptomatic treatment is available for Alzheimer disease. Three acetylcholinesterase inhibitor medications (donepezil, rivastigmine, and galantamine) are available that slow the decline of Alzheimer disease rather than improve cognition. In addition, the N-methyl-D-aspartate receptor antagonist (NMDA) memantine has been approved for treatment of moderate-to-severe Alzheimer disease. Other medications are often used to control some of the behavioral symptoms noted in these patients. Atypical neuroleptic agents can be used for agitation, hallucinations, delusions, and unusual behaviors, but their use should be restricted when nonpharmacological interventions are insufficient for behavioral control. Selective serotonin reuptake inhibitors seem to work well for depression and are fairly well tolerated. Anxiety and excessive motor activities may respond to the atypical neuroleptic agents or low doses of benzodiazepines. In general, all medications should be started at low doses and increased slowly.

SELECTED REFERENCES

Biller J, ed. *Practical neurology*, 4th ed. Philadelphia: Lippincott Williams & Wilkins, Wolters Kluwer Health, 2012.

Knopman DS, DeKosky ST, Cummings JL, et al. Practice parameter: diagnosis of dementia (an evidence-based review). Report of the Quality Standards Subcommittee of the American Academy of Neurology. *Neurology* 2001;56:1143–1153.

McKhann GM, Knopman DS, Chertkow H, et al. The diagnosis of dementia due to Alzheimer's disease: recommendations from the National Institute on Aging-Alzheimer's Association workgroups on diagnostic guidelines for Alzheimers disease. *Alzheimers Dement* 2011;7(3):263–269.

SEE QUESTIONS: 86, 106, 107, 109, 110, 174

CASE 33

DEMENTIA WITH LEWY BODIES

OBJECTIVES

- To discuss the clinical features of dementia with Lewy bodies.
- To distinguish dementia with Lewy bodies from other forms of neurodegenerative dementia.
- To discuss treatment of the behavioral manifestations of dementia with Lewy bodies.

VIGNETTE

This 76-year-old man developed right-hand tremor followed by hypophonia, slowed gait, and stooped posture, 7 years prior to presentation. He had also gotten lost several times when driving and needed help to find his way back home from some errands. Treatment with pramipexole within the first 6 months led to paranoia and visual hallucinations and needed to be discontinued. Similar complication occurred as he was introduced to levodopa, which was worsened by olanzapine, initiated after a visit to the emergency room. Over the next years, his balance worsened and he had falls, some associated with postural light-headedness. His sleep was complicated by dream enactment behaviors, with thrashing and shouting. After 6 years from symptom onset, he needed help with dressing, bathing, and shaving. A walker was used for ambulation to minimize the risk of falls. His hallucinations were few and far between with clozapine, but he had episodes where he would mistake his wife for an impostor.

CASE SUMMARY

 This man's examination demonstrated moderate to severe dementia (Montreal Cognitive Assessment [MoCA] = 9/30; MMSE = 13/28; Frontal Assessment Battery = 5/18) associated with agraphia, agraphesthesia, astereognosis, ideomotor apraxia, and frontal release signs (positive glabellar, snout, and grasp reflexes) in the setting of advanced parkinsonism, shown in the video as stooped posture, shuffling gait, and impaired postural reflexes). The reliance on a walker only 6 years from symptom onset belies a faster speed of progression than that of Alzheimer disease.

The presence of cognitive impairment at or shortly after the onset of a parkinsonian phenotype, along with the historic presence of early hallucinations and dream enactment behaviors indicative of comorbid REM sleep behavior disorder, strongly suggested the diagnosis of dementia with Lewy bodies (DLB) (Table 33.1). The patient died 9 years after symptom onset, and DLB was confirmed at autopsy (prominent Lewy bodies in the temporal lobe and amygdala were the presumed correlates of visual hallucinations).

DLB should always be suspected in cases where dementia occurs before or within 1 year from the onset of any parkinsonian motor features. Visual but also auditory and, more rarely, olfactory and tactile hallucinations are among the earliest behavioral manifestations. Recurrent visual hallucinations are a core feature in DLB and, unlike Parkinson disease (where psychosis occurs more commonly with dopamine agonists than with levodopa), develop regardless of treatment with dopaminergic or anticholinergic treatments. Hallucinations are important clinical clues in predicting Lewy body over other pathologies. Another important feature is the marked sensitivity to neuroleptic drugs. Psychotic bouts with visual hallucinations, delusions, and paranoia can worsen when treated in an emergency setting with atypical, let alone typical, antipsychotics.

Two key cognitive features raise the stakes for DLB compared to other forms of dementia. First, fluctuating levels of overall cognition, especially in attention, within the same day, can give these patients the same erratic behavioral flavor of metabolic and infectious encephalopathies. Second, a striking visuospatial disorientation translates early on into episodes of "getting lost" when driving or having overall difficulty finding a way around hitherto familiar places. The clinical pearl is that these patients are orientation impaired early on, at a time when memory may be intact, opposite to the cognitive profile of Alzheimer disease (Table 33.2). This visuospatial disorientation is also expressed as

TABLE 33.1 IMPORTANT FEATURES OF DLB

Behaviors	Recurrent Visual Hallucinations and Delusions
Temporal pattern	Prominent fluctuations in cognition and attention (periods of confusion interspersed with periods of lucidity) that must be differentiated from toxic/metabolic encephalopathy and delirium of other causes
Temporal association with parkinsonism	Dementia occurring within 1 y from onset of parkinsonism (Patients are classified as having PD dementia when dementia features appear >1 y after the onset of parkinsonism)
Treatment response	Hypersensitivity to neuroleptics, sometimes fatal

TABLE 33.2   COGNITIVE FEATURES COMPARING DLB AND AD

DBL is Better than AD	DLB as Affected as AD	DLB is Worse than AD
• Episodic memory (day-to-day events)	• Semantic memory[a] • Language (verbal fluency)	• Visuospatial orientation • Working memory • Attention

[a]In pictorial semantic memory, DLB fare worse than AD.
From Espay and Biller. *Concise neurology.* Philadelphia: Lippincott Williams & Wilkins, 2011.

constructional apraxia (drawing disturbance) whereby the task of drawing intersecting pentagons is much worse early on in DLB than in other dementias.

The case study highlighted above also demonstrated Capgras syndrome, a delusional belief that a person has been replaced by an impostor. This delusional misidentification syndrome is unique to DLB compared to Parkinson disease dementia (PDD), unlike the lesser specificity of other psychiatric features such as delusions of persecution, theft, or spousal infidelity, which are seen in both DLB and, less frequently, in PDD.

Another distinctive clinical presentation of DLB is that of the posterior cortical atrophy syndrome. Superimposed on a phenotype of parkinsonism and visual hallucinations, patients demonstrate simultanagnosia, ocular apraxia, and optic ataxia, elements of the Balint syndrome, as illustrated in the second video, which suggest involvement of the dorsal–occipitoparietal visual pathway (Fig. 33.1). Besides DLB, the narrow diagnostic differential of the posterior cortical atrophy syndrome includes the "visual variant" of Alzheimer disease, which is its most common pathology, corticobasal degeneration, and Creutzfeldt-Jakob disease.

The management of DLB rests in using levodopa rather than dopamine agonists (ropinirole, pramipexole, and rotigotine) as the first line of treatment for the parkinsonian features and approaching the treatment of the associated psychosis with nonpharmacological measures first. Psychotic bouts are first managed by ruling out metabolic or infectious processes and by simplifying the medication regimen through the reduction or discontinuation of anticholinergic medications (benztropine, and trihexyphenidyl), amantadine, dopamine agonists, and MAO-B inhibitors, in sequence as necessary. Pharmacologic treatment hinges on the use of low doses of either of two atypical antipsychotics. Quetiapine can be given at 25 mg at bedtime, increasing by 25-mg increments every

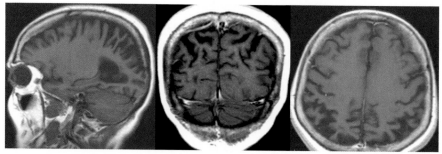

Figure 33.1   Brain MRI of a patient with the posterior cortical atrophy presentation of dementia with Lewy bodies, highlighting the prominent biparieto-occipital atrophy.

week until reaching clinical efficacy or intolerable side effects, whichever comes first. Bear in mind, though, that the efficacy of quetiapine in DLB is modest and the "neuroleptic sensitivity" of DLB can apply to this drug. In this situation, clozapine may be the only feasible antipsychotic, given at 12.5 mg/day, increasing by 12.5 mg/week as needed and tolerated. Clozapine is the only treatment recommended for the drug-induced psychosis of PDD and, naturally, is considered the best option for the treatment of psychosis in DLB, although at the inconvenience of setting up a system for weekly or biweekly monitoring for agranulocytosis. Olanzapine, risperidone, aripiprazole, and ziprasidone have all been associated with worsening of the parkinsonism and are not recommended. Rivastigmine, a cholinesterase inhibitor approved for PDD, has been found beneficial for the cognitive and behavioral abnormalities of DLB, presumably because of the greater cholinergic loss compared to AD.

▶ **Case 33, Video 2:** A 71-year-old man with parkinsonism, dementia, and prominent hallucinations, with probable dementia with Lewy bodies, demonstrating full Balint syndrome due to a posterior-predominant cortical atrophy pattern of atrophy. Optic ataxia and simultanagnosia are prominent. Ocular apraxia is not shown. (Taken with permission from Espay and Lang. *Common movement disorders pitfalls: case-based teaching.* New York: Cambridge University Press, 2012.)

SELECTED REFERENCES

Biller J, ed. *Practical neurology*, 4th ed. Philadelphia: Lippincott Williams & Wilkins, Wolters Kluwer Health, 2012.

Espay A, Biller J. *Concise neurology*. Philadelphia: Lippincott Williams & Wilkins, 2011:Chapter 6.

Josephs KA. Capgras syndrome and its relationship to neurodegenerative disease. *Arch Neurol* 2007;64(12):1762–1766.

Williams DR, Warren JD, Lees AJ. Using the presence of visual hallucinations to differentiate Parkinson's disease from atypical parkinsonism. *J Neurol Neurosurg Psychiatry* 2008;79(6):652–655.

SEE QUESTIONS: 284, 285, 286

SECTION 4

CEREBROVASCULAR

CASE 34

ASYMPTOMATIC CAROTID ARTERY STENOSIS

OBJECTIVES

- To review epidemiological data on asymptomatic carotid artery bruits and carotid artery stenosis.
- To review current understanding on the management of patients with asymptomatic carotid artery stenosis.

VIGNETTE

A 67-year-old man with diabetes, arterial hypertension, and coronary artery disease was found to have a left carotid bruit. He had no retinal or hemispheric ischemic events.

CASE SUMMARY

Our patient had an asymptomatic carotid artery bruit. Noninvasive studies (carotid ultrasound and magnetic resonance angiography [MRA]) showed bilateral 50% to 79% internal carotid artery stenosis.

Approximately 4% of adults have asymptomatic neck bruits. However, a carotid bruit is a poor predictor of carotid artery disease or high-grade carotid artery stenosis. Although screening for carotid artery stenosis is advocated by some, the U.S. Preventive Service Task Force does not recommend routine screen for stroke prevention because more patients with asymptomatic carotid artery stenosis will experience cardiovascular events than stroke. Moreover, the sensitivity of carotid bruits in detecting carotid artery stenosis greater than 70% is low.

The estimated annual stroke risk among individuals with asymptomatic carotid bruits is 1.5% at 1 year and 7.5% at 5 years. The incidence of ischemic events correlates with the progression of carotid artery stenosis. Asymptomatic carotid artery stenosis less than equal to 75% carries a stroke risk of 1% to 2% annually. When the carotid artery stenosis is greater than equal to 75%, the annual stroke rate is about 5% to 6%.

Data from six randomized clinical trials (RCTs) on the efficacy of carotid endarterectomy (CEA) in patients with asymptomatic carotid artery stenosis are now available. The Carotid Artery Surgery Asymptomatic Narrowing Operation Versus Aspirin (CASANOVA) trial included asymptomatic patients with 50% to 90% carotid artery stenosis. Patients with greater than 90% stenosis were excluded on the basis of presumed surgical benefit. All patients were treated with 330 mg of aspirin and 75 mg of dipyridamole three times daily. Overall, the CASANOVA trial showed no differences in outcomes between the medical and surgical groups.

The Mayo Asymptomatic Carotid Endarterectomy (MACE) trial was prematurely terminated due to a significantly higher number of myocardial infarctions (MIs) and transient ischemic attacks (TIAs) in the surgical group. The Veterans Affairs Asymptomatic Carotid Endarterectomy Trial compared outcomes of surgery and medical treatment among 444 asymptomatic patients with angiographically proven 50% to 99% carotid artery stenosis. Results showed a reduction in the relative risk of ipsilateral neurological events with surgery only when TIAs and stroke were included as composite endpoints. However, when ipsilateral stroke was considered alone, only a nonsignificant trend favoring surgery was noted, but for the combined outcome of stroke and death, no significant differences were found between the two treatment arms.

The Asymptomatic Carotid Atherosclerosis Study (ACAS) compared CEA, aspirin therapy, and medical risk factor management in asymptomatic patients younger than 80 years who had 60% to 99% carotid artery stenosis. Based on a 5-year projection, ACAS concluded that CEA reduced the absolute risk of stroke by 5.9% (absolute risk reduction of only 1.2% per year) and the relative risk of stroke and death by 53%. The favorable outcome of surgery over aspirin was partly dependent on a low aggregate perioperative stroke and death rate of only 2.3%, including a permanent arteriographic complication rate of 1.2%. Similar results were reported by the Asymptomatic Carotid Surgery Trial (ACST), a European trial of highly selected patients with greater than 60% carotid artery stenosis by ultrasound and no prior history of cerebrovascular disease. In the ACST study, the 5-year stroke risk for surgery was 6.4% compared with 11.8% for medical therapy for the endpoints of fatal or nonfatal stroke, but the benefits were not substantiated for patients older than 75 years of age and the perioperative risks were much lower than in routine clinical practice (1.5%). Neither ACAS nor ACST showed increasing benefit from surgery with increasing degree of stenosis from 60% to 99%.

A systematic review of three RCTs (5,223 patients) found that patients with asymptomatic carotid artery stenosis who underwent CEA had a reduced risk of preoperative stroke, death, or subsequent ipsilateral stroke over 3 to 4 years compared to those who received medical therapy alone. However, the absolute risk reduction was small (approximately 1% per year during the first few years).

Carotid artery angioplasty and stenting (CAS) has been proposed as an alternative treatment to CEA. The Carotid Revascularization Endarterectomy Versus Stenting Trial (CREST) showed that among patients with either symptomatic or asymptomatic carotid artery stenosis, the risk of stroke, MI, or death was not statistically different between those patients who underwent CEA and CAS.

SELECTED REFERENCES

Biller J, Thies WH. Carotid endarterectomy is warranted in selected symptomatic patients. *Am Fam Phys* 2000;61:400–406.

Brott TG, Hobson RW II, Howard G, et al. Stenting versus endarterectomy for treatment of carotid-artery stenosis. *N Engl J Med* 2010;363:11–23.

Chambers BR, Domman GA. Carotid endarterectomy for asymptomatic carotid stenosis. *Cochrane Database Syst Rev* 2005:CD001923.

Fleck JD, Biller J. Choices in medical management for prevention of acute ischemic stroke. *Curr Neurol Neurosci Rep* 2001;1(Jan):33–38.

SEE QUESTIONS: 32, 89, 93

CASE 35

VERTEBROBASILAR TIAs: BASILAR ARTERY STENOSIS

OBJECTIVES

- To review clinical manifestations of vertebrobasilar circulation transient ischemic attack (TIAs).
- To review clinical manifestations of carotid circulation TIAs.
- To review therapeutic strategies for symptomatic basilar artery stenosis.

VIGNETTE

Over the course of 1 year, this 78-year-old hypertensive man developed recurrent, brief, nonpositional spells of slurred speech, double vision, circumoral numbness, left-sided weakness, and imbalance. He initially received platelet antiaggregants. Subsequently, he was treated with warfarin without resolution of his spells.

CASE SUMMARY

The most common causes of ischemic strokes and TIAs are atheromatous disease of large- and medium-sized extracranial and/ or intracranial arteries, small vessel disease, and cardiac embolism. Intracranial atherosclerosis is an important cause of ischemic stroke, especially among African-Americans and Asians. Our patient had recurrent episodes of vertebrobasilar ischemia, associated with a high-grade basilar artery stenosis. He had angioplasty and stenting of the basilar artery, as he had disabling refractory episodes of vertebrobasilar ischemia, despite several antiplatelet agents alone or in combination, and warfarin therapy.

The brainstem, cerebellum, and labyrinths are supplied by the vertebrobasilar arterial system. The basilar artery is formed by the vertebral arteries at the level of the pontomedullary junction. Three branches on each side provide blood supply to the cerebellum; the posterior inferior cerebellar artery (PICA) usually originates from the intracranial

TABLE 35.1   CLINICOANATOMICAL CORRELATION OF DISORDERS OF NEUROVASCULAR FUNCTION

	Neurovascular	Cerebral	Cranial Nerves	Motor/ Reflexes Cerebellar/Gait	Sensory
Carotid TIA	Carotid bruit, decreased carotid pulse	Transient aphasia and dysarthria	Ipsilateral amaurosis fugax, contralateral HH	Transient contralateral weakness or clumsiness	Transient contralateral loss
Vertebrobasilar TIA	Vertebral or basilar bruit	Normal	Transient CN findings— diplopia, dysarthria	Transient bilateral weakness or clumsiness	Transient bilateral or crossed loss

HH, homonymous hemianopia; CN, cranial nerves.

segment of the vertebral artery, whereas the anterior inferior cerebellar artery (AICA) and the superior cerebellar artery (SCA) arise from the basilar artery.

A TIA is a transient and acute episode of focal neurological or retinal dysfunction secondary to impaired blood supply. The attacks usually last less than 24 hours leaving no residual deficits. Because the episodes usually last less than 60 minutes (most often less than 20 minutes), patients often lack clinical manifestations by the time they present to medical attention. However, this time-based definition of TIAs is inadequate, because infarctions are sometimes evident on diffusion-weighted (DW) magnetic resonance imaging (MRI). Thus, a "tissue-based" definition of TIAs has been proposed: brief episodes of neurological dysfunction caused by focal retinal or brain ischemia with symptoms typically lasting less than 60 minutes and without evidence of infarction.

Manifestations of TIAs in the carotid and vertebrobasilar territories are outlined in Table 35.1. Transient vertigo, diplopia, dysarthria, or dysphagia in isolation is insufficient to establish a diagnosis of vertebrobasilar TIAs (Table 35.2). Isolated drop attacks seldom result from vertebrobasilar ischemia. Approximately 10% to 30% of patients with ischemic stroke have preceding TIAs. The annual risk of stroke after a TIA is 3% to 4%. The risk of stroke is three times greater for individuals who have had a TIA compared to those individuals who have not experienced a TIA.

TABLE 35.2   SYMPTOMS SUGGESTIVE OF VERTEBROBASILAR TRANSIENT ISCHEMIC ATTACKS

- Usually bilateral weakness or clumsiness but may be unilateral or shifting
- Bilateral, shifting, or crossed (ipsilateral face and contralateral body) sensory loss or paresthesias
- Bilateral or contralateral homonymous visual field defects or binocular vision loss
- Two or more of the following symptoms: vertigo, diplopia, dysphagia, dysarthria, and ataxia
- Symptoms not acceptable as evidence of vertebrobasilar transient ischemic attack:
  Syncope, dizziness, confusion, urinary or fecal incontinence, or generalized weakness
  Isolated vertigo, diplopia, dysphagia, ataxia, tinnitus, amnesia, drop attacks, or dysarthria

Although early studies advocated intracranial angioplasty and stenting as a promising therapy for patients with symptomatic intracranial arterial stenosis, a randomized study of symptomatic patients with 70% to 99% stenosis of a major intracranial artery demonstrated the superiority of aggressive medical management over the use of the Wingspan stent system.

SELECTED REFERENCES

Albers GW, Caplan LR, Easton JD, et al. Transient ischemic attack: proposal for a new definition. *N Engl J Med* 2002;347:1713–1716.

Chimowitz MI. Angioplasty or stenting is not appropriate as first line treatment of intracranial stenosis. *Arch Neurol* 2001;58:1690–1692.

Chimowitz MI, Lynn MJ, Derdeyn CP, et al. Stenting versus aggressive medical therapy for intracranial arterial stenosis. *N Engl J Med* 2011;365:993–1003.

SEE QUESTIONS: 46, 47, 49, 50, 64, 65

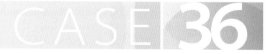

CASE 36

DYSPHAGIA/IMBALANCE: VERTEBRAL ARTERY STENOSIS

OBJECTIVES

- To review the important morbidity associated with dysphagia.
- To discuss different pathogenetic mechanisms of dysphagia and dysarthria.
- To illustrate potential risks of catheter cerebral angiography.

VIGNETTE

A 71-year-old man with a history of coronary artery bypass graft (CABG), left carotid endarterectomy (CEA), abdominal aortic aneurysm (AAA) repair, bilateral femoral artery bypass, hypertension, and cigarette smoking was evaluated because of a 9-month history of slurred speech, swallowing difficulties, and tongue weakness. He also had headaches and posterior neck pain. Once, he had a "passing out" spell. Since that event, he had balance difficulties.

CASE SUMMARY

Swallowing is a complex process that involves efferent and afferent fibers from the nuclei of cranial nerves (CN) V, VII, IX, X, and XII. Disorders of swallowing and articulation can be acute, subacute, chronic, persistent, or episodic and can be caused by a variety of central nervous system and neuromuscular disorders. Our patient had multiple vascular risk factors. He consulted because of subacute progressive and persistent swallowing and speech difficulties, imbalance, and posterior neck pain. Other symptoms of possible vertebrobasilar ischemia such as vertigo, diplopia, or visual field defects were lacking. Although our patient had a "passing out" spell, it was not characteristic of syncope due to glossopharyngeal or vagal dysfunction. The most worrisome concern was his oropharyngeal dysphagia. He had no evidence of hoarseness. His dysphagia resulted in considerable weight loss.

Examination was remarkable for dysarthria, hypernasal voice, impaired tongue movements, asymmetric and brisk lower extremity muscle stretch reflexes, and a left Babinski sign. He had no evidence of emotional incontinence, muscle atrophy, muscle weakness, or fasciculations. Gait was normal.

Early identification and systematic evaluation of dysphagia is extremely important. In particular, elderly patients with dysphagia have a high risk of aspiration pneumonia. Furthermore, dysphagia may result in malnutrition, dehydration, and airway obstruction. Because bedside dysphagia testing may not be reliable at detecting silent aspiration, fiberoptic evaluation or fluoroscopic examination is recommended for severe dysphagia.

Ancillary investigations showed no evidence of muscle or neuromuscular junction abnormalities or motor neuron disease. There was no evidence of multiple cranial neuropathies, basal ganglia disease, or evidence of intrinsic brainstem lesions at the level of the glossopharyngeal and vagus nerves. However, there was extrinsic encroachment of the oblongated medulla by an atherosclerotic tortuosity and elongation involving the vertebrobasilar arterial system. This arterial elongation is characteristic of vertebrobasilar dolichoectasia, a vasculopathy of unclear etiology that may cause hemodynamic changes (leading to thrombosis or microembolization) but also brainstem compression, explaining the dysphagia and dysarthria in our patient. Besides ischemic stroke, other potential presentations for vertebrobasilar dolichoectasia include cervicomedullary junction compression, cerebellar dysfunction, central sleep apnea, and hydrocephalus.

The vertebrobasilar circulation supplies blood to the brainstem, cerebellum, occipital lobes, and labyrinths via the paired vertebral arteries, which converge to form the basilar artery at the pontomedullary junction. Atherothrombotic disease in the vertebrobasilar system has a predilection for the distal vertebral artery and the lower or middle basilar artery. Clinical manifestations of vertebrobasilar dolichoectasia result from compression of adjacent cranial nerves and brainstem structures.

Catheter cerebral angiography is an invasive investigation with an overall combined minor and major complication (primarily stroke) rate of approximately 1.0%. Access site hematoma is the most commonly observed complication. Fortunately, the majority of neurologic complications are transient or reversible. Following catheter cerebral angiography, our patient underwent endovascular coil occlusion of the dolichoectatic vessel, which was complicated with a small cerebellar and occipital lobe infarction. He had a complete recovery.

SELECTED REFERENCES

Biller J, ed. *Practical neurology,* 4th ed. Philadelphia: Lippincott Williams & Wilkins, Wolters Kluwer Health, 2012.

Dray TG, Hillel AD, Miller RM. Dysphagia caused by neurological deficits. *Otolaryngol Clin North Am* 1998;31:507–523.

Kaufmann TJ, Huston J III, Mandrekan JN, et al. Complications of diagnostic cerebral angiography: evaluation of 19,826 consecutive patients. *Radiology* 2007;243:812–819.

Ramsey DJ, Smithard DG, Kalra L. Early assessment of dysphagia and aspiration risk in acute stroke patients. *Stroke* 2003;34:1252–1257.

SEE QUESTION: 50

CASE 37

PURE MOTOR HEMIPARESIS DUE TO CAPSULAR LACUNAR INFARCTION

OBJECTIVES

- To review the clinical characteristics of pure motor hemiparesis, the most common lacunar syndrome.
- To discuss the importance of careful follow-up of patients with lacunar stroke.
- To review risk factors for stroke recurrence.

VIGNETTE

Several years prior to this assessment, this 82-year-old left-handed woman with hypertension and hyperlipidemia had sudden onset of right-sided weakness and slurred speech. On admission, she was also found to have an inferior wall myocardial infarction.

CASE SUMMARY

Most ischemic strokes result from disease of large- and medium-sized extracranial or intracranial arteries, cardiac embolism, or small vessel disease (lacunar infarctions). Rare causes of ischemic stroke include cervicocephalic arterial dissections and other non-atherosclerotic vasculopathies, border-zone infarcts due to arterial hypotension and poor cerebral perfusion, and hypercoagulable states. Approximately 20% of strokes are due to lacunar infarctions. The risk of recurrent stroke is lowest for lacunar strokes; the overall stroke recurrence rate among patients with lacunar infarctions within 3 months is 1.2%, but this rate may increase up to 10% among those with poorly controlled hypertension and diabetes (an association not shared by hyperlipidemia). Patients with a lacunar stroke index event are equally likely to have recurrent small or large vessel ischemic strokes.

The most frequent clinical lacunar syndromes are (1) pure motor hemiparesis (PMH), (2) pure sensory stroke, (3) sensorimotor stroke, (4) clumsy hand dysarthria, and (5) homolateral ataxia and crural paresis.

Our patient had a PMH caused by an internal capsule lacunar infarction. She initially received prophylactic antiplatelet therapy, but then, she developed atrial fibrillation and was switched to warfarin (target INR = 2.0 to 3.0). Atrial fibrillation is an important preventable cause of ischemic stroke. The relative risk of stroke in patients with nonvalvular atrial fibrillation is at least fivefold greater than that in patients with normal sinus rhythm. Warfarin therapy reduces the rate of stroke by 68% [95% confidence interval (CI), 50% to 79%], while aspirin reduces the rate of stroke by 21%. When balanced against the risk for major hemorrhage (1.3% for warfarin, 1.0% per year for aspirin), warfarin therapy was justified in our patient. She subsequently required a pacemaker due to a high-degree atrioventricular (AV) block.

PMH, the most common lacunar syndrome, may also be caused by a basis pontis or corona radiata lacuna. PMH is characterized by contralateral hemiparesis or hemiplegia involving the face, the arm, and to a lesser extent the leg. There may be mild dysarthria, particularly at onset of stroke. Patients show no evidence of aphasia, apraxia, or agnosia, and lack of sensory, visual, or other higher cortical disturbances. Multiple lacunar infarctions may result in a pseudobulbar syndrome and vascular dementia.

SELECTED REFERENCES

Arboix A, Font A, Garro C, et al. Recurrent lacunar infarction following a previous lacunar stroke: a clinical study of 122 patients. *J Neurol Neurosurg Psychiatry* 2007;78(12):1392–1394.

Biller J, ed. *Practical neurology,* 4th ed. Philadelphia: Lippincott Williams & Wilkins, Wolters Kluwer Health, 2012.

Brazis PW, Masdeu JC, Biller J. *Localization in clinical neurology,* 6th ed. Philadelphia: Lippincott Williams & Wilkins, Wolters Kluwer Health, 2011.

Kappelle LJ, van Latum JC, van Swieten JC, et al. Recurrent stroke after transient ischemic attack or minor ischaemic stroke: does the distinction between small and large vessel disease remain true to type? Dutch TIA Trial Study Group. *J Neurol Neurosurg Psychiatry* 1995;64:771–776.

Moroney JT, Bagiella E, Paik MC, et al. Risk factors for early recurrence after ischemic stroke: the role of stroke syndrome and subtype. *Stroke* 1998;29:2118–2124.

SEE QUESTIONS: 32, 36, 70, 87, 88, 95, 148, 149, 167, 233, 372

CASE 38

ATAXIC HEMIPARESIS DUE TO PONTINE INFARCTION

OBJECTIVES

- To describe the clinical characteristics of ataxic hemiparesis.
- To review the pathogenesis of lacunar infarcts.
- To highlight the many localizations responsible for ataxic hemiparesis (homolateral ataxia and crural paresis).
- To review variants of this syndrome.

VIGNETTE

A 75-year-old woman with hypertension and hyperlipidemia had sudden onset of dizziness followed by slurred speech and right-sided weakness.

CASE SUMMARY

Every year at least 795,000 Americans experience a new or recurrent stroke. Strokes result from either ischemia or hemorrhage. Ischemic strokes resulting from small vessel or penetrating artery disease (lacunes) have unique clinical, radiological, and pathological features. Lacunar infarcts are small ischemic infarctions involving the deep regions of the brain or brainstem ranging in diameter from 0.5 to 15.0 mm resulting from occlusion of a single perforating artery, chiefly the anterior choroidal, middle cerebral, posterior cerebral, and basilar arteries. Lacunes usually occur in patients with long-standing arterial hypertension or diabetes mellitus. Lacunar infarcts could also be the result of occlusion of penetrating arteries by atherosclerosis of the parent artery or by microembolism from extracranial arterial or cardiac sources. The most frequent sites of lacunes are the putamen, pontis, thalamus, posterior limb of the internal capsule, and caudate nucleus.

Lacunar syndromes are highly predictive of lacunar infarcts. While there are well over twenty described lacunar syndromes, the five that have been best described include pure motor hemiparesis, pure sensory stroke, mixed sensorimotor stroke, dysarthria–clumsy hand syndrome, and ataxic hemiparesis (homolateral ataxia and crural paresis) (Table 38.1). These lacunar syndromes have been described with ischemic lacunar infarctions as well as with discrete hemorrhages.

Ataxic hemiparesis is often due to a lacune affecting either the contralateral posterior limb of the internal capsule or, as in our patient, the contralateral basis pontis. This syndrome has also been described with lesions of the contralateral thalamocapsular region, contralateral red nucleus, corona radiata, and lentiform nucleus. Ataxic hemiparesis has been associated with superior cerebellar artery territory infarcts, and with superficial anterior cerebral artery territory infarcts involving the paracentral region.

Ataxic hemiparesis is characterized by mild to moderate hemiparesis, predominantly involving the lower extremity, and an ipsilateral cerebellar type of incoordination of the arm and leg out of proportion to the weakness. There is usually an extensor plantar response. Dysarthria and facial involvement are rare. Cortical signs or visual field deficits are absent.

The spectrum of the ataxic hemiparesis syndrome has been expanded to include the hemiataxia–hypesthesia syndrome, painful ataxic hemiparesis, hypesthetic ataxic hemiparesis, ataxic hemiparesis accompanied by contralateral sensorimotor or motor trigeminal weakness, dysarthria hemiataxia, and quadrataxic hemiataxia.

TABLE 38.1 LACUNAR SYNDROMES AND THEIR LOCALIZATION

Lacunar Syndrome	Classic Neurologic Deficits	Localization
Pure motor stroke	Hemiparesis, including face (arm > leg weakness), dysarthria	Internal capsule (posterior limb) Corona radiata Basis pontis
Pure sensory stroke	Hemisensory loss	Thalamus (VPL nucleus)
Mixed sensorimotor stroke	Hemiparesis and ipsilateral hemisensory loss	Thalamus (VPL nucleus) and adjacent internal capsule (posterior limb)
Dysarthria–clumsy hand	Supranuclear facial weakness, tongue deviation, dysphagia, dysarthria, and impaired hand fine motor control	Basis pontis Internal capsule (genu)
Ataxic hemiparesis	Homolateral ataxia and crural paresis (leg > arm weakness)	Internal capsule (posterior limb) Thalamocapsular region Lenticulocapsular region Basis pontis Corona radiata

VPL, ventroposterolateral.

SELECTED REFERENCES

Biller J, ed. *Practical neurology*, 4th ed. Philadelphia: Lippincott Williams & Wilkins, Wolters Kluwer Health, 2012.

Brazis PW, Masdeu JC, Biller J. *Localization in clinical neurology*, 6th ed. Philadelphia: Lippincott Williams & Wilkins, Wolters Kluwer Health, 2011.

SEE QUESTIONS: 30, 88, 95, 148, 149, 167

CASE **39**

LEFT INTERNAL CAROTID ARTERY DISSECTION

OBJECTIVES

- To review the clinical manifestations of extracranial internal carotid artery dissections.
- To briefly discuss the pathophysiology of cervicocephalic arterial dissections.
- To review common associations predisposing to cervicocephalic arterial dissections.
- To analyze current ancillary tests used in the evaluation of cervicocephalic arterial dissections.
- To discuss management strategies for patients with extracranial internal carotid artery dissections.

VIGNETTE

A 45-year-old man was sitting at his desk when he suddenly became disoriented, followed by inability to talk, right-sided weakness, and a scotoma on the visual field of his left eye. Visual acuity was 20/20-1 OD and 20/70-3 OS; unchanged with pinhole testing. There was a partial right inferior homonymous hemianopia. In addition, in both eyes he had paracentral scotomas on the left field. Pupils were 7 mm in diameter with normal reactivity. There was no relative afferent pupillary defect (RAPD).

CASE SUMMARY

Our patient had a spontaneous left extracranial internal carotid artery (ICA) dissection resulting in left hemispheric and left retinal ischemia. He was treated with intra-arterial thrombolysis.

Cervicocephalic arterial dissections are an important cause of stroke in young adults. A dissection is produced by subintimal or subadventitial (or both) penetration of blood in a cervicocephalic vessel with subsequent longitudinal extension of the intramural hematoma between its layers. The extracranial ICA is the site of most cervicocephalic arterial dissections. Vertebrobasilar and intracranial carotid artery dissections are less common. Intracranial dissections are usually subintimal and may cause subarachnoid hemorrhage. Multivessel cervicocephalic arterial dissections are rare. After the first month, the recurrence rate of cervicocephalic arterial dissections is approximately 1% per year. The risk is higher in young patients and among those with family history of arterial dissections.

Cervicocephalic arterial dissections are either spontaneous or result from blunt or penetrating trauma. Intraoral and peritonsillar trauma are important causes in children. Dissections have also been associated with fibromuscular dysplasia, Marfan syndrome, vascular Ehlers-Danlos syndrome, pseudoxanthoma elasticum, Menkes disease, osteogenesis imperfecta type I, coarctation of the aorta, adult polycystic kidney disease, cystic medial necrosis, reticular fiber deficiency, accumulation of mucopolysaccharides, elevated arterial elastase content, atherosclerosis, extreme vessel tortuosity or redundancy, moyamoya disease, homocystinuria, pharyngeal infections, luetic arteritis, α_1-antitrypsin deficiency, sympathomimetic drug abuse, and lentiginosis.

Cervicocephalic arterial dissections should be considered in the differential diagnosis of TIAs or cerebral infarction in young adults, particularly when traditional vascular risk factors are missing. Other signs and symptoms associated with extracranial ICA dissections include hemicranial headaches plus a Horner syndrome (without anhidrosis); an isolated Horner syndrome; hemicranial headaches plus delayed hemispheric or retinal ischemia; head, orbital, face, or neck pain; scalp tenderness; scintillations; subjective audible bruit; tinnitus; light-headedness or syncope; and cranial nerve palsies. In addition to a postganglionic Horner syndrome, other neuro-ophthalmological manifestations of ICA dissections include central or branch retinal artery occlusion, ophthalmic artery occlusion, ischemic optic neuropathy, homonymous hemianopia, and cranial nerve palsies.

The diagnosis of cervicocephalic arterial dissection is often based on arteriographic findings. Arteriographic features include the presence of a pearl and string sign; double lumen sign; short, smooth, tapered occlusion; or pseudoaneurysm formation. High-resolution magnetic resonance imaging (MRI), magnetic resonance angiography (MRA), and ultrafast spiral CT (3D CT angiography) provide valuable noninvasive information and have replaced catheter angiography. MRI demonstrates the intramural hematoma and the false lumen of the dissected artery. Ultrasound studies are helpful in monitoring the course and treatment of the disease.

Intravenous tissue plasminogen activator (tPA) should be considered in selected patients with extracranial cervicocephalic arterial dissections associated with acute ischemic strokes within 4.5 hours of onset of symptoms. Randomized clinical trials comparing anticoagulant therapy versus antiplatelets in patients with extracranial cervicocephalic arterial dissections have not been completed. The Cervical Artery Dissection in Stroke Study (CADISS) is an ongoing randomized multicenter open-treatment trial comparing anticoagulant and antiplatelet therapy for acute (within 7 days) symptomatic extracranial carotid or vertebral artery dissection. Anticoagulation should be withheld in patients with intracranial dissections because of the risk of subarachnoid hemorrhage. Endovascular interventions have been used in some patients.

SELECTED REFERENCES

Biller J, ed. *Practical neurology*, 4th ed. Philadelphia: Lippincott Williams & Wilkins, Wolters Kluwer Health, 2012.

Love BB, Biller J. Stroke in young adults. In: Samuels MA, Keske SF, eds. *Office practice of neurology*, 2nd ed. New York: Churchill Livingstone, 2003:337–358.

SEE QUESTIONS: 29, 43, 44, 45, 46, 70, 89, 95, 112, 167, 233

CASE 40

WALLENBERG SYNDROME SECONDARY TO VERTEBRAL ARTERY DISSECTION

OBJECTIVES

- To review clinical manifestations of the lateral medullary syndrome (Wallenberg syndrome).
- To briefly discuss clinical manifestations of vertebrobasilar dissections.
- To review common associations predisposing to vertebrobasilar dissections.

VIGNETTE

A 33-year-old man had sudden onset of severe posterior neck pain, dizziness, unsteadiness, nausea, and vomiting. Computed tomography (CT) was normal. He was a block mason whose work involved heavy lifting.

CASE SUMMARY

Our patient had classical symptoms and signs of a lateral medullary syndrome (Wallenberg syndrome) due to a vertebral artery dissection. These included left pupillary myosis and ptosis (Horner syndrome), horizontal left-beating nystagmus in primary position and on left gaze, left facial sensory loss with ipsilateral hemiataxia and lateropulsion, and contralateral hemihypesthesia. Whereas *ipsilesional* lateropulsion with crossed hypalgesia (and other brainstem signs such as Horner syndrome and dysarthria) suggest Wallenberg due to vertebral artery stroke, lateropulsion and dysmetria *contralesional* to the nystagmus are most often due to infarcts in the medial branch of the posterior inferior cerebellar artery (PICA), which is also often associated with central vertigo.

This syndrome was first described in 1895 by Wallenberg, who demonstrated it to result from damage to the dorsolateral medulla. Wallenberg syndrome is most often caused by occlusion of the ipsilateral intracranial vertebral artery and less commonly of the PICA. Its onset may be preceded by occipital or neck pain hours, days, or months in advance. The classic dorsolateral medullary syndrome is recognized by the presence of crossed sensory loss with ipsilateral facial hypesthesia to pain and temperature (trigeminal nucleus lesion) with contralateral arm and leg hypesthesia to the same sensory modalities (lateral spinothalamic tract lesion). Variable accompanying signs and symptoms include vertigo, nystagmus, Horner syndrome, dysphagia, and dysarthria. Of interest, severe hiccups are one of the most unique symptoms in Wallenberg syndrome, as demonstrated in the latter part of the video. These can last for weeks and interfere with eating, sleeping, and carrying on conversations.

Vertebrobasilar artery dissection is an underrecognized etiology of stroke in young adults and children. Signs and symptoms associated with vertebrobasilar dissections include occipital or posterior neck pain, mastoid pain, vertebrobasilar transient ischemic attacks, variations of the lateral or medial medullary infarction, cerebellar infarction, and posterior cerebral artery distribution infarction.

SELECTED REFERENCES

Brazis PW, Masdeu JC, Biller J. *Practical neurology*, 6th ed. Philadelphia: Lippincott Williams & Wilkins, Wolters Kluwer Health, 2011.

Love BB, Biller J. Stroke in young adults. In: Samuels MA, Keske SF, eds. *Office practice of neurology*, 2nd ed. New York: Churchill Livingstone, 2003:337–358.

SEE QUESTIONS: 19, 35, 36, 38, 95

CASE 41

MULTIPLE CEREBRAL INFARCTIONS DUE TO ANTIPHOSPHOLIPID ANTIBODY SYNDROME

OBJECTIVES

- To review the main manifestations of the antiphospholipid antibody syndrome (APAS).
- To discuss nosologic entities associated with the secondary type of APAS.
- To summarize therapeutic guidelines for arterial thrombosis associated with APAS.

VIGNETTE

Several years prior to this evaluation, this 45-year-old woman, with history of pregnancy-induced hypertension and preeclampsia, had her first stroke, affecting her left hemibody. The patient was treated with warfarin. Two years later, while on warfarin, she lost consciousness and was diagnosed with acute obstructive hydrocephalus due to a pineal gland hemorrhage requiring placement of a ventriculoperitoneal shunt. This was followed a year later by two additional hemispheric strokes. The patient received aspirin. Seven years on, she had an episode of vomiting, diarrhea, right-hand weakness, and difficulty speaking and was treated with aspirin and dipyridamole.

CASE SUMMARY

Our patient was diagnosed with the APAS. APAS is an acquired pro-thrombotic syndrome characterized by recurrent arterial or venous thromboembolism, unexplained fetal loss usually within the first 10 weeks of gestation, and thrombocytopenia, with the presence of circulating antiphospholipid antibodies. Primary APAS is an immune-mediated coagulopathy associated with cerebral ischemia in young adults, the etiology of which remains unknown. Secondary APAS can occur within the context of several diseases, mainly autoimmune or rheumatologic disorders, infections, malignancy, and drugs.

Antiphospholipid antibodies are a heterogeneous group of autoantibodies directed against phospholipid-binding proteins. Several antiphospholipid antibodies have been described; the most thoroughly studied subsets include lupus anticoagulant (LA) and anticardiolipins (aCL) IgG, IgA, and IgM isotypes. The mechanism of anticoagulation by aCL includes the formation of a complex between aCL and beta-1 glycoprotein 1 antibody (β2GPI), leading to a dysfunctional protein C pathway.

APAS may be primary, or secondary, to underlying diseases such as systemic lupus erythematosus (SLE), rheumatoid arthritis, Sjögren syndrome, Sneddon syndrome (livedo reticularis and ischemic cerebrovascular disease), malignancies, syphilis, acute and chronic infections including AIDS, inflammatory bowel disease, administration of certain drugs, liver transplantation, and early-onset severe preeclampsia.

Antiphospholipid antibodies cause cerebral and ocular ischemia, myocardial infarction, peripheral arterial thromboembolism, as well as venous thrombosis and pulmonary emboli. Multiple cerebral infarctions (as in our patient) are common in patients with APAS; a subset of patients may present with vascular dementia or an acute ischemic encephalopathy. Although only ischemic stroke is an accepted neurologic diagnostic criterion for the syndrome, other neurologic conditions have been associated with APAS, most commonly migraine, and various movement disorders, most particularly chorea.

Pathologically, there is evidence of a chronic thrombotic microangiopathy, but no evidence of vasculitis. Patients with antiphospholipid antibodies also have an increased frequency of mitral and aortic vegetations resembling verrucous endocarditis (Libman-Sacks endocarditis).

Treatment for arterial thrombosis associated with APAS is not well established. It is accepted that oral anticoagulation with moderate-intensity warfarin (target INR 2.0 to 3.0) is the preferred treatment of venous thromboembolic events. Warfarin is replaced by low molecular weight heparin or unfractionated heparin during pregnancy. Aspirin is also a reasonable alternative for patients who have APAS and first ischemic stroke in the absence of other underlying etiology for the ischemic event.

SELECTED REFERENCES

Biller J, ed. *Practical neurology*, 4th ed. Philadelphia: Lippincott Williams & Wilkins, Wolters Kluwer Health, 2012.

Cuadrado MJ, Hughes GRV. Antiphospholipid (Hughes) syndrome. *Rheum Dis Clin North Am* 2001;27:507–524.

Levine SR, Welch KMA. The spectrum of neurologic disease associated with antiphospholipid antibodies. Lupus anticoagulants and anticardiolipin antibodies. *Arch Neurol* 1987;44:876–883.

Lin W, Crowther MA, Eikelboom JW. Management of antiphospholipid antibody syndrome. A systematic review. *JAMA* 2006;295(9):1050–1057.

SEE QUESTIONS: 20, 54, 71, 94, 96, 97, 160, 161

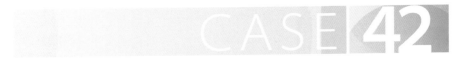

PSEUDOBULBAR PALSY (MULTIPLE STROKES)

OBJECTIVES

- To review clinical characteristics of pseudobulbar palsy.
- To discuss pathogenetic mechanisms of pseudobulbar palsy.
- To describe nonvascular etiologies of pseudobulbar palsy.

VIGNETTE

A 48-year-old man with history of arterial hypertension, cigarette smoking, prior strokes, a left atrial appendage thrombus, and heterozygosity for the factor V Leiden was admitted for evaluation of increasing difficulties with speaking and swallowing. He also had a 40-pound weight loss.

CASE SUMMARY

 Our patient had multiple vascular risk factors. Hypertension is the single most important modifiable risk factor for ischemic stroke. An estimated 40% to 90% of stroke patients are diagnosed with hypertension before their index event. Smokers have a four- to sixfold increased risk of stroke compared to patients who never smoked; the risk declines significantly 2 to 4 years after quitting, although it takes several decades to return to the risk level of someone who has never smoked.

His dysphagia resulted in considerable weight loss. Examination was remarkable for dysarthria, hypernasal voice, automatic-voluntary dissociation of facial movements, primitive reflexes, asymmetric and brisk muscle stretch reflexes, and a small-stepped gait (marche à petit pas). He also reported emotional incontinence with pathological laughing and crying, features suggestive of pseudobulbar palsy. Our patient's pseudobulbar palsy resulted from multiple subcortical infarctions. Other less common vascular etiologies of pseudobulbar palsy include the antiphospholipid antibody syndrome and embolism from atrial myxomas. Pseudobulbar palsy has also been associated with a variety of inflammatory, infectious, demyelinative, neoplastic, iatrogenic (chemotherapeutic agents, such as cytosine arabinoside), and neurodegenerative disorders (such as amyotrophic lateral sclerosis and progressive supranuclear palsy) and has also been reported after posterior fossa surgery in children.

SELECTED REFERENCES

Biller J, ed. *Practical neurology*, 4th ed. Philadelphia: Lippincott Williams & Wilkins, Wolters Kluwer Health, 2012.

Brazis PW, Masdeu JC, Biller J. *Localization in clinical neurology*, 6th ed. Philadelphia: Lippincott Williams & Wilkins, Wolters Kluwer Health, 2011.

Mancardi GL, Romagnoli P, Tassinari T, et al. Lacunae and cribriform cavities of the brain. Correlations with pseudobulbar palsy and parkinsonism. *Eur Neurol* 1988;28(1):11–17.

SEE QUESTIONS: 33, 88, 148

CASE 43

WATERSHED INFARCTS

OBJECTIVES

■ To review clinical characteristics of watershed infarctions.
■ To discuss pathogenetic mechanisms of watershed infarctions.

VIGNETTE

A 65-year-old woman with a T4, N1, M0 squamous cell carcinoma of the left retromalar trigone and mandible had a composite resection with modified radical neck dissection and tracheostomy followed by a free flap reconstruction. On the morning after surgery, the patient appeared slightly less responsive and remained ventilated. Eventually she became more responsive; however, she continued to have poor movements of all her extremities.

CASE SUMMARY

Our patient had a perioperative watershed stroke due to a combination of arterial hypotension and carotid artery stenosis. Arterial hypotension and poor cerebral perfusion are important factors in the production of perioperative strokes. Patients with severe carotid artery disease are at high risk of perioperative watershed infarction.

The watershed cortical areas are the first to be deprived of sufficient blood flow in instances of cerebral hypoperfusion. Watershed infarcts occur in the border zone between adjacent arterial perfusion beds. Although most authors suggest that watershed infarctions arise from hemodynamic derangements, they may also result from cerebral embolism, as there is preferential distribution of emboli in the arterial border-zone regions.

During or after cardiac surgery or after an episode of sustained and severe arterial hypotension after cardiac arrest, prolonged hypoxemia, or bilateral severe carotid artery disease (as in our patient), ischemia may occur in the watershed areas between the major circulations. Unilateral watershed infarcts occur in the context of hemodynamic failure in patients with underlying severe arterial stenosis or occlusion and a noncompetent circle of Willis. Watershed infarcts may also be associated with microembolism, hyperviscosity states, and near-drowning events.

Ischemia in the border-zone territory of the anterior cerebral artery (ACA) and middle cerebral artery (MCA) may result in transcortical motor aphasia, impaired saccadic eye movements due to injury to the frontal eye fields, and bibrachial cortical sensorimotor impairment (man in a barrel).

Ischemia in the border-zone territory between the ACA and posterior cerebral artery (PCA) results in bilateral parietooccipital infarcts, which yield a variety of visual manifestations, including impairments in depth perception, in visual navigation (optic ataxia), and in oculomotor initiation (ocular apraxia) and a number of abnormalities ranging from alexia, dyscalculia, dysgraphia, and cortical blindness.

Watershed infarcts are also recognized between the territorial supply of the posterior inferior cerebellar artery (PICA), anterior inferior cerebellar artery (AICA), and superior cerebellar artery (SCA). Watershed infarcts may also involve the internal watershed region of the centrum semiovale alongside and slightly above the body of the lateral ventricles, as well as spinal cord.

SELECTED REFERENCES

Biller J, ed. *Practical neurology*, 4th ed. Philadelphia: Lippincott Williams & Wilkins, Wolters Kluwer Health, 2012.

Brazis PW, Masdeu JC, Biller J. *Localization in clinical neurology*, 6th ed. Philadelphia: Lippincott Williams & Wilkins, Wolters Kluwer Health, 2011.

Caplan LR, Hennerici M. Impaired clearance of emboli (washout) is an important link between hypoperfusion, embolism, and ischemic stroke. *Arch Neurol* 1998;55(11):1475–1482.

Graeber MC, Jordan JE, Mishra SK, et al. Watershed infarction on computed tomographic scan. An unreliable sign of hemodynamic stroke. *Arch Neurol* 1992;49:311–313.

SEE QUESTIONS: 20, 116, 117, 118, 119, 120, 121, 122, 123, 138, 139, 179

CASE 44

MOYAMOYA SYNDROME ASSOCIATED WITH DOWN SYNDROME

OBJECTIVES

- To review the basic pathophysiology of moyamoya disease.
- To review clinical characteristics of moyamoya disease.
- To discuss ancillary diagnostic tests in moyamoya disease.
- To review management principles in moyamoya disease.

VIGNETTE

At the age of 18, this boy experienced transient right upper extremity weakness associated with dysarthria and right facial weakness.

CASE SUMMARY

Our patient had specific facial features, brachiocephaly, up-slanted and narrow palpebral fissures, shortened digits, hypotonia, and joint hyperextensibility, characteristic of trisomy 21 or Down syndrome. He also had hypothyroidism and sleep apnea but no underlying congenital heart disease. His stroke was due to moyamoya syndrome.

Moyamoya (Japanese for "puff of smoke") disease is a progressive, nonatherosclerotic, noninflammatory, occlusive cerebral arteriopathy of unknown etiology with particular involvement of the terminal portions of the internal carotid arteries (ICAs) and the circle of Willis. Moyamoya is characterized by stenosis or occlusion of the distal intracranial ICA or the adjacent anterior, middle, or posterior cerebral arteries, along with the development of basal, parenchymal, leptomeningeal, or dural collaterals. Moyamoya disease has a bimodal age distribution with a peak in the first and fourth decades of life. Half of the affected patients present before 10 years of age. Familial occurrence has been reported. Pathologically, there is fibrocellular thickening of the intima, waving of the internal elastic lamina, and attenuation of the media.

Proposed criteria for the diagnosis of moyamoya disease include bilateral stenosis or occlusion of the ICA bifurcation (C1) proximal portions of the anterior cerebral (A1) and middle cerebral (M1) arteries, and an unusual netlike (puff of smoke) appearance of collateral arteries arising from the circle of Willis.

Many disease states have been associated with moyamoya. These include neonatal anoxia, trauma, basilar meningitis, tuberculous meningitis, leptospirosis, cranial irradiation therapy for optic pathway gliomas, neurofibromatosis type 1 (von Recklinghausen disease), tuberous sclerosis, complex, brain tumors, fibromuscular dysplasia, polyarteritis nodosa, Marfan syndrome, pseudoxanthoma elasticum, hypomelanosis of Ito, Williams syndrome, Turner syndrome, Alagille syndrome, cerebral dissecting and saccular aneurysms, sickle cell anemia, β thalassemia, aplastic anemia, Fanconi anemia, Apert syndrome, factor XII deficiency, type I glycogenosis, NADH-coenzyme Q reductase deficiency, renal artery stenosis, coarctation of the aorta, and Down syndrome.

Young adults with moyamoya disease may present with hemiparesis, monoparesis, alternating hemiparesis, early morning headaches and nausea, seizures, involuntary (mostly choreiform) movements, intellectual decline, intellectual disabilities, cerebral infarction, and intracranial hemorrhage. In adults, the most common symptoms are caused by subarachnoid, subependymal, or intraventricular hemorrhage. Ischemic strokes may be multiple and recurrent and predominantly involve the carotid circulation. The infarcts may be superficial or deep and often involve watershed territories.

Routine hematological, biochemical, and serologic investigations are unrevealing except for reports of elevated cerebrospinal fluid (CSF) fibroblastic growth factor. Diagnosis is based on the distinct arteriographic appearance previously described. MRA or CTA may preclude the need for conventional angiography if surgery is not anticipated.

Optimal treatment for moyamoya disease has not yet been determined. Platelet antiaggregants, calcium channel blockers, corticosteroids, and vasodilators have been used. Various surgical procedures involving direct or indirect anastomosis have been recommended in the management of the ischemic complications of childhood moyamoya. Revascularization surgery is less useful in patients presenting with intracranial hemorrhage.

SELECTED REFERENCES

Hoffman H. Moyamoya disease and syndrome. *Clin Neurol Neurosurg* 1997;99:S39–S44.
Pearson E, Lenn NJ, Cail WS. Moyamoya and other causes of stroke in patients with Down syndrome. *Pediatr Neurol* 1985;1(May–Jun):174–179.

SEE QUESTIONS: 29, 30, 46, 78, 141, 203

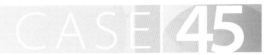

TAKAYASU ARTERITIS

OBJECTIVES

- To review the basic pathophysiology of the vasculitides.
- To review the clinical characteristics of Takayasu arteritis.
- To discuss ancillary diagnostic tests in Takayasu arteritis.
- To review management principles in Takayasu arteritis.

VIGNETTE

A 36-year-old woman with a history of erythema nodosum, left-eye uveitis, and bilateral episcleritis experienced flulike symptoms for 3 years, including generalized fatigue and soreness in her shoulders, hips, and back. She also developed episodes of effort-induced left arm pain and weakness and episodes of visual "whiteouts" whenever exposed to bright light. Examination showed her blood pressure to be 140/90 mm Hg on the right arm and unobtainable on the left arm. The left radial pulse was not palpable. There was a harsh right-sided cervical bruit. She was seen by numerous physicians without a conclusive diagnosis. She was noted to be anemic, and further investigations were undertaken to evaluate her gastrointestinal tract.

CASE SUMMARY

The vasculitides are characterized by blood vessel inflammation and necrosis. Four basic types of immunopathogenetic mechanisms have been proposed: I, anaphylactic type; II, cytotoxic/cell-activating type; III, immune complex type; and IV, cell-mediated type. Injury can also occur by other pathways including cytokine mediated, neutrophil involvement, infectious, or environmental/chemical injury. More than one mechanism is likely to be involved in a particular vasculitis. Diagnosis of vasculitis is often inferential, based on clinical presentation, presence of multisystem organ involvement, and abnormal serologic tests.

Takayasu arteritis (TA) is a chronic, large vessel panarteritis localized to the aortic arch or its branches, the ascending thoracic aorta, the abdominal aorta, or the entire aorta. TA, also known as pulseless disease, is more common among young women. The disorder has two distinctive phases: a prepulseless (inflammatory or systemic) phase and a pulseless phase. Systemic symptoms of TA include fatigue, weight loss, low-grade fever, arthralgias, thoracic back pain, and new-onset arterial hypertension. Other systemic-related symptoms include vertigo when looking upwards, syncope, convulsions, dementia, claudication in one arm or leg, ischemia of the extremities, ischemic optic neuropathy, and decreased visual acuity. Widespread arterial bruits, a weak or absent radial pulse, and differences in blood pressure between both arms are helpful clinical clues. Jaw claudication and atrophy of the facial musculature may be evident.

Diagnosis of TA is confirmed by aortic angiography or 3D CT angiography. MRI and MRA are valuable noninvasive diagnostic tools. There may be anemia, leukocytosis, increased erythrocyte sedimentation rate (ESR), elevated C-reactive protein (CRP), and hypergammaglobulinemia. ^{18}F-FDG PET coregistered with enhanced CT images may also demonstrate the distribution and inflammatory activity in the affected vessels in causes of active TA.

Management includes glucocorticoids. Antiplatelet therapy is often used to prevent thrombus formation. Surgical reconstructive methods or percutaneous transluminal angioplasty is often needed for the chronic arterial lesions of TA.

SELECTED REFERENCES

Fraga A, Mint G, Valle L, et al. Takayasu's arteritis: frequency of systemic manifestations (study of 22 patients) and favorable response to maintenance steroid therapy with adrenocorticosteroids (12 patients). *Arthritis Rheum* 1977;15:617–624.

Kobayashi Y, Ishii K, Oda K, et al. Aortic wall inflammation due to Takayasu arteritis imaged with ^{18}F-FDG PET coregistered with enhanced CT. *J Nucl Med* 2005;46:917–922.

Lupi-Herrera E, Sanchez-Torres G, Marcushamer J, et al. Takayasu's arteritis. Clinical study of 107 cases. *Am Heart J* 1977;93:94–103.

SEE QUESTIONS: 29, 45, 94

CASE 46

RECURRENT FACIAL PALSIES (VZV) FOLLOWED BY CEREBRAL INFARCTION

OBJECTIVES

- To review the clinical characteristics of Ramsay Hunt syndrome (herpes zoster oticus).
- To analyze different vasculopathies associated with varicella-zoster virus (VZV) infection.

VIGNETTE

A 47-year-old left-handed man had chickenpox at approximately 7 years of age. Since then, he had intermittent painful blisters on his right hand, as well as painful blisters on the right posterior neck associated with unilateral right-sided headaches. At the age 41, he had a cerebral infarction. He was found to have an occluded right ICA and 90% left ICA stenosis. He had a left CEA. A year later, he developed a right peripheral facial palsy associated with right ear vesicles. Over the subsequent years, he had recurrent episodes right hand and posterior neck vesicular rashes. He also had a recurrent left peripheral facial paralysis a few years after his initial stroke.

CASE SUMMARY

Our patient had acute facial paralysis associated with herpetic vesicles on the skin of the external auditory canal. A diagnosis of Ramsay Hunt syndrome (aka: herpes zoster oticus, geniculate neuralgia, or nervus intermedius neuralgia) was made. Subsequently, he had a hemispheric cerebral infarction probably associated with varicella-zoster virus (VZV) infection. Besides acute peripheral facial paralysis and intense otalgia on the affected side, patients with Ramsay Hunt syndrome may experience vertigo, ipsilateral tinnitus, and ipsilateral hearing loss. The herpetic vesicles may also involve the pinna, tympanic membrane, soft palate, and anterior two-thirds of the tongue (Fig. 46.1).

VZV infection may be associated with a large or small vessel vasculopathy. It may also cause a necrotizing arteritis similar to CNS granulomatous angiitis. A large vessel vasculitis developing between 4 and 6 weeks after herpes zoster ophthalmicus is the most common VZV vasculitis. Cerebral angiography often demonstrates unilateral segmental narrowing of the proximal segments of the MCA, ACA, or, less commonly, the PCA or ICA. CSF may show a discrete lymphocytic pleocytosis. Uncommonly, a postvaricella angiopathy of small and large vessels may develop.

Intravenous acyclovir is the treatment of choice for complicated VZV infections. Other options include valacyclovir, famciclovir, or ganciclovir.

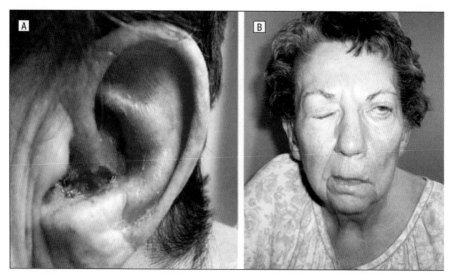

Figure 46.1 **Ramsay Hunt Syndrome. A:** Well-circumscribed erythematous rash on the left ear. Dry exudate from vesicular lesions can be appreciated. **B:** Peripheral left facial paralysis with Bell phenomenon (normal upward rolling of the ipsilateral eye when patient is asked to occlude the eyes). (With permission from Espay AJ, Bull RL. Petrositis in Ramsay Hunt Syndrome with multiple cranial neuropathies. *Arch Neurol* 2005;62(11):1774–1775.)

SELECTED REFERENCES

Espay AJ, Bull RL. Petrositis in Ramsay Hunt syndrome with multiple cranial neuropathies. *Arch Neurol* 2005;62(11):1774–1775.

Hilt DC, Buchholz D, Krumholz A, et al. Herpes zoster ophthalmicus and delayed contralateral hemiparesis caused by cerebral angiitis: diagnosis and management approaches. *Ann Neurol* 1983;14:543–553.

Robillard RB, Hilsinger RL, Adour KK. Ramsay Hunt facial paralysis: clinical analyses of 185 patients. *Otolaryngol Head Neck Surg* 1986;95:292–297.

SEE QUESTIONS: 83, 87, 148, 152, 157, 158, 164, 165

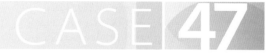

CASE 47

MULTIPLE LOBAR HEMORRHAGES DUE TO CEREBRAL AMYLOID ANGIOPATHY

OBJECTIVES

- To review clinical characteristics of lobar intracerebral hemorrhages.
- To discuss nonhypertensive causes of intracerebral hemorrhages.
- To illustrate a unique form of cerebral angiopathy.

VIGNETTE

A 56-year-old normotensive man had recurrent lobar intracerebral hemorrhages.

CASE SUMMARY

 Our patient had multiple, bilateral, recurrent, lobar posterior intracerebral hemorrhages. *Intracranial hemorrhage* is defined as any bleed occurring within the cranial cavity. An intracranial hemorrhage may be epidural, subdural, subarachnoid, parenchymal, or intraventricular. Intracerebral hemorrhage is one of the most deadly stroke subtypes and accounts for 10% to 15% of all strokes in Western countries. Arterial hypertension is the most common cause of nontraumatic intracerebral hemorrhage in adults. Other major causes include intracranial aneurysms, CNS vascular malformations, bleeding diatheses, anticoagulant therapy, thrombolytic therapy, cerebral amyloid angiopathy (CAA), brain tumors, vasculitides, and drug abuse. Hypertensive hemorrhages often involve the putamen, thalamus, subcortical white matter, cerebellum, or pons.

Brain hemorrhages often occur during activity. Headaches are present in half of the patients. Nausea and vomiting are present in over half of the patients. The level of alertness may be variably compromised. Seizures rarely occur at onset of bleeding. Signs of meningeal irritation signs may result if bleeding extends to the subarachnoid space. Fundoscopy may show retinal hemorrhages.

Hematoma location, size, direction of spread, and rate of bleeding play a major role in ultimately determining clinical presentation and outcome. A lobar intracerebral hemorrhage refers to bleeding parenchymatous bleeding involving the subcortical supratentorial white matter and located outside the deep nuclear structures. Frontal lobar hemorrhages often result in contralateral hemiparesis and abulia. Conjugate eye deviation towards the side of the hematoma may occur. Bifrontal headache is frequently reported. Parietal lobe hemorrhages result in contralateral hemisensory loss and neglect of the contralateral visual field. Variable degrees of contralateral homonymous hemianopia, mild hemiparesis, and anosognosia may be present. Dominant temporal lobe hemorrhages result in Wernicke aphasia. Left temporoparietal hematomas result in conduction or global aphasia. Temporal lobe hemorrhages may also result in contralateral visual field defects, or agitated delirium. Occipital lobe hemorrhages are associated with ipsilateral orbital pain and contralateral homonymous hemianopsia.

Patients suspected of having an intracerebral hemorrhage deserve a thorough evaluation. Unenhanced CT is still the safest and most common imaging modality to evaluate these patients. MRI is an important tool for identifying bleeding lesions such as vascular malformations and/or tumors. Gradient echo MRI sequences are extremely useful in detecting small petechial hemorrhages or areas of hemosiderin deposition. Catheter cerebral angiography is indicated if there is reason to suspect an aneurysm, arteriovenous malformation, vasculitis, or moyamoya disease and in patients with atypical location for hypertensive hemorrhage.

Additional investigations are employed to exclude most common causes of recurrent lobar intracerebral hemorrhage. In our patient, based on cortical involvement, multiplicity of lesions in space and time, bilaterality, and the recurrent nature of the intracerebral hemorrhages, we suspect sporadic CAA as the most likely etiology. Hemorrhages secondary to CAA are usually lobar, large, and multiple. As in our patient, there is a predilection for the parietooccipital regions.

CAA is characterized by amyloid beta ($A\beta$) deposition in the media and adventitia of leptomeningeal, cortical, and subcortical medium and small-sized arteries and arterioles. Unlike the predominant accumulation of $A\beta1$-42 in the senile plaques of patients with Alzheimer disease, $A\beta1$-40 accumulates in the cerebral arterioles of patients with CAA, mostly of the periventricular white matter. Pathologically, amyloid is stained pink with Congo red and demonstrates a characteristic yellow-green birefringence under polarized light. Different biochemical types of amyloid have been identified. The amyloid peptide (A4), a cleavage product of amyloid precursor protein on chromosome 21, is usually found in patients with Alzheimer disease, Down syndrome, or in older but otherwise healthy individuals.

CAA is also found in the Dutch variant of hereditary cerebral hemorrhage with amyloid angiopathy (HCHWA-D), in the Icelandic type of hereditary cerebral hemorrhage with amyloidosis, and in a rare variant associated with nonneuritic plaques and dementia. The Icelandic type is related to a mutation of the cystatin C gene. CAA is also associated with dementia pugilistica, cerebellar ataxia, granulomatous angiitis, rheumatoid vasculitis, giant cell arteritis, postradiation necrosis, and vascular malformations. Intracerebral hemorrhage, in patients with CAA associated with apolipoprotein E epsilon 4 (APOE-epsilon 4) allele, occurs at an earlier age.

Severe CAA can cause lobar intracerebral hemorrhage, vascular dementia, and transient neurological deficits. CAA is the most common cause of lobar hemorrhages among older normotensive individuals. It has been estimated that approximately 20% of patients with CAA eventually have intracerebral bleeding. CAA-associated hemorrhages often involve the cortical surface and often rupture into the subarachnoid space. Cerebellum or pontine involvement is exceptional. Subdural hematomas and subarachnoid hemorrhage can occur. Unusual variants of CAA-related inflammation (nonvasculitic and vasculitic) have been effectively treated with corticosteroid therapy.

Effective therapy of intracerebral hemorrhage due to CAA is currently not available. Platelet antiaggregants and nonsteroidal anti-inflammatory drugs should be avoided.

SELECTED REFERENCES

Greenberg SM. Genetics of primary intracerebral hemorrhage. *Semin Cerebrovasc Dis Stroke* 2002;2:59–65.

Izumihara A, Ishihara T, Iwamoto N, et al. Postoperative outcome of 37 patients with lobar intracerebral hemorrhage related to cerebral amyloid angiopathy. *Stroke* 1999;30:29–33.

Kase CS, Williams JP, Wyatt DA, et al. Lobar intracerebral hematomas: clinical and CT analysis of 22 cases. *Neurology* 1982;32:1146.

Kloppenberg RP, Richard E, Sprengers MES, et al. Steroid responsive encephalopathy in cerebral amyloid angiopathy: a case report and review of evidence for immunosuppressive treatment. *J Neuroinflammation* 2010;7:18.

Pendlebury WW, Iole ED, Tracy RP, et al. Intracerebral hemorrhage related to cerebral amyloid angiopathy and tPA. *Ann Neurol* 1991;29:210–213.

SEE QUESTIONS: 52, 66, 71, 93, 104, 178, 188, 216, 217, 220, 221, 223

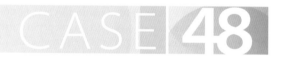

PURE SENSORY STROKE DUE TO THALAMIC HEMORRHAGE

OBJECTIVES

- To describe the clinical characteristics of pure sensory stroke (pure hemisensory or paresthetic stroke).
- To highlight the fact that discrete hemorrhages can account for this and other lacunar syndromes.

A 61-year-old African-American woman with a history of poorly controlled arterial hypertension was evaluated because of acute onset of left hemibody numbness. Her blood pressure was 204/100 mm Hg.

► **CASE SUMMARY** ◄

Acute stroke is one of the leading causes of morbidity and mortality in the world. The World Health Organization estimates that approximately 15 million new strokes occur each year worldwide. Stroke is a clinical diagnosis that requires prompt diagnostic treatment. Differentiation between brain infarction and hemorrhage is paramount. In the Western world, of all strokes, 87% are ischemic. Hemorrhagic strokes account for the remaining. A thorough history and physical examination are essential in guiding a rational and cost-effective management.

Our patient had uncontrolled arterial hypertension and presented to the emergency room fully alert after sudden onset of hemisensory deficits. Initial interpretation of her deficits suggested a subcortical ischemic lesion. However, the head CT showed a small hypertensive thalamic hemorrhage. Pure sensory stroke (also reported as pure hemisensory or paresthetic stroke) is characterized by unilateral numbness, paresthesias, and a hemisensory deficit involving the face, arm, trunk, and leg. Subjective complaints may be out of proportion to objective findings. Lacunae in the ventroposterolateral nucleus of the thalamus may cause this syndrome. Pure sensory stroke can also be due to ischemic infarctions in the corona radiata or in the parietal cortex.

Small ischemic strokes involving the internal capsule/corona radiata, subthalamus, midbrain, or parietal cortex may also cause a pure sensory stroke, as may pontine lacunes involving the medial lemniscus or paramedian dorsal pons. In these cases, distal sensory manifestations are common in the form of cheiro–oral, cheiro–pedal, or cheiro–oral–pedal syndromes. Only rarely are sensory manifestations restricted to proximal body segments.

Differentiation of a pontine pure sensory syndrome from a thalamic pure sensory syndrome may be challenging. Brainstem pure sensory strokes often show a discrepancy between superficial and deep sensations. In pontine pure sensory stroke, vibration and position sense are often reduced on the paresthetic side, whereas sensation to pinprick and temperature are preserved. Conversely, in cases of pure sensory stroke involving the thalamus, internal capsule, or corona radiata, both spinothalamic and medial lemniscal modalities are compromised. Likewise, ipsilateral impairment of smooth pursuit and vestibuloocular reflex may indicate a pontine lesion in patients with hemisensory stroke. A pure sensory deficit affecting pain and temperature sensation may also be due to a small hemorrhage in the dorsolateral midbrain.

In a report of 21 patients with pure sensory stroke, 11 patients had thalamic strokes, 7 patients had lacunes or hemorrhages in the leticulocapsular region or corona radiata, 2 had pontine tegmental strokes, and 1 had a small cortical infarct. Hemisensory deficits of all modalities usually were associated with a relatively large lacune or hemorrhage in the lateral thalamus, whereas tract-specific or restricted sensory changes suggested very small strokes in the sensory pathway from the pons to the parietal cortex.

SELECTED REFERENCES

Biller J, ed. *Practical neurology*, 4th ed. Philadelphia: Lippincott Williams & Wilkins, Wolters Kluwer Health, 2012.

Brazis PW, Masdeu JC, Biller J. *Localization in clinical neurology*, 6th ed. Philadelphia: Lippincott Williams & Wilkins, Wolters Kluwer Health, 2011.

SEE QUESTIONS: 35, 39, 47, 55, 71, 93, 104, 188, 216, 217, 233

CASE 49

LACUNAR HEMICHOREOATHETOSIS

OBJECTIVE

- To demonstrate a hyperkinetic presentation of a lacunar stroke.

VIGNETTE

This 56-year-old woman with history of uncontrolled arterial hypertension had sudden onset of left hemibody paresthesias, followed by left upper and lower extremity weakness, and adventitious movements of her left upper extremity.

CASE SUMMARY

 Our patient had sudden left hemibody numbness and mild weakness, followed by random jerking, involuntary movements of her left hand and arm. Her adventitious movements disappeared during sleep. She did not have facial grimacing or tongue protrusion. MRI showed a lacunar infarction of the contralateral putamen and caudate nucleus with sparing of the anterior limb of the internal capsule. Random blood sugar and thyroid function tests were normal. Remainder of ancillary investigations were unremarkable.

Lacunar infarcts involve deep regions of the brain or brainstem. The most frequent sites of involvement are the putamen, basis pontis, thalamus, posterior limb of the internal capsule, and caudate nucleus. Multiple lacunae are associated strongly with arterial hypertension and diabetes mellitus. Lacunar infarcts are often associated with *in situ* occlusion of a single perforating vessel or thickening of the arteriolar wall. Lacunar infarcts can also be caused by a different etiology than hypertensive small vessel cerebral disease, including cardiac embolism, and embolism from artery to artery atheroma or intracranial arterial stenosis.

Overall, lacunar infarcts have a relatively favorable prognosis as they are usually associated with a good functional recovery, a lower recurrence rate, and a higher survival rate than other types of ischemic strokes. However, this has been debated, as the prognosis of lacunar infarcts is not always favorable. Although there are over 20 described lacunar syndromes, those that have been best described are pure motor hemiparesis (PMH), pure sensory stroke (PSS), sensorimotor stroke (SMS), ataxic hemiparesis (AH), and dysarthria–clumsy hand syndrome (DCHS). Hemichorea/hemiballismus (HH), the most frequently reported movement disorder associated with acute stroke, is an uncommon presentation of a lacunar infarction. Some degree of dystonia may be mixed in, yielding a phenotype referred to as athetosis or choreoathetosis (slower forms of chorea, within the spectrum of hyperkinetic disorders).

Discrete or hemorrhagic lesions of the caudate nucleus or putamen, thalamus, subthalamic nucleus, and corona radiata may be associated with contralateral hyperkinetic motor activity confined to one side of the body. Lesions in or near the subthalamic nucleus produce contralateral hemiballismus. Hemiballismus may also result from lesions in the caudate, putamen, globus pallidus, precentral gyrus, or thalamic nuclei. Destruction of the corticospinal tract ipsilateral to the subthalamic nucleus prevents the development of hemiballismus. Small unilateral lesions of the anteroventral portion of the caudate cause contralateral choreoathetosis. Unilateral lesions of the globus pallidus may result in contralateral hemidystonia. Unilateral pallidal–putaminal lesions may present with sudden falling to the contralateral side while sitting, standing, or walking. Unilateral lateral-posterior thalamic strokes have been associated with delayed onset of a contralateral hyperkinetic syndrome (chorea and dystonia or choreoathetosis, with or without action-induced tremor).

Repetitive involuntary movements (hemichorea and hemiballismus) have been reported with basal ganglia lacunar infarcts and with carotid artery occlusive disease. Hemichorea and hemiballismus have also been reported in association with nonketotic hyperglycemia. Rarely bilateral choreiform movements have been reported with lacunar infarcts involving the corpus striatum. Brainstem lacunar infarctions may result in involuntary tonic limb spasms. Focal hand dystonia has been observed in patients with lacunar infarctions of the lenticular or caudate nucleus, whereas posthemiplegic athetosis may develop after ischemic or hemorrhagic lesions of the contralateral putamen and globus pallidus.

SELECTED REFERENCES

Ghika-Schmid F, Ghika J, Regli F, et al. Hyperkinetic movement disorders during and after stroke: the Lausanne Stroke Registry. *J Neurol Sci* 1997;146(2):109–116.

Kase CS, Maulsby GO, de Juan E, et al. Hemichorea-hemiballism and lacunar infarction in the basal ganglia. *Neurology* 1981;31:452–455.

Kim JS. Delayed onset mixed involuntary movements after thalamic stroke. Clinical, radiological and pathophysiological findings. *Brain* 2000;124(2):299–305.

Lee B-C, Hwang S-H, Chang GY. Hemiballismus-hemichorea in older diabetic women: a clinical syndrome with MRI correlation. *Neurology* 1999;52:646–648.

Mead GM, Lewis SC, Wardlaw JM, et al. Severe ipsilateral carotid stenosis and middle cerebral artery disease in lacunar ischemic stroke: innocent bystanders? *J Neurol* 2002;249:266–271.

Sacco S, Marini C, Totaro R, et al. A population study of the incidence and prognosis of lacunar stroke. *Neurology* 2006;66:1335–1338.

SEE QUESTIONS: 189, 200

CASE 50

ALEXIA WITHOUT AGRAPHIA DUE TO BIOPSY-NEGATIVE PRIMARY CNS ANGIITIS

OBJECTIVES

- To briefly discuss management of primary CNS angiitis.
- To review an unusual cause of alexia without agraphia.

VIGNETTE

A 39-year-old right-handed schoolteacher was evaluated for recurrent ischemic strokes and inability to read.

CASE SUMMARY

Six months prior to her evaluation, our patient noticed anxiety and inability to sleep. She had increased blood pressure and felt "not herself." She also complained of "inability to see well" and of a "slow thought processing." A month later, she could not find words, and her speech became slurred. She realized she had difficulty with reading but not with writing.

Her brain MRI showed areas of restricted diffusion in the left cerebral hemisphere and splenium of the corpus callosum. There was subtle enhancement on the left hippocampus anteriorly as well as high T2 and FLAIR signal abnormalities in the posterior lateral aspect of the left thalamus and probably a few small foci on the right cerebral hemisphere. MRA showed scattered vessel irregularity with multiple areas of narrowing involving the ACA, MCA, and PCA bilaterally, with more severe stenosis involving the proximal portion of the left PCA and the proximal portion of the A1 segment of the left ACA. The cervical carotid artery bifurcations were normal. Cerebrospinal fluid and numerous additional ancillary investigations were negative for systemic vasculitis, hypercoagulable states, or cardioembolic disorders. Catheter cerebral angiography showed multiple areas of segmental arterial narrowing in the distal left MCA and left ACA branches; multiple areas of segmental arterial narrowing in the distal right MCA and right ACA branches; and segmental arterial narrowing of both PCAs, worse on the left P1 and P2 segments, with 70% stenosis associated with reduced flow in the PCAs, left greater than right (Fig. 50.1).

A brain biopsy (right frontal) was unrevealing. She was treated with high-dose IV methylprednisolone and received one dose of intravenous cyclophosphamide (500 mg/m²) and was then started on prednisone and nimodipine.

A month later, symptomatic worsening was associated with interval occurrence of a new left occipital–parietal infarct and a new left callosal infarct (Fig. 50.2). Neurologic examination was remarkable for congruous right homonymous hemianopsia, alexia without agraphia, dyschromatopsia, and impaired verbal memory. She had some word finding and naming difficulties. There was no optic ataxia. Visual memory was in the low average range. Facial recognition memory was normal.

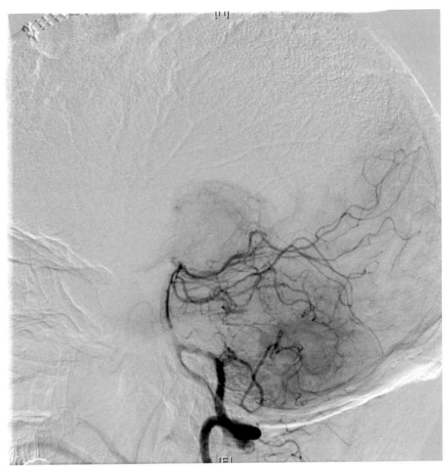

Figure 50.1   Cerebral Angiogram. Left vertebral contrast injection shows multiple segmental arterial narrowing and stenosis of both PCAs, left greater than right.

Because of her clinical presentation, the diffuse vascular irregularity with alternating areas of stenosis and dilatation on angiogram, and the sequential appearance new punctate areas of restricted diffusion in several lobar arterial distributions, a diagnosis of primary CNS angiitis was made.

In the context of left inferior occipital and occipital–temporal strokes (which also interrupt the outflow of the splenium of the corpus callosum), our patient developed alexia without agraphia and associated conditions including impaired visual confrontation naming of concrete entities, colors, and actions; impaired acquisition of declarative verbal material; mild visual object agnosia; and mild color agnosia. Our patient also demonstrated two somewhat more unusual features in her neuropsychological profile. The first of these, which is somewhat reminiscent of the phenomenon known as "deep dyslexia," was her tendency to generate semantic paralexic associations. The second of these more unusual features was her ability to acquire and retain memory for words that she was not able to read, when tested with a forced-choice recognition task.

Primary angiitis of the CNS (aka: isolated CNS vasculitis, primary CNS vasculitis, or granulomatous angiitis of the nervous system) is a rare, noninfectious,

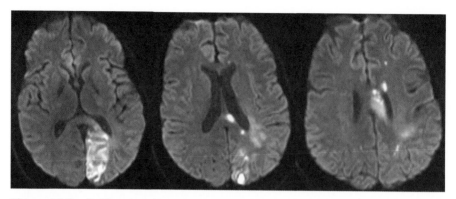

Figure 50.2   FLAIR and axial brain MRI sequences show new strokes in the distribution of the left PCA, affecting, among other regions, the left occipital lobe and splenium of the corpus callosum.

granulomatous, necrotizing angiopathy of unknown cause. Primary angiitis of the CNS is characterized by predominant or exclusive involvement of the CNS. Men are more commonly affected than women (M:F = 7:3). Usual symptoms include headaches and altered mental status. Symptoms of predominant small- and medium-sized cerebral blood vessel involvement may present as a mass lesion or as a multifocal encephalopathy. Small vessel strokes may occur over weeks to many months. Intracerebral hemorrhage and subarachnoid hemorrhage have been reported. The ESR is usually normal or minimally elevated. Other acute phase reactants are characteristically normal. CSF abnormalities include increased opening pressure, increased protein, normal glucose, and a lymphocytic pleocytosis rarely exceeding 250 cells/mm³. In some cases, oligoclonal bands can be detected. Contrast-enhanced MRI studies are abnormal in over 90% of cases. Prominent leptomeningeal enhancement may be present. MRA lacks adequate resolution to show the medium-sized and small cerebral blood vessel involvement in this disorder. Catheter arteriography may show segmental arterial narrowing, vascular occlusions, peripheral aneurysms, vascular shifts, and avascular areas. Brain/leptomeningeal biopsy is the gold standard of diagnosis. There is segmental inflammation and necrosis of leptomeningeal and parenchymal blood vessels. Leptomeningeal vessels are predominantly involved. Skipped lesions are not uncommon. Thus, because of its focal nature, a negative biopsy result does not preclude the diagnosis of primary CNS angiitis. Early recognition and management is essential because of its progressive and often fatal course if untreated. Therapy consists of combined immunosuppressive therapy with long-term treatment with high-dose corticosteroids, with the addition of intermittent cyclophosphamide.

SELECTED REFERENCES

Biller J, Adams HP. Non-infectious granulomatous angiitis of the central nervous system. In: Toole JF, ed. *Handbook of clinical neurology*. Amsterdam, The Netherlands: Elsevier Science Publishers, 1989:387–400.

Biller J, Grau RG. Cerebral vasculitis. In: Adams HP Jr ed., *Handbook of cerebrovascular diseases* (revised and expanded), 2nd ed. New York: Marcel Dekker, 2005:653–680, Chapter 28.

Cupps TR, Moore PM, Fauci AS. Isolated angiitis of the central nervous system. *Am J Med* 1983;74:97–105.

Lott SN, Friedman RB. Can treatment for pure alexia improved letter-by-letter reading speed without sacrificing accuracy. *Brain Lang* 1999;67:188–201.

SEE QUESTION: 327

CASE 51

SUPERIOR SAGITTAL SINUS THROMBOSIS

OBJECTIVES

- To discuss the clinical presentation of cerebral venous thrombosis.
- To discuss the management of superior sagittal sinus (SSS) thrombosis.
- To discuss the management of anticoagulant therapy in pregnancy.

VIGNETTE

A 30-year-old woman was evaluated 3 years earlier due to severe bifrontal headaches and dizziness. After 3 days, she noted that her left leg became "limp." Then, her left arm also became weak. She also had slurred speech and left facial weakness. She then had a spell characterized by turning of her head to the left associated with jerking of her left limbs with secondary generalization. A diagnosis of SSS thrombosis was made. She was found to have elevated IgA antiphosphatidylethanolamine antibody. She was treated with intravenous and fractionated heparin and was discharged on warfarin (target INR 2.0 to 3.0). Three years later, while on warfarin, she became pregnant.

CASE SUMMARY

At the age of 27, our patient suddenly experienced severe right frontal headaches associated with left leg weakness. CT showed a small right frontal lobar hemorrhage. MRI showed a hemorrhagic infarction involving the right frontoparietal lobe and the left posterior parietal lobe. Magnetic resonance venography (MRV) and catheter cerebral angiography documented an occlusion of the anterior portion of the SSS. Subsequently, the patient had a single seizure characterized by head deviation to the left, followed by rhythmic clonic movements of the left arm and leg, followed by loss of consciousness. She received intravenous phenytoin and was referred for further evaluation and management.

Past medical history was fairly unremarkable except for abruptio placenta at 8 months of gestation. She smoked a pack of cigarettes daily and was not on oral contraceptives. Physical examination showed extensive livedo reticularis. There was residual weakness of her left hamstrings, foot dorsiflexors, and plantar flexors. Patellar and ankle reflexes were brisk (left greater than right). Ancillary investigations showed persistent elevation of IgA antiphosphatidylethanolamine titers. She was treated with intravenous unfractionated heparin followed by warfarin. She also received oral phenytoin and folic acid.

Three years later, while still on warfarin, she became pregnant. She discontinued warfarin on the first day she recognized she was late for her menses. A fetal ultrasound was normal. Neurologic examination was stable.

The patient was treated with 81 mg of aspirin daily and subcutaneous enoxaparin (initially 60 mg twice daily and then 80 mg twice daily). She also received folic acid, prenatal vitamins, vitamin D, and calcium supplements. On her 37th week of gestation, enoxaparin was discontinued and she received subcutaneous unfractionated heparin. Following an unremarkable delivery, she was allowed to breast-feed her baby, and warfarin was restarted.

TABLE 51.1   CAUSES OF CEREBRAL VENOUS THROMBOSIS

Category of Disease	Etiologies
Infectious	Facial/orbital/paranasal sinuses/middle ear infections
	Sepsis
	Trichinosis
	Syphilis
	Varicella-zoster virus infections
Coagulopathic disorders	Pregnancy and puerperium
	Carcinoma
	Dehydration
	Neoplasm (meningioma, metastasis, glomus tumors)
	Antiphospholipid antibody syndrome
	Disseminated intravascular coagulation
	Nephrotic syndrome
	AT deficiency
	Protein S deficiency
	Protein C deficiency
	Combined deficiencies (proteins C, S, and AT)
	Activated protein C resistance
	Factor V Leiden mutation
	Prothrombin G20210A mutation
	Persistent elevations of factor VIII, IX, or XI
	Heparin-induced thrombocytopenia
	Hypoplasminogenemia
	Afibrinogenemia
	Cryofibrinogenemia
	Budd-Chiari syndrome
	Polycythemia vera
	Essential thrombocythemia
	Sickle cell disease and trait
	Paroxysmal nocturnal hemoglobinuria
	Microangiopathic hemolytic anemia (TTP/HUS/DIC)
	Familial histidine-rich glycoprotein deficiency
	Maternal coagulopathy (twin transfusion reaction)
	Marasmus
Rheumatologic disorders	Polyarteritis nodosa
	Systemic lupus erythematosus
	Wegener granulomatosis
	Behcet disease
	Inflammatory bowel disease
	Sarcoidosis
	Sturge-Weber syndrome
	Kohlmeier-Degos disease
Metabolic disorders	Diabetes mellitus
	Homocystinuria
	Iron deficiency anemia
Iatrogenic	1-Asparaginase
	Androgen
	Cisplatin and etoposide
	Epsilon-aminocaproic acid
	Medroxyprogesterone
	Intravenous catheters, cardiac pacemakers
	Head injury

Intracranial sinovenous occlusive disease is an infrequent cause of all strokes (0.5% to 1%). Most common symptoms of cerebral venous sinus thrombosis are headaches, seizures, focal neurologic deficits, and altered consciousness. Funduscopic examination may show bilateral papilledema secondary to raised intracranial pressure. The SSS is most frequently involved; imaging studies often reveal parasagittal lesions. MRI combined with MRV remains the most sensitive neuroimaging technique to diagnose cerebral venous thrombosis.

Proper diagnosis, evaluation, and treatment of patients with cerebral venous sinus thrombosis are of utmost importance. It is crucial to determine whether the intracranial venous thrombosis is aseptic or the result of a local infection as septic venous thromboses require specific antimicrobial treatment. Cerebral venous thrombosis has been associated with many disorders (Table 51.1).

Treatment of aseptic SSS targets the underlying pathology and predisposing risk factors. Currently, there is consensus supporting the use of either intravenous unfractionated heparin or subcutaneous low molecular weight heparin. Warfarin anticoagulation is recommended for long-term use in patients with an underlying hypercoagulable state. Because warfarin is teratogenic, it is not used during pregnancy. The highest risk of warfarin embryopathy occurs in infants exposed between the 6th and 12th weeks of gestation. Subcutaneous heparin is often used in pregnant women requiring anticoagulation.

However, there are risks associated with the use of heparin during pregnancy including osteoporosis, heparin-induced thrombocytopenia (with or without thrombosis), hypoaldosteronism, and alopecia. Calcium and vitamin D should be supplemented because of the risk of osteoporosis. The dose of heparin is often increased in the later stages of pregnancy and may need to be adjusted by measuring the activated partial thromboplastin time (aPTT). Low molecular weight heparins can be used as a replacement for heparin. Low-dose aspirin (81 mg) may be added to heparin, especially in patients with APAS. Warfarin may be resumed postpartum.

Antiepileptic drugs (AEDs) are used for seizure prevention. Appropriate treatment for raised intracranial pressure is used when necessary. Endovascular thrombolysis can be considered in selected instances.

SELECTED REFERENCES

Bousser MG, Russel RR. *Cerebral venous thrombosis (Monograph)*. London: WB Saunders, 1996.

Carhuapoma JR, Mitsias O, Levine SR. Cerebral venous thrombosis and anticardiolipin antibodies. *Neurology* 1997;28:2363–2369.

Guyatt GH, Akl EA, Crowther M, et al. Executive summary: antithrombotic therapy and prevention of thrombosis, 9th ed: American College of Chest Physicians Evidence-Based Clinical Practice Guidelines. *Chest* 2012;141:7S–47S.

Kaplan JM, Biller J, Adams HP Jr. Outcome in non-septic spontaneous superior sagittal sinus thrombosis in adults. *Cerebrovasc Dis* 1991;1:231–234.

Rosene-Montella K, Ginsberg J. Thromboembolic disease in pregnancy. In: Elkayam U, Gleicher N, eds. *Cardiac problems in pregnancy*. New York: Wiley-Liss, 1998:223–235.

SEE QUESTIONS: 71, 104, 145, 220, 221, 227

SECTION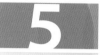

MOVEMENT DISORDERS

CASE 52

RESTING TREMOR (AND A "STROKE OF LUCK")

OBJECTIVES

- To review the clinical features of parkinsonian tremor.
- To illustrate the unusual subsequent occurrence of a subcortical infarct that abated the patient's tremor.

VIGNETTE

This 72-year-old woman consulted us because of tremors.

CASE SUMMARY

Our patient had an asymmetric oscillation (about 4 Hz) of her relaxed left hand, with a predominant pronation–supination pattern, characteristic of parkinsonian tremor. Tremor consists of rhythmic, oscillating movements of agonist and antagonist muscles, in an alternating (such as in Parkinson disease) or co-contracting fashion (such as in dystonic tremor). A predominant resting tremor is typical of Parkinson disease and drug-induced parkinsonism, though it can be seen less often in atypical parkinsonisms.

The cardinal features of Parkinson disease (PD) are rest tremor, rigidity, bradykinesia, and gait and/or postural instability unrelated to visual, proprioceptive, cerebellar, or vesticular dysfunction. In PD, the classical tremor consists of rhythmic pronation–supination movements of the forearm, extended onto the hand in the form of alternating opposition of the thumb and fingers (pill-rolling movements).

Parkinsonian tremor is often markedly asymmetric, or purely unilateral at onset, and mainly involves the distal aspect of the upper limb. The more rare resting tremor of the distal leg is almost exclusive of PD rather than any other parkinsonian disorder. Occasionally the resting tremor reappears when the hands are held in an outstretched posture (reemergence tremor). The tremor may also involve the chin, jaw, eyelids, or tongue. The tremor disappears during sleep and worsens with anxiety and stress. Rest tremor rarely involves the head. Tremor-dominant PD represents approximately 25% to 40% of cases.

Following a subcortical infarction in the distribution of the right anterior choroidal artery, not causing hemiparesis, our patient's unilateral left hand resting tremor ceased. We hypothesized that this clinical observation is somewhat similar to Dr. Irving Cooper's pioneering observations, who treated some patients with tremors by creating deep lesions with either anterior choroidal artery ligation or cryogenic thalamotomy.

SELECTED REFERENCES

Biller J, ed. *Practical neurology*, 4th ed. Philadelphia: Lippincott Williams & Wilkins, Wolters Kluwer Health, 2012.

Brazis PW, Masdeu JC, Biller J. *Localization in clinical neurology*, 6th ed. Philadelphia: Lippincott Williams & Wilkins, Wolters Kluwer Health, 2011.

Rosenow J, Das K, Rovit RL, et al. Irving S. Cooper and his role in intracranial stimulation for movement disorders and epilepsy. *Stereotact Funct Neurosurg* 2002;78:95–112.

SEE QUESTIONS: 40, 41, 42, 52, 60, 107, 125, 126, 169, 170, 234

CASE 53

ESSENTIAL TREMOR

OBJECTIVES

- To review the clinical features of essential tremor.
- To discuss the differential diagnosis of essential tremor.
- To summarize medical and surgical management options for essential tremor.

VIGNETTE

This 72-year-old man complained of bilateral hand tremors since his teenage years, very slowly progressive. It had only been over the last 5 years that he felt the tremor had affected his dexterity and begun to interfere with his social life, his ability to play the guitar, and put together airplane models, one of his hobbies. He occasionally spilled coffee and had to shave with an electrical razor to avoid cuts. He had difficulty operating the computer mouse and did very little handwriting given the illegibility of his notes. His voice may occasionally quiver. He was not aware of head movements, which had been brought to his attention by others. He continued to work full-time in an executive position. Alcohol attenuated the severity of his tremor. He denied anosmia, constipation, or depression. He had been on no treatments for his tremor but wished to pursue some. A prior trial with low-dose propranolol was discontinued for lack of efficacy. His mother had tremor and two of his six children also did.

CASE SUMMARY

 Tremors are rhythmic, oscillatory behaviors whereby a set of agonist and antagonist muscles activate in an alternating (as in the case of essential tremor and Parkinson disease, for instance) or synchronous fashion (as in the case of dystonic tremor). Our patient had the characteristic features for essential tremor, exemplified by a long history of slowly progressive, alcohol-response, often familial, postural, and kinetic tremor (Fig. 53.1). The examination also showed normal arm swinging during walking and macro- rather than micrographia, nullifying the possibility of Parkinson disease and no jerky, irregular, position-specific, action-induced tremor that would have supported dystonic tremor instead.

Essential tremor most commonly affects both arms, with potential spread into the head and vocal cords, but virtually never into the legs. The predominantly flexion–extension oscillations differ from the predominantly pronation–supination oscillations of Parkinson disease, in those cases when a postural tremor component arises. The tremor is characteristically absent at rest, present with maintained posture, and most evident at the end of a goal-directed movement. Over time, however, a resting component may appear. The jaw is rarely involved. Though often symmetric, asymmetry in its appearance is not unusual.

Essential tremor is the most common movement disorder, with a population prevalence of 0.4% to 6%. The disorder affects men and women equally. Age of onset is bimodal with peaks in the second and sixth decades, or unimodal, peaking in the fifth decade. Essential tremor may be sporadic or hereditary. Essential tremor is familial in 50% to 70% of cases, with most patients inheriting the disorder through an autosomal dominant gene. Responsiveness to alcohol occurs in 50% of the familial cases. Despite its frequency, there remains uncertainty as to its underlying neuropathology and genetics, possibly because such conditions as dystonic tremor and even Parkinson disease may be misdiagnosed as essential

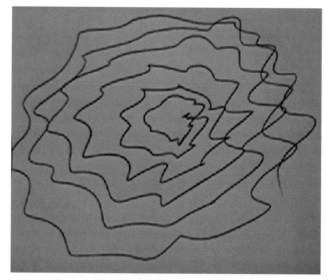

Figure 53.1   Spiral Drawing in This Patient. Note the sinusoidal waveform pattern, particularly more clear when the speed of hand displacement was slower, in the right half of the figure (as shown in the video). In dystonic tremor, the waveform is less sinusoidal and more variable, exhibiting a seesaw or jagged pattern.

tremor. Tremorogenic drugs, such as lithium and valproate, and metabolic disorders such as liver disease and hyperthyroidism can exacerbate an underlying essential tremor.

Primidone and propranolol are the only two first-line therapies for essential tremor. Propranolol is usually favored for younger patients and primidone for older individuals. Many other medications such as gabapentin and topiramate have been reported to be of benefit, but the strength of evidence is less robust. Botulinum toxin may be useful in some patients with drug-resistant head tremor, vocal tremor, or geniospasm, conditions that may represent focal dystonias. For patients with medically refractory and disabling upper extremity tremor, deep brain stimulation of the ventralis intermedius nucleus of the thalamus can be highly effective.

▶ **Case 53, Video 2:** Patient is shown performing the spiral drawing and writing tasks. These tasks allowed and supported the clinical diagnosis of essential tremor rather than dystonic tremor and parkinsonian tremor, always of importance in the differential diagnosis.

SELECTED REFERENCES

Biller J, ed. *Practical neurology*, 4th ed. Philadelphia: Lippincott Williams & Wilkins, Wolters Kluwer Health, 2012.

Elble RJ. Diagnostic criteria for essential tremor and differential diagnosis. *Neurology* 2000;11 (Suppl 4):S2–S6.

Koller WC, Hristova A, Brin M. Pharmacologic treatment of essential tremor. *Neurology* 2000;11 (Suppl 4):S30–S38.

Pahwa R, Lyons K, Koller WC. Surgical treatment of essential tremor. *Neurology* 2000;11(Suppl 4):S39–S44.

SEE QUESTIONS: 60, 107, 125, 126, 169, 234

CASE **54**

DYSTONIC TREMOR

OBJECTIVES

- To review the clinical features of a patient with dystonic tremor.
- To highlight the distinguishing features of dystonic tremor versus essential tremor and parkinsonian tremor.
- To discuss the management of dystonic tremor.

VIGNETTE

This 69-year-old woman has noted "head shakes" for about 3 years. These were originally brought to her attention by her husband. She has remained largely unaware of the tremor. When questioned further, she also admits to tremor of her voice but not of her hands or feet. She felt her job performance at a school cafeteria was not compromised. She could carry big food trays without any shaking. She was worried that she had developed a tremor like her mother's at a younger age than she did (her mother, still alive in her early 90s, has a dystonic hand tremor).

CASE SUMMARY

 Our patient had jerky tremor of the face, head (torticollis), and voice (adductor-type spasmodic dysphonia), consistent with segmental adult-onset dystonia. The etiology is likely genetic as her mother is also known to have dystonia (see second video). There was no clear spread into her arms and no hand dystonic tremor was noted (Fig. 54.1). The rest of the examination was normal.

A jerky, irregular, action-induced, position-sensitive (and sometimes task-specific) tremor defines dystonic tremor. Sometimes the dystonic phenomenology is in another body part (e.g., torticollis and hand tremor, a category also known as *tremor associated with dystonia*) (Fig. 54.2). The relative clumsy movements give the appearance of bradykinesia, but the lack of decrementing amplitude or speed (fatiguing) with rapid alternating movements, such as those elicited during the finger-tapping task, suggest the disorder is not within the category of parkinsonism.

Essential tremor (ET) is an overused diagnostic label. Anywhere from 40% to 50% of those diagnosed with essential tremor may actually have other conditions, most often dystonia (dystonic tremor, DYT) or Parkinson disease (PD) (Table 54.1). Although neither response to alcohol nor family history reliably distinguish ET from DYT, certain features may be more common in one compared to the other (Table 54.2). Still, some clinical features of ET, PD, and dystonic tremor overlap. For example, ET tremor can present unilaterally and at rest, becoming potentially misdiagnosed as PD, or with a jerky handwriting and be misdiagnosed as dystonic tremor. Dystonia, as the second most common source of "false ET," tends to produce a tremor that, when in full bloom, should be very different from ET: asymmetric, dysrhythmic, irregular in amplitude and periodicity, directional (i.e., more overt in a given direction), and *exacerbated by muscle contraction*. Dystonia is easier to identify when the tremor appears or increases only on certain positions or tasks, when overt

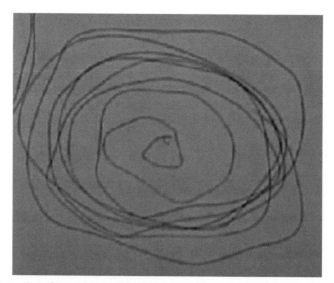

Figure 54.1   Spiral Drawing in This Patient. Lacking overt hand tremor, there are instead multiple patterns of superimposed fluctuations in direction and speed.

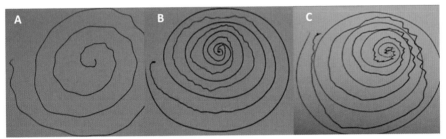

Figure 54.2   Spiral Drawing in Her Mother. Initially, the drawing task showed minimal tremor activity **(A)**, which became more pronounced **(B)** when she was asked to complete the task within a premade spiral, trying to avoid the "walls" of the spiral. The spiral drawing of another patient with dystonic tremor **(C)** shows a clearer "focal" waveform between 12 and 3 (as if it were the face of a clock). This directional preponderance, which suggests the same muscle groups are consistently involved, is an expression of the position-dependent nature of the tremor, a feature of dystonic but not of essential tremor.

posturing develops (e.g., "spooning" of the hands, i.e., wrist flexion with hyperextension of the fingers when arms are outstretched), and in the setting of clear sensory tricks (e.g., touching the more affected hand with the contralateral one to lessen the amplitude of the tremor). *Isolated* tremor in the legs, head, facial muscles, voice, jaw, or tongue is considered atypical for ET and most often indicative of parkinsonism or dystonia.

The management of focal dystonias, including dystonic hand tremor, is based on chemodenervation with botulinum toxin injections as first line of therapy. When the dystonia is severe and segmental (rarely generalized in adults), anticholinergic drugs, such as trihexyphenidyl or benztropine are indicated. Tetrabenazine may also be helpful.

▶ **Case 54, Video 2:** Mother of patient shown in prior video. This 91-year-old woman

started exhibiting mild head tremor at the age of 80 years, progressing relatively slowly over time. Examination showed cervical and limb position-dependent postural-and-action tremor with mild right torticollis and no evidence of rigidity or any other parkinsonian features. Her lack of anosmia, constipation, dream-enactment behaviors, and depression were strong historic evidence against Parkinson disease, despite a "resting" component of her tremor (likely an artifact of insufficient relaxation).

TABLE 54.1   **RED FLAGS IN "ESSENTIAL TREMOR"**

Signs	Most Likely ET-Like Disorder
Unilateral tremor	Parkinson disease
Rest tremor	Parkinson disease
Bradykinesia	Parkinson disease
Gait disturbance	Cerebellar tremor, Parkinson disease
Sudden onset	Psychogenic tremor
Isolated head tremor	Dystonic tremor
Abnormal head, trunk, or hand posture	Dystonic tremor
Exposure to tremorogenic drugs	Iatrogenic tremor

TABLE 54.2   **ESSENTIAL TREMOR VERSUS DYSTONIC TREMOR: DISTINGUISHING FEATURES**

More Common in ET	ET ≅ DYT	More Common in DYT
Younger age at onset (longer disease course)	Response to alcohol	Older age at onset (shorter disease course at diagnosis)
Combined head, arms, and voice tremor	Family history	_Isolated_ head tremor
		Isolated voice tremor*

*Voice tremor was nonsignificantly more common among "atypical" tremor (e.g., dystonia) in the Schrag et al. series.
ET, essential tremor; DYT = dystonic tremor.
Adapted from Espay AJ, Lang AE. _Common movement disorders pitfalls: case-based teaching._ New York: Cambridge University Press, 2012.

SELECTED REFERENCES

Bain PG. The management of tremor. _J Neurol Neurosurg Psychiatry_ 2002;72(Suppl 1):i3–i9.

Espay AJ, Lang AE. _Common movement disorders pitfalls: case-based teaching._ New York: Cambridge University Press, 2012.

Jain S, Lo SE, Louis ED. Common misdiagnosis of a common neurological disorder: how are we misdiagnosing essential tremor? _Arch Neurol_ 2006;63(8):1100–1104.

Jedynak CP, Bonnet AM, Agid Y. Tremor and idiopathic dystonia. _Mov Disord_ 1991;6(3):230–236.

Schrag A, Munchau A, Bhatia KP, et al. Essential tremor: an overdiagnosed condition? _J Neurol_ 2000;247(12):955–959.

SEE QUESTIONS: 287, 288, 289, 290, 291

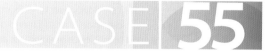

PARKINSON DISEASE

OBJECTIVES

- To review the clinical features of Parkinson disease (PD).
- To list the differential disorders that can be confused with PD.
- To summarize treatment options for PD.

VIGNETTE

A 56-year-old man had progressive right-sided weakness, lack of dexterity, slowness, and micrographia. He also noted a muffled character in his voice and frequently was asked to repeat statements. On occasions, he also had difficulty swallowing medications but not food. He also noted urinary urgency, a weak urinary stream, and mild nocturia. He had no cognitive problems.

CASE SUMMARY

Our patient presented with a 3- to 4-year history of slowly progressive functional impairment of the right arm and leg. Initially, he had difficulties using the gas and brake pedals while driving. Subsequently, he had difficulty brushing his teeth, combing his hair, and buttoning clothes. While walking, he noted he would drag his right foot and hold his right arm in an elevated position.

Neurological examination demonstrated bradykinesia with facial hypomimia, decreased eyelid blink frequency, and hypophonia with a soft mumbling and monotonous speech. There was an overall paucity of spontaneous movements and decreased amplitude of movements. Handwriting was small (micrographia) and effortful. No tremor was present at rest or with the arms outstretched. There was asymmetric oscillating cogwheel rigidity (right > left) detected by passive movements of the limbs. Gait showed short stride and reduced arm swing (right > left). He had no difficulty with initiating walking. There was mild postural instability.

PD is a progressive neurodegenerative disorder characterized by a number of motor and nonmotor features. The cardinal features of PD are as follows:

1. Rest tremor
2. Rigidity
3. Bradykinesia
4. Loss of postural reflexes

The former feature (tremor) may be absent in over 40% of patients. The latter feature (loss of postural reflexes) does not occur until later stages of the disease: its presence at the onset should suggest an atypical parkinsonism, such as progressive supranuclear palsy. The diagnosis of PD is often suspected by simple observation of the patient while walking as the steps tend to be short and at times shuffling, associated with a stooped posture and reduced arm swing as part of an overall impairment of associated movements. Small handwriting (micrographia) is another common feature. Other motor manifestations include facial hypomimia, dysarthria, dysphagia, and sialorrhea.

Nonmotor manifestations may include anosmia, paresthesias, pain, sleep abnormalities, and autonomic dysfunction. Cognitive impairment and dementia may occur in moderate to advanced stages and seems particularly more common in the akinetic-rigid rather than tremor-dominant form of the disease.

Differential diagnosis of PD is extensive. Alternative diagnosis to PD were identified in 24% of cases in the UK Brain Bank criteria, including cases of progressive supranuclear palsy (PSP), multiple system atrophy (MSA), corticobasal syndrome (CBS), and vascular (lacunar) parkinsonism. Early falls, early dementia, early and marked autonomic features, and sudden onset of symptoms should suggest an alternative diagnosis. Patients receiving neuroleptics for psychiatric disease and those receiving antiemetics such as prochlorperazine (Compazine), or metoclopramide (Reglan), should have these medications reduced or, ideally, discontinued. Patients with recent viral encephalitis, exposure to manganese, and carbon monoxide poisoning, or those with normal pressure hydrocephalus, may demonstrate features of parkinsonism, though careful examination should help distinguish these from PD.

PSP is invariably associated with parkinsonism, but there are several distinctive features. Patients have a supranuclear gaze palsy initially affecting volitional downgaze. As the disease progresses, upgaze and eventually horizontal volitional gaze are affected. In contrast to PD, PSP patients have more prominent axial or proximal rigidity, less tremor, and a disproportionate degree of speech, swallowing, and balance involvement. Other prominent features in PSP are early falls, motor perseveration, dysexecutive-predominant dementia, facial dystonia, apraxia of eyelid opening, and erect posture with retrocollis. Olfaction is normal in PSP.

MSA is another akinetic-rigid syndrome presenting with parkinsonism in combination with dysautonomia. MSA with predominant parkinsonian features (MSA-P) was formerly known as striatonigral degeneration. MSA with predominant cerebellar features (MSA-C) was formerly known as olivopontocerebellar atrophy. MSA with predominant autonomic features (MSA-A) was formerly known as Shy-Drager disease.

CBS may also resemble PD. Patients with CBS have additional features including asymmetric or unilateral parietal lobe deficits (alien hand, impaired sensation including astereognosis and agraphesthesia, as well as prominent apraxia and dystonia). Lower limb onset results in early postural instability and backward falls. CBS can be due to various pathologies including corticobasal degeneration (CBD), Alzheimer disease, PSP, and frontotemporal dementia. Olfactory dysfunction is not a major feature of CBD or PSP.

Dementia with Lewy bodies (DLB) may present with parkinsonism and any of the following: early-onset dementia, fluctuating cognitive impairment, syncope, visual hallucinations, delusions, psychosis, and neuroleptic sensitivity. The development of dementia within a year from the onset of parkinsonian features is a critical diagnostic criterion for the diagnosis of DLB.

Therapeutic options for PD include a variety of drugs having dopaminergic or anticholinergic effects. Levodopa/carbidopa typically produces striking immediate improvement in patients with PD. Early PD patients with mild motor deficits may respond sufficiently to dopamine agonists, amantadine, or the selective MAO-B inhibitors selegiline and rasagiline. Catechol O-methyltransferase inhibitors (entacapone and, to a greater extent, tolcapone) are capable of extending the duration of action of Levodopa once motor fluctuations (wearing off) develops. Patients remain responsive to levodopa but may develop disabling motor fluctuations despite optimization of therapy. In these individuals, deep brain stimulation of the subthalamic nucleus or internal portion of the globus pallidus can be considered, assuming dementia has not developed and any psychiatric complications (hallucinations and severe depression), if present, are well controlled.

SELECTED REFERENCES

Biller J, ed. *Practical neurology*, 4th ed. Philadelphia: Lippincott Williams & Wilkins, Wolters Kluwer Health, 2012.

Espay AJ, Biller J. *Concise neurology*. Philadelphia: Lippincott Williams & Wilkins, Wolters Kluwer Health, 2012.

Hughes AJ, Daniel SE, Blankson S, et al. A clinicopathologic study of 100 cases of Parkinson's disease. *Arch Neurol* 1993;50:140–148.

SEE QUESTIONS: 40, 41, 42, 125, 126, 169, 170

CASE 56

MULTIPLE SYSTEM ATROPHY, PARKINSONIAN TYPE

OBJECTIVES

- To illustrate the clinical presentation of multiple system atrophy, parkinsonian type.
- To describe the typical imaging abnormalities.
- To highlight distinguishing features with Parkinson disease.

VIGNETTE

This 57-year-old woman noticed right toe curling when running or jogging about 8 years prior to this evaluation, followed, within a year, by right arm stiffness and micrographic handwriting. Her hand was noted as having a reddish discoloration in the mornings, and her dexterity for various fine tasks became impaired. By her second year of symptoms, she developed fainting spells when standing, her walking slowed with reduced arm swinging. She had early substantial response to levodopa for about 12 to 18 months, but subsequent titration efforts failed to curb her progressive postural impairment and increasing rate of falls, most of which were backward. Over the prior year, she needed a walker while at home to minimize the risk of falls. Her speech became hypophonic and effortful and she developed a "thick tongue" sensation and starting chokes almost daily with liquids more than solids. She developed constipation, dream-enactment behaviors, and urinary stress incontinence. She believed her sense of smell was normal.

CASE SUMMARY

The patient presented with a tremorless but asymmetric parkinsonism associated with atypical features for Parkinson disease (PD), including a relatively rapid accrual of disability, initial but transient responsiveness to levodopa, early development of dysautonomia (neurogenic bladder, Raynaud phenomenon, and orthostatic hypotension) and, on exam, stimulus-sensitive axial myoclonus, hyperreflexia, lower limb spasticity, and striatal toes with extensor plantar responses. These findings were highly suspicious for the parkinsonian variant of multiple system atrophy (MSA-P). The diagnosis was further supported by the finding of slit hyperintensity in the lateral putamen on T2-weighted brain magnetic resonance imaging (MRI) (Fig. 56.1).

MSA-P is an akinetic-rigid syndrome with prominent cerebellar, autonomic, and pyramidal involvement, typically developing at an earlier age than PD and associated with worse overall prognosis. Corticospinal involvement manifests as extensor plantar response with hyperreflexia. Cerebellar impairment results in gait or limb ataxia, ataxic dysarthria, and sustained gaze-evoked nystagmus. Dysautonomic features include orthostatic hypotension (drop of 20 mm Hg systolic or 10 mm Hg diastolic upon standing), urinary incontinence, erectile dysfunction, anhidrosis, and respiratory dysfunction (sleep apnea, snoring, and inspiratory stridor). Compared to the peripheral dysautonomia of PD, in MSA the pathology is preganglionic or central while the peripheral autonomic system is spared.

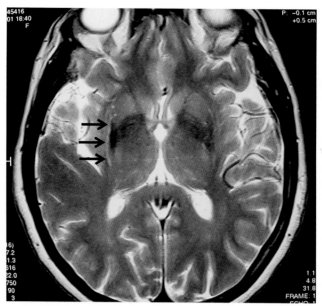

Figure 56.1 Classical Neuroimaging Finding in MSA-P (from a different Patient). Axial T2-weighted brain MRI demonstrating a slitlike area of hyperintensity bordered by increased hypointensity (from iron deposition) in the putamen, worse on the right (*arrows*). The putaminal atrophy is always greater on the opposite side to the more affected hemibody.

Unlike other atypical parkinsonisms, dementia is not a feature of early MSA, but frontal lobe dysfunction usually develops. "Softer" MSA features include rapid eye movement (REM) sleep behavior disorder, cold mottled hands (Raynaud phenomenon), action and stimulus-sensitive myoclonus of hands and face, dystonic anterocollis, severely hypophonic speech, and "Pisa syndrome" (axial dystonia, causing leaning of the trunk to one side). Response to levodopa can be marked but transient and an unusual pattern of dyskinesias, involving the lower face and feet, may complicate its use.

In addition to optimizing motor function with levodopa (while avoiding dopamine agonists or MAO-B inhibitors), management of MSA is heavily demanding in the control of orthostatic hypotension, which becomes a major source of disability in most patients. Nonpharmacologic options include liberalizing salt intake, use of elastic thigh-high stocking, and head elevation at night. Pharmacologic interventions are fludrocortisone (Florinef, volume expander by decreasing natriuresis, 0.1 to 0.3 mg/d) and midodrine (ProAmatine, peripheral α1-adrenergic receptor agonist, 15 to 30 mg/d). The latter may cause piloerection, scalp pruritus, urinary retention, and supine hypertension.

SELECTED REFERENCES

Biller J, ed. *Practical neurology*, 4th ed. Philadelphia: Lippincott Williams & Wilkins, Wolters Kluwer Health, 2012.

Espay AJ, Biller J. *Concise neurology*. Philadelphia: Lippincott Williams & Wilkins, Wolters Kluwer Health, 2012.

Quinn N. Multiple system atrophy—the nature of the beast. *J Neurol Neurosurg Psychiatry* 1989;52(Suppl):78–79.

SEE QUESTIONS: 292, 293

CASE

CORTICOBASAL SYNDROME (CORTICOBASAL DEGENERATION)

OBJECTIVES

- To illustrate the clinical presentation of corticobasal syndrome.
- To discuss corticobasal degeneration and other disorders presenting as a corticobasal syndrome.
- To describe localizing features of the various forms of alien limb phenomenon.

VIGNETTE

This 81-year-old man noted that he "lost use of my left arm" 3 years prior to this evaluation.

It started with tremor and posturing but evolved into progressive difficulties with moving the left arm at will, and eventually, it interfered with the action of the opposite hand. Over time, he also noted that the left leg became weak and incoordinated. Two years into his illness, he needed a walker and, shortly thereafter, a wheelchair for ambulation. His speech volume softened and his swallowing slowed, requiring him to clear his throat often. Prior medication trials with levodopa, amantadine, tizanidine, and baclofen failed due to the development of light-headedness or drowsiness.

CASE SUMMARY

The presence of a rapidly progressive and profoundly asymmetric akinetic-rigid syndrome with severe arm dystonia and rigidity, postural tremor, stimulus-sensitive myoclonus, and historic evidence of arm levitation (alien limb syndrome), in the setting of sensory extinction and severe position loss in the left arm suggested the presence of a corticobasal syndrome (CBS). Cognitive impairment meeting criteria for mild dementia was detected at by bedside screening (Mini-Mental State Examination [MMSE] = 21/30; Frontal Assessment Battery = 16/18; abnormal clock drawing). The brain magnetic resonance imaging (MRI) demonstrated asymmetric focal atrophy, greater in the right parietal and, to a lesser extent, temporal lobes, with corresponding mild ex vacuo enlargement of the occipital horn of the right lateral ventricle.

Major features of CBS are early postural and gait impairment, asymmetric bradykinesia, rigidity, dystonia (with or without an "alien limb" phenomenon), postural and kinetic tremor, and later cortical deficits (progressive ideomotor apraxia, aphasia, astereognosis, and agraphesthesia). Our patient's high-frequency, high-amplitude unilateral tremor, occurring intermittently at rest and on posture, suggested a pathology of corticobasal degeneration (CBD), which is absent in all cases of CBS due to pathology-proven AD, a major cause of CBS (Fig. 57.1) (see second video). The other clinical features of CBS, including ideomotor and limb kinetic apraxia (confirmed before dystonia and rigidity become severe) and action and stimulus-sensitive myoclonus, have been reported in a range of disorders including vascular parkinsonism, AD, progressive supranuclear palsy

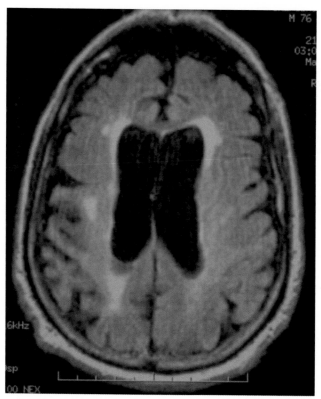

Figure 57.1   Axial fluid attenuated inversion recovery (FLAIR) brain MRI showing asymmetric hemispheric atrophy, predominantly right parietal, in a patient with corticobasal syndrome due to Alzheimer disease pathology.

(PSP), Creutzfeldt-Jakob disease, dementia with Lewy bodies, and frontotemporal dementia. In fact, most cases of CBS are due to PSP rather than CBD pathology. These CBS–PSP cases tend to have delayed onset of vertical supranuclear gaze palsy (greater than 3 years after onset of first symptom) and rarely have predominant downgaze abnormalities.

The alien limb in CBS due to CBD or AD pathology is of a "posterior variant," whereby an object cannot be released from grasp without the contralateral hand "peeling" the fingers away from the grasped object. There may be an associated "instinctive avoidance reaction," in which the digits extend and the hand pulls away from approaching objects. Postacute presentations of the posterior alien limb syndrome may result from strokes in the nondominant parietotemporal area, often associated with hemianesthesia, hemianopia, or even anosognosia. In contrast, the "frontal variant" alienlike behavior most closely resembles exploratory reaching, grasping reflex, manual groping, and other utilization behaviors and may be more commonly seen as a severe form of grasp reflex in the setting of left anteromedial frontal lobe degeneration. The "frontal" alien reflects frontotemporal lobar degeneration pathology in chronic progressive cases and left anterior cerebral artery stroke in late manifestations of an acute vascular event.

These posterior and frontal variants are to be distinguished from the *callosal* alien hand syndrome, in which there is intermanual conflict and manual interference of the nondominant hand.

▶ **Case 57, Video 2:** This 76-year-old left-handed man presented with a 2-year history of micrographia, hypophonia, and decreased left arm swing. His family reported that initially his left hand would sometimes "wander" and go into his pocket or grab his shirt, without him intending to do so. Carbidopa/levodopa was initiated soon after symptom onset with no noticeable benefits. Over time, his balance worsened and he tended to lean to the left. He developed freezing of gait, difficulty with depth perception, and ultimately the need for assistance with dressing, grooming, and eating. He is shown to have prominent ideational apraxia, left greater than right. His left arm was held in a flexed dystonic posture at his side. He had moderate to severe rigidity, left greater than right; spontaneous and stimulus-sensitive myoclonus in the left arm; and extensor plantar responses bilaterally. MRI showed moderate cortical atrophy, with predominant involvement of the temporal and parietal lobes (right greater than left) and mild periventricular and subcortical leukoaraiosis (Fig. 57.1). His symptoms progressed rapidly. Over the next 4 years, he became mute and wheelchair bound. He succumbed to his condition 6 years after symptom onset, at age 80. A brain autopsy confirmed Alzheimer disease, with a focal presentation in the form of CBS. (Case courtesy of Dr. Andrew Duker, University of Cincinnati.)

SELECTED REFERENCES

Biller J, ed. *Practical neurology*, 4th ed. Philadelphia: Lippincott Williams & Wilkins, Wolters Kluwer Health, 2012.

Espay AJ, Biller J. *Concise neurology*. Philadelphia: Lippincott Williams & Wilkins, Wolters Kluwer Health, 2012.

Ling H, O'Sullivan SS, Holton JL, et al. Does corticobasal degeneration exist? A clinicopathological re-evaluation. *Brain* 2010;133(Pt 7):2045–2057.

Wadia PM, Lang AE. The many faces of corticobasal degeneration. *Parkinsonism Relat Disord* 2007;13 (Suppl 3):S336–S340.

Whitwell JL, Jack CR Jr, Boeve BF, et al. Imaging correlates of pathology in corticobasal syndrome. *Neurology* 2010;75(21):1879–1887.

SEE QUESTIONS: 38, 39

CASE **58**

PROGRESSIVE SUPRANUCLEAR PALSY

OBJECTIVES

- ■ To illustrate the clinical presentation of progressive supranuclear palsy.
- ■ To discuss progressive supranuclear palsy and pathologies presenting with a similar syndrome.
- ■ To highlight the importance of oculomotor exam in the diagnosis of this form of parkinsonism.

This 59-year-old woman reported balance impairment and falls (at least four), within the last year. Her husband also noted slowness in the movement of the eyes and walking while "looking at the floor," which she never did before. More recently, her speech became slurred, slow, and with poor enunciation, and she started having choking spells. She admitted to lifelong anosmia but denied constipation or urinary problems, skin discoloration, excessive sweating, or postural light-headedness. She used to play golf but felt that her game was not up to expectations. She was involved in three motor vehicle accidents within this year, which raised concerns regarding her driving safety.

CASE SUMMARY

 The presence of postural impairment leading to falls close to symptom onset, associated with a tremorless symmetric parkinsonism, with axial-predominant rigidity, facial dystonia (furrowing the forehead and deepening of the nasolabial folds are obvious on inspection), dysphagia, dysarthria with "hypobradyphonia," apraxia of eyelid opening, square-wave jerks, supranuclear vertical gaze palsy, and a positive "applause sign" (an evidence of motor perseveration) were highly suggestive of the classical form of progressive supranuclear palsy (PSP) or Richardson syndrome. There was no apraxia or cortical sensory loss, nor dysautonomic features. Although no overt cognitive impairment was documented at the initial visit (MMSE = 28/30; Frontal Assessment Battery = 16/18; normal clock drawing test), a dysexecutive frontal-predominant form of dementia eventually developed. The patient succumbed to her illness within 5 years from symptom onset. PSP was confirmed at autopsy.

Described by Steele, Richardson, and Olszewski in 1964, PSP is about 1/100 as prevalent as Parkinson disease (PD), but just as common as myasthenia gravis and Huntington disease (about 3 to 4:1,000,000). Hence, every neurologist will encounter this atypical parkinsonian disorder in their practice. In its classic form, PSP is suspected when poor levodopa response and supranuclear vertical gaze restriction are present in a tremorless and posturally impaired parkinsonian patient who has had early loss of postural reflexes with backward falls within 1 year of disease onset. Other features may be prominent dysphagia, dysarthria, facial dystonia with decreased blinking rate (giving the face its characteristic "concerned staring" appearance), apraxia of eyelid opening, square-wave jerks, erect posture with retrocollis, and executive dysfunction. These features should make this disorder easier to distinguish from PD than multiple system atrophy (MSA) or corticobasal degeneration (CBD).

Because gait can be affected early on, PSP can also be confused with another "lower body parkinsonism" disorder, normal pressure hydrocephalus, in part because ventricular enlargement may be associated. Importantly, when the extent of dysexecutive dementia is prominent, the PSP phenotype could develop within the spectrum of a frontotemporal lobar degeneration (FTLD–PSP), as demonstrated in the second video. In that video, a patient is shown with similar facial, ocular, and postural features as shown by the index case, but with more severe dementia and with palilalia, a feature of advanced PSP and other disorders affecting the globus pallidus. The brain magnetic resonance imaging (MRI) demonstrated hydrocephalus (ex vacuo, as judged by the extent of surrounding parenchymal atrophy) and the typical tegmental midbrain atrophy, yielding the hummingbird sign on midsagittal cuts (Fig. 58.1).

PSP may present under a number of atypical presentations including PSP–parkinsonism or "benign" (early on, indistinguishable from PD; falls occur after the first year of symptoms), pure akinesia (without rigidity), primary progressive freezing of gait, corticobasal syndrome, and frontotemporal dementia. Nondegenerative diseases that can present

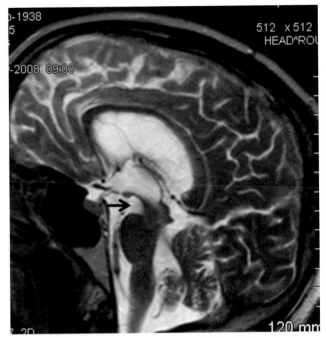

Figure 58.1   Brain MRI of Patient 2, Whose PSP Phenotype Fit within the FTLD–PSP Spectrum. There is substantial frontal-predominant atrophy expressed as thinning of the anterior portion of the corpus callosum and ex vacuo hydrocephalus. Only the hummingbird sign resulting from midbrain atrophy (*arrow*) was present in the original case.

as a PSP syndrome are multi-infarct state, mesencephalic tumors, Whipple disease, Niemann-Pick disease type C (vertical supranuclear gaze abnormality, ataxia, and parkinsonism), neurosyphilis, mitochondrial myopathy, and myasthenia gravis.

Amantadine and amitriptyline can ameliorate gait and rigidity in PSP. Botulinum toxin injections into the orbicularis oculi muscles can alleviate apraxia of eyelid opening. Cholinergic striatal interneuron loss limits the efficacy of cholinesterase inhibitors for cognitive enhancement.

▶ **Case 58, Video 2:** Another patient once worked up as "normal pressure hydrocephalus," with axial-predominant akinetic-rigid syndrome with severe gait and postural impairment, hyperreflexia, distal sensory loss, and dementia affecting executive functioning, language (echolalia, and palilalia), and memory domains (MMSE = 14/30; Frontal Assessment Battery = 4/18; ideomotor apraxia). Some utilization behavior is demonstrated during the finger-to-nose task. His pathology was consistent with frontotemporal lobar degeneration due to an MAPT mutation (FTLD-Tau/MAPT), which expressed as a PSP syndrome with frontotemporal dementia.

SELECTED REFERENCES

Biller J, ed. *Practical neurology*, 4th ed. Philadelphia: Lippincott Williams & Wilkins, Wolters Kluwer Health, 2012.

Espay AJ, Biller J. *Concise neurology*. Philadelphia: Lippincott Williams & Wilkins, Wolters Kluwer Health, 2012.

Williams DR, Holton JL, Strand K, et al. Pure akinesia with gait freezing: a third clinical phenotype of progressive supranuclear palsy. *Mov Disord* 2007;22(15):2235–2241.

Williams DR, Lees AJ. Progressive supranuclear palsy: clinicopathological concepts and diagnostic challenges. *Lancet Neurol* 2009;8(3):270–279.

SEE QUESTIONS: 40, 41, 42

CASE 59

CERVICAL DYSTONIA

OBJECTIVES

- To illustrate the clinical presentation and diagnosis of cervical dystonia.
- To outline common types of focal dystonia.
- To summarize treatment options for disabling focal dystonia.

VIGNETTE

A 50-year-old woman was referred for evaluation of painful spasms of her neck and right shoulder.

CASE SUMMARY

The patient presented with marked left torticollis and left shoulder elevation, a set of involuntary, relatively sustained, and patterned muscular contractions producing an abnormal neck posture and referred to as cervical dystonia. In general, dystonia can express as sustained (presenting as fixed posturing or tonic spasms) or intermittent muscle contractions (presenting as spasmodic torticollis or dystonic tremor). Placement of patients' own hand or fingers on the affected region has the potential of temporarily attenuating the dystonia, a phenomenon referred to as sensory tricks or geste antagonistique, highlighting the disruption of the motor program by a closed-loop sensory feedback. Dystonia may be *generalized* as is the case with *primary*, typically inherited, childhood-onset dystonias (such as DYT1 dystonia); *focal* (as in most *secondary* or adult-onset dystonias); or *segmental* (such as in acute dystonic reactions from use of dopamine-blocking drugs). Although secondary dystonias are usually focal or segmental, diffuse brain lesions can lead to generalized dystonia, such in cerebral palsy. Unlike childhood-onset primary dystonias, which affect the lower extremities first and then generalizing, adult-onset primary dystonias most often begin in the neck, face, or arms and rarely generalize. Adult-onset dystonia affecting the feet and childhood-onset dystonia affecting the upper body first should raise suspicion for a secondary rather than primary form of dystonia. In these cases, further diagnostic testing, such as brain imaging, becomes warranted.

TABLE 59.1 AUTOSOMAL DOMINANT PRIMARY DYSTONIAS

	DYT	Type	Chr	Gene
Pure Dystonia	DYT1	Generalized	9q	TOR1A
	DYT4	Whispering dysphonia	—	—
	DYT6	Cranio-cervical, laryngeal, arm	8p	THAP1
	DYT7	Cranio-cervical or arm	18p	—
	DYT13	Cranio-cervical or arm	1p	—
Dystonia Plus	DYT5a	Foot dystonia (DRD)	14q	GCH1
	DYT11	Arm, shoulders, neck (M-D)	7q	SGCE
	DYT12	Cranio-bulbar to arm-PKN (RDP)	19p	ATP1A3
	DYT15	Arm, shoulders, neck (M-D)	18p	—
Paroxysmal Dystonia	DYT8	Generalized (PNKD)	2q	PNKD1/M FR1
	DYT9	PNKD + ataxia and spasticity	1p	—
	DYT10	Generalized (PKD)	16p	—
	DYT18	Foot dystonia (PED)	1p	SLC2A1

The autosomal dominant disorders presenting or associated with cervical dystonia are shown in red font.
Modified from Breakefield XO, Blood AJ, Li Y, et al. The pathophysiological basis of dystonias. *Nat Rev Neurosci* 2008;9(3): 222–234; and Müller U. The monogenic primary dystonias. *Brain* 2009;132:2005–2025.

Genetic types of dystonia are illustrated on Tables 59.1 and 59.2. The most common early-onset primary dystonia affecting the cervical region is DYT6, and recent studies suggest it may be more common than DYT1, which tends to become symptomatic in the feet first.

Cervical dystonia is a form of focal dystonia, most often sporadic, which results in either isolated head tremor (e.g., "no–no" head movements) or pulling of the head in the form of turning (right or left torticollis), tilting (right or left laterocollis), flexing (antero-collis), extending (retrocollis), or a combination thereof. Therefore, the old nomencla-ture "spasmodic torticollis" is discouraged as it only describes one of many presenting forms of cervical dystonia. Other focal dystonias include blepharospasm, writer's cramp,

TABLE 59.2 AUTOSOMAL RECESSIVE AND X-LINKED DYSTONIAS

	DYT	Type	Chr	Gene
Pure Dystonia	DYT2	Generalized or limbs (Spanish Romani family)	—	—
	DYT17	Cervical becoming segmental or generalized (Lebanese family)	20p	—
Dystonia Plus-AR	DYT5b	Dystonia and parkinsonism	11p	TH
	DYT16	Dystonia and parkinsonism	2q	PRKRA
Dystonia Plus-X-linked	DYT3	Dystonia and parkinsonism (Lubag)	Xq	TAF1/DYT3

The autosomal recessive disorders presenting or associated with cervical dystonia are shown in red font.
Modified from Breakefield XO, Blood AJ, Li Y, et al. The pathophysiological basis of dystonias. *Nat Rev Neurosci* 2008;9(3):222–234; and Müller U. The monogenic primary dystonias. *Brain* 2009;132:2005–2025.

TABLE 59.3 **CERVICAL DYSTONIA MIMICS**

- **Rotational atlantoaxial subluxation**
- **Congenital Klippel-Feil anomaly**
- **Chiari malformation**
- **Posterior fossa tumor**
- **Trochlear nerve palsy**
- **"Vestibular" torticollis**
- **Congenital muscular torticollis (fibromatosis colli)**
- **Schwartz-Jampel syndrome** (generalized myotonia, blepharospasm, blepharophimosis, dwarfism, pinched face with low-set ears, joint limitation, contractures, and bone dysplasia)
- **Sandifer syndrome** (paroxysmal torticollis, occasionally with opisthotonos, that occur during feeding in infants with GERD often associated with hiatal hernia)
- **Spasmus nutans** (combination of horizontal or vertical head tremor or nodding, torticollis, and pendular and asymmetric nystagmus)

---

spasmodic dysphonia, and oromandibular dystonia. Not uncommonly, segmental spread can occur in patients affected by either of these focal dystonias (e.g., cervical and oromandibular dystonia or cervical dystonia and writer's cramp).

All forms of dystonia are aggravated by stress, anxiety, and fatigue and improve with rest. There may be some degree of fluctuation throughout the day or from week to week, but in general symptoms are steady. In cases of new-onset dystonia, particularly if presenting as retrocollic cervical dystonia or jaw-opening oromandibular dystonia, it is imperative to look for recent or concurrent exposure to a dopamine-blocking drug. Young patients with focal dystonia should be screened for Wilson disease. Chemodenervation with botulinum toxin injections is the first line of therapy for patients with cervical dystonia. Response can be excellent, as demonstrated in the second video. Extensive segmental spread may demand the concurrent or alternative use of anticholinergic drugs with or without benzodiazepine. A number of cervical dystonic mimics must be kept in the differential diagnosis in atypical cases (young onset, failure to respond to chemodenervation, associated neurological findings, etc.) (Table 59.3).

▌ **Case 59, Video 2:** Patient shown after the third cycle of EMG-guided botulinum toxin type A (OnabotulinumtoxinA) injections on the right sternocleidomastoid, left splenius capitis, and left trapezius.

SELECTED REFERENCES

Biller J, ed. *Practical neurology*, 4th ed. Philadelphia: Lippincott Williams & Wilkins, Wolters Kluwer Health, 2012.

Breakefield XO, Blood AJ, Li Y, et al. The pathophysiological basis of dystonias. *Nat Rev Neurosci* 2008;9(3):222–234.

Espay AJ, Biller J. *Concise neurology*. Philadelphia: Lippincott Williams & Wilkins, Wolters Kluwer Health, 2012.

Müller U. The monogenic primary dystonias. *Brain* 2009;132:2005–2025.

SEE QUESTIONS: 204, 254, 255, 290, 291, 300, 301, 302

CASE **60**

CEREBRAL PALSY/DYSTONIA

OBJECTIVES

- To define cerebral palsy.
- To define dystonia.
- To discuss the treatment of dystonia.

VIGNETTE

A 19-year-old man with cerebral palsy developed jerky tremor and abnormal posture of the head.

CASE SUMMARY

This young man had a history of microcephaly, developmental delay, static encephalopathy, spastic quadriparesis, and complex partial seizures with secondary generalization. Neuroimaging studies showed left hemispheric atrophy, diffuse ventricular enlargement, and cerebellar atrophy. On examination, he had intermittent head turning to the right representing cervical dystonia with a dystonic tremor component. He received botulinum toxin injections into both sternocleidomastoid muscles, right and left splenius capitis muscles, left levator scapula, and right cervical trapezius.

Cerebral palsy is a static encephalopathy of prenatal or perinatal origin resulting in spasticity, hypotonia, ataxia, athetosis, chorea, or a combination thereof. Diagnosis is based on a history of delayed motor milestones and on clinical examination. Intellectual impairment and seizures are fairly common. Although the term "static" implies lack of progression, patients remain vulnerable to the development of abnormal neurologic features, such as dystonia, which rarely progress beyond the degree of severity shown in the video. Cerebral palsy can be mimicked by metabolic disorders such as Lesch-Nyhan syndrome, glutaric aciduria type 1, pyruvate dehydrogenase deficiency, argininemia, cytochrome oxidase deficiency, and female carriers of ornithine transcarbamylase deficiency. Several clues can help in distinguishing these disorders. For instance, an athetoid cerebral palsy–type phenotype with corpus callosum agenesis and cystic lesions in the basal ganglia, cerebellum, and brainstem on magnetic resonance imaging (MRI) are typical of the X-linked pyruvate dehydrogenase deficiency.

Dystonia is a disorder consisting of intermittent or sustained, often painful, twisting repetitive muscle spasms that may occur in one part of the body or throughout the entire body. In particular, cervical dystonia, previously referred to as one of its primary examples, spasmodic torticollis, consists of intermittent involuntary spasms of selected cervical muscles and is often associated with pain. This is the most common form of focal, adult-onset dystonia. It is often asymmetric, abates during sleep, and increases with stress or anxiety. Several abnormal head postures may occur (often in combination): rotation (torticollis), lateral tilt (laterocollis), hyperextension of the head (retrocollis), and forward flexion of the head (anterocollis). Torticollis and laterocollis are the two most common head positions.

Chemodenervation with botulinum toxin injections is the first line of therapy for cervical dystonia. Potential side effects of botulinum toxin injections include transient weakness of the injected muscles, dry mouth, and a local hematoma. Although less effective, oral anticholinergics, dopaminergic and antidopaminergic medications, benzodiazepines, antidepressants, and some anticonvulsants can also be used in isolation (when dystonia has spread beyond two body segments) or as adjunctive treatment to botulinum toxin injections. Intrathecal baclofen may be considered for patients with secondary spastic dystonia, dystonia of trunks and legs, and "dystonic storm."

SELECTED REFERENCES

Biller J, ed. *Practical neurology*, 4th ed. Philadelphia: Lippincott Williams & Wilkins, Wolters Kluwer Health, 2012.

Brashear A. The botulinum toxins and the treatment of cervical dystonia. *Semin Neurol* 2001;21:85–90.

Nass R. Developmental disabilities. In: Bradley WG, Daroff RB, Fenichel GM, et al., eds. *Neurology in clinical practice*. Philadelphia: Butterworth-Heineman, 2000:1585–1594.

SEE QUESTIONS: 189, 204, 304, 305

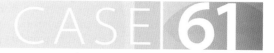

PALATAL TREMOR DUE TO MEDULLARY INFARCTION

OBJECTIVES

- To discuss the disorder of palatal tremor (formerly, palatal myoclonus).
- To distinguish the essential from symptomatic forms of palatal tremor.
- To briefly review the main features of the medial medullary syndrome.

VIGNETTE

This 59-year-old man with diabetes mellitus, arterial hypertension, and prior coronary artery bypass graft (CABG) had a history of multiple strokes.

CASE SUMMARY

 Our patient had multiple supratentorial and infratentorial ischemic strokes. He was confined to a wheelchair due to severe gait unsteadiness. Examination showed mild head titubation, dysarthria, asymmetric horizontal–torsional jerk nystagmus, and continuous rhythmic contractions affecting the palate. He did not complain of objective tinnitus or an ear click. Magnetic resonance imaging (MRI) showed multiple supratentorial and infratentorial infarcts including a right medial medullary infarction. There was hyperintensity in the inferior

TABLE 61.1 **DISTINGUISHING FEATURES BETWEEN ESSENTIAL AND SYMPTOMATIC PALATAL TREMORS**

	Essential Palatal Tremor	**Symptomatic Palatal Tremor**
Ear clicks	Present	Absent
Palatal involvement	Proximal soft palate	Distal soft palate
Nerve affected	Tensor veli palatini	Levator veli palatini
Extrapalatal movements	No extrapalatal movements	Pharynx, larynx, diaphragmatic, and ocular muscles
Ataxia	Absent	Often present
Brain MRI	Normal	Lesions anywhere in the Guillain-Mollaret triangle and resulting olivary hypertrophy

olivary nuclei, suggesting early development of pseudohypertrophy. Magnetic resonance angiography (MRA) showed no evidence of vertebrobasilar dolichoectasia.

Examination showed asymmetric horizontal–torsional jerk nystagmus indicative of dysfunction of the vestibulocerebellar pathways. The continuous rhythmic contractions of his soft palate and uvula were characteristic of palatal tremor, formerly known as palatal myoclonus. Palatal tremor is a rare neurological condition characterized by continuous and synchronous contractions of the soft palate and other oropharyngeal muscles occurring at frequencies of 1 to 2 Hz. Palatal tremor is subdivided into primary or *essential palatal tremor*, where ear clicking is a prominent feature and no lesions are detectable on brain MRI, and secondary or *symptomatic palatal tremor*, which is associated with cerebellar or brainstem lesions, invariably detected on brain MRI (Table 61.1). In *symptomatic* palatal tremor, there usually are concomitant contractions of other muscles including the larynx, extraocular muscles, neck, diaphragm, tongue, and face, and patients may complain of dysphagia and even respiratory difficulty.

Symptomatic palatal tremor manifests as sleep-resistant, 1- to 2-Hz rhythmic movements of the distal soft palate due to contractions of the vagally innervated levator veli palatini. It results from lesions disrupting the pathways between the red nucleus, inferior olivary nucleus, and contralateral dentate nucleus (dentato–rubro–olivary pathway or Guillain-Mollaret triangle). In this setting, there is common development of a hyperintense, swollen, non–contrast-enhanced olivary nucleus in the medulla on T2-weighted brain MRI sequences, due to deafferentation from transsynaptic degeneration of inhibitory dentato–olivary GABAergic neurons. The causative lesion of this olivary pseudohypertrophy is located in the ipsilateral pons or upper medulla (involving the central tegmental tract), or, less often, in the contralateral superior cerebellar peduncle or dentate nucleus. The symptomatic palatal tremor associated with either of these tends to be contralateral to a lesion in the pons or upper medulla and ipsilateral to a lesion in the superior cerebellar peduncle. It must be noted that while symptomatic palatal tremor is often associated with hypertrophic olivary degeneration, the opposite is not true. Indeed, hypertrophic olivary degeneration resulting from lesions in the dentate nucleus may yield a tremor that spares the palato-pharyngo-laryngo-oculo-diaphragmatic region.

Symptomatic palatal tremor may result from cerebrovascular, demyelinating, neoplastic, encephalitic, postinfectious, traumatic, or neurodegenerative etiologies. It has also been associated with extrinsic compression of the inferior olive by an ectatic vertebral artery. An autosomal dominant form of palatal tremor with histopathologic features resembling Alexander disease has been described. An unusual subtype of sporadic progressive ataxia and palatal tremor should suggest possible diagnosis of MSA-C. Palatal tremor should be distinguished from the oculomasticatory myorhythmia of Whipple disease.

Palatal tremor is usually resistant to pharmacologic interventions. Baclofen, sodium valproate, clonazepam, benzodiazepines, lamotrigine, phenytoin, and piracetam have been attempted with variable results. Botulinum toxin injections have been used in an attempt to treat the tinnitus.

Our patient also had multiple supratentorial and infratentorial ischemic infarcts. MRI demonstrated a right medial medullary infarction. The medial medullary syndrome may result from occlusion of the vertebral artery, a branch of the vertebral artery, the lower basilar artery, or vertebrobasilar dolichoectasia. Classic manifestations consist of ipsilateral lower motor neuron paralysis of the tongue, contralateral paralysis of the arm and leg, and contralateral hemibody loss of tactile, vibratory, and position sense.

SELECTED REFERENCES

Deuschl G, Mischke G, Schenck E, et al. Symptomatic and essential rhythmic palatal myoclonus. *Brain* 1990;113:1645–1672.

Espay AJ, Revilla FJ. Cerebellar limb tremor and inferior olivary hypertrophy. *Neurology* 2006;67(7):1250.

Meyer MA, David CE, Chahin NS. Palatal myoclonus secondary to vertebral artery compression of the inferior olive. *J Neuroimaging* 2000;10(4):221–223.

Okamoto Y, Mitsuyama H, Jonosono M, et al. Autosomal dominant palatal myoclonus and spinal cord atrophy. *J Neurol Sci* 2002;195(1):71–76.

Samuel M, Torum N, Tuite PJ, et al. Progressive ataxia and palatal tremor (PAPT). Clinical and MRI assessment with review of palatal tremor. *Brain* 2004;127(Pt 6):1252–1268.

SEE QUESTIONS: 47, 50, 88, 308, 309

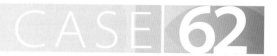

HEMICHOREA–HEMIBALLISM

OBJECTIVES

- To demonstrate a hyperkinetic complication of a metabolic derangement.
- To discuss the differential diagnosis of hemichorea–hemiballism.

VIGNETTE

This 37-year-old man had insulin-dependent diabetes mellitus since age 5 with end-stage renal disease requiring kidney and pancreas transplant by the age of 30 years. He was admitted to the hospital for diabetic ketoacidosis. His calculated serum osmolarity fluctuated from 304 to 287 over a 6-hour period. Serum glucose reached 528 mg/dL (normal, 70 to 105 mg/dL). His mental status normalized in 2 days after insulin and intravenous hydration. Three weeks later, he noted a "fidgety" right arm and right leg, rapidly growing in intensity.

 (**CASE SUMMARY**)

Our patient had right hemichorea with a ballistic component associated with increased T1-weighted signal in the contralateral putamen and a T2-weighted central pontine hyperintensity sparing of the corticospinal fibers (Fig. 62.1). He was diagnosed with hemichorea–hemiballism (HC/HB) due to diabetic ketoacidosis, which was also complicated with osmotic demyelination expressed as a central pontine myelinolysis. He responded to haloperidol, which was discontinued after 1 month without hemichorea relapse. At the 3-month reevaluation, despite symptomatic resolution, serial brain magnetic resonance imaging (MRI) studies continued to demonstrate similar imaging abnormalities.

Lesions in or near the subthalamic nucleus can result in contralateral HC/HB, including lesions in the caudate, putamen, globus pallidus, precentral gyrus, or thalamic nuclei. Destruction of the corticospinal tract ipsilateral to the subthalamic nucleus prevents the development of hemiballismus. Small unilateral lesions of the anteroventral portion of the caudate cause contralateral choreoathetosis. Unilateral lesions of the globus pallidus may result in contralateral hemidystonia. Unilateral pallidal–putaminal lesions may present with sudden falling to the contralateral side while sitting, standing, or walking.

Unilateral basal ganglia hyperintensity on T1-weighted MRI is largely an imaging domain of HC/HB due to nonketotic hyperglycemia, the most common metabolic complication among diabetics. Unlike T2 signal abnormalities, high T1 signal is uncommon and, when present, virtually always bilateral, due in most cases to hypermagnesemia, such as in acquired hepatolenticular degeneration, methcathinone toxicity, and long-term total

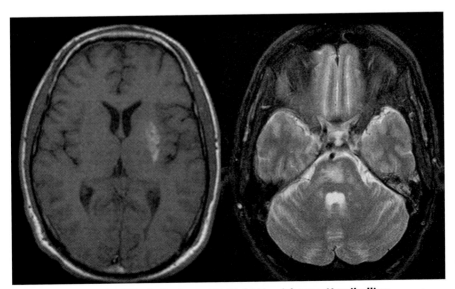

Figure 62.1   Brain MRI of a Patient with Right Hemichorea–Hemiballism.
T1-weighted hyperintensity in the left putamen and a T2-weighted central pontine hyperintensity, sparing of the corticopontine and corticospinal fibers.

parenteral nutrition. Bilateral T1-weighted hyperintensities in the basal ganglia have also been variably reported in neurofibromatosis and calcification.

Most cases of chorea are of slow onset and include infectious or autoimmune central nervous diseases, estrogen replacement (birth control pills), levodopa therapy for Parkinson disease patients, hyperthyroidism, pregnancy (chorea gravidarum), and polycythemia rubra. Acute HC/HB only results from vascular events (typically lacunar striatal strokes) and metabolic disorders (most often, nonketotic diabetic hyperglycemia). Hemichorea usually develops within hours to several days as a complication of stroke and within days to weeks as a complication of diabetic hyperglycemia, probably because of downstream neuroplastic changes.

Two additional disorders need to be considered in the differential diagnosis of HC/HB: (1) recurrent limb-shaking syndrome transient ischemic attack (TIA), due to carotid-occlusive disease and resulting cerebral hypoperfusion and (2) epilepsia partialis continua. These disorders should be thought of in the context of neck hyperextension or other maneuvers affecting the carotid lumen in the former or as rhythmic or semirhythmic movements rather than random, dancelike movements in the latter.

Finally, this case demonstrated that diabetic ketoacidosis can generate concurrent but pathophysiologically distinct lesions: putaminal hyperintensities on T1-weighted brain MRI and pontine hyperintensities on T2-weighted sequences, usually representing central pontine myelinolysis (fortunately not associated with quadriparesis). The contributory osmotic shifts for both lesions may be generated by rapid serum glucose changes without necessarily any sodium changes. The HC/HB associated with nonketotic hyperglycemia typically resolves over 6 months (often with resolution of the T1-weighted hyperintensity), although both the chorea and putaminal hyperintensity can persist, the latter for up to 6 years.

SELECTED REFERENCES

Duker AP, Espay AJ. Images in clinical medicine: hemichorea–hemiballism after diabetic ketoacidosis. *N Engl J Med* 2010;363(17):e27.

Ghika-Schmid F, Ghika J, Regli F, et al. Hyperkinetic movement disorders during and after stroke: the Lausanne Stroke Registry. *J Neurol Sci* 1997;146(2):109–116.

Kase CS, Maulsby GO, de Juan E, et al. Hemichorea-hemiballism and lacunar infarction in the basal ganglia. *Neurology* 1981;31:452–455.

Kaufman DK, Brown RD, Karnes WE. Involuntary tonic spasms of a limb due to a brainstem lacunar infarction. *Stroke* 1994;25:217–219.

Oh SH, Lee KY, Im JH, et al. Chorea associated with non-ketotic hyperglycemia and hyperintensity basal ganglia lesion on T1-weighted brain MRI study: a meta-analysis of 53 cases including four present cases. *J Neurol Sci* 2002;200:57–62.

Postuma RB, Lang AE. Hemiballism: revisiting a classic disorder. *Lancet Neurol* 2003;2:661–668.

SEE QUESTIONS: 189, 200, 310

CASE 63

PARANEOPLASTIC CHOREA/SENSORY NEURONOPATHY

OBJECTIVES

- To illustrate an important cause of adult-onset chorea.
- To review the causes of sensory neuronopathy and outline an appropriate diagnostic evaluation.

VIGNETTE

A 63-year-old retired coal miner complained of left upper extremity burning pain and numbness followed by weakness of both upper extremities. At the time of the video, the patient had difficulty chewing and could not clean his dentures because of impaired hand dexterity. He could not drive because he had inadequate control of the steering wheel. He also could not write due to inability to properly hold a pen.

CASE SUMMARY

Our patient had a striking combination of progressive sensory disturbance of the limbs resulting in large fiber sensory dysfunction and subsequent ataxia. In addition, he had involuntary movements of the hands and face consistent with chorea, although it is plausible that some of the hyperkinetic phenomenology may be due to proprioceptive deprivation ("pseudoathetosis").

Most distal sensory peripheral neuropathies initially involve the feet, eventually spreading to the hands. Predominant symptoms involve small sensory fibers dealing with pain and temperature. However, there are rare sensory neuron diseases beginning with symmetric symptoms involving the upper extremities and subsequently spreading to the lower extremities. These conditions affect the dorsal root ganglia or nerve roots (sensory neuronopathies or ganglionopathies) and include the following disorders: iatrogenic neuropathies, such as vincristine, carboplatin, or cisplatin neuropathy; vitamin related, such as pyridoxine intoxication or nicotinic acid deficiency; subacute combined system degeneration from vitamin B_{12} deficiency, Sjögren sensory neuronopathy, immune-mediated or postinfectious polyradiculopathy, or sensory ganglionopathy; and paraneoplastic (bronchial carcinoma, small cell lung cancer, Hodgkin lymphoma, breast cancer, ovarian cancer, sarcoma, and neuroendocrine tumors), and paraneoplastic subacute/chronic sensory neuronopathy associated with anti-Hu or CV2/CRMP-5 antibodies.

Chorea is an unusual paraneoplastic central nervous system disorder. However, paraneoplastic chorea has been reported in patients with anti-CRMP-5 IgG antibodies in serum or cerebrospinal fluid (CSF) and in association with chest malignancies, such as small cell lung cancer (SCLC) or thymomas. Paraneoplastic chorea has also been reported in association with anti-Hu antibodies. In our case, high titers of IgG CRMP-5 immunoglobulin were detected in serum and CSF.

Although less than 1% of patients with cancer have a clinically significant paraneoplastic syndrome, antibodies against CRMP-5 are present in up to 30% to 40% of paraneoplastic chorea.

Management of paraneoplastic sensory neuronopathy can be quite challenging. As with most paraneoplastic syndromes, the primary goal is to appropriately treat the underlying malignancy. The second strategy applied to a broad spectrum of paraneoplastic syndrome is immunotherapy.

Several movement disorders have been associated with specific paraneoplastic antibodies. Besides chorea and anti-CRMP5, parkinsonism has been associated with anti-Ma, cerebellar ataxia and tremor with anti-Yo, and ataxia and pseudoathetosis with anti-Hu. In the nonparaneoplastic autoimmune category, chorea, stereotypies, and dystonia are often seen in patients with encephalitis due to anti-*N*-methyl-D-aspartate receptor (anti-NMDAR) antibodies, rigidity is seen in patients with antiglutamic acid decarboxylase or antiamphiphysin antibodies (stiff person syndrome), and neuromyotonia is common in patients with voltage-gated potassium channels binding to CASPR2 antigens and opsoclonus–myoclonus–ataxia due to unknown antibodies.

SELECTED REFERENCES

Kinirons P, Fulton A, Keoghan M, et al. Paraneoplastic limbic encephalitis (PLE) and chorea associated with CRMP-5 neuronal antibody. *Neurology* 2003;61(11):1623–1624.

Panzer J, Dalmau J. Movement disorders in paraneoplastic and autoimmune disease. *Curr Opin Neurol* 2011;24(4):346–353.

Posner JB. *Neurologic complications of cancer. Contemporary neurology series 45.* Philadelphia: F.A. Davis, 1995:353–385.

Sghirlazoni A, Pareyson D, Lauria G. Sensory neuron diseases. *Lancet Neurol* 2005;4:349–361.

Tremont-Lukats IW, Fuller GN, Ribalta T, et al. Paraneoplastic chorea: case study with autopsy confirmation. *Neuro Oncol* 2002;4:192–195.

SEE QUESTIONS: 186, 189, 200, 228, 230, 241, 311

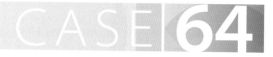

HEMIFACIAL SPASM

OBJECTIVES

- To present an example of hemifacial spasm.
- To discuss the differential diagnosis of unilateral involuntary facial movements.
- To summarize current management strategies for hemifacial spasm.

VIGNETTE

This 67-year-old man had twitching of his left face for about 20 years. Over the last 2 years, he experienced increased frequency and severity of jerking, which affected his ability to teach accounting, his profession. He underwent resection of a large right frontal meningioma 15 years ago, with reintervention due to regrowth a year later. He had been on antiseizure prophylaxis with phenytoin first and lamotrigine later. Only one seizure developed when he was rapidly discontinued from phenytoin. He had no tinnitus, vertigo, or disequilibrium, and no previous facial palsy or facial trauma. He had an extensive set of normal investigations, including brain magnetic resonance imaging/magnetic resonance angiography (MRI/MRA) and electroencephalography (EEG).

CASE SUMMARY

Our patient had an insidious onset of brief, painless, unilateral clonic contractions of the facial musculature beginning in the orbicularis oculi that gradually spread to involve other facial muscles and evolved from a mild clonic to a predominantly tonic recurrent phenomenon. His wife had noted that the facial movements persisted during sleep. He had no history of Bell palsy or traumatic facial injury. A diagnosis of sporadic idiopathic hemifacial spasm was made. The patient had an excellent response to botulinum toxin injections into the involved muscles.

Hemifacial spasm has been classically attributed to vascular loop compression of the facial nerve at the root exit zone from the pons by an aberrant blood vessel (e.g., branches of the vertebral artery or anterior inferior cerebellar artery). Other causes include tortuous basilar artery, vertebral artery dolichoectasia, vertebrobasilar junction dissecting aneurysms, cerebellopontine angle mass lesions, Paget disease of the bone, idiopathic intracranial hypertension, multiple sclerosis plaque, basilar meningitis, and parotid gland tumors. Hemifacial spasm may also follow Bell palsy (postparalytic hemifacial spasm with synkinesias) or traumatic facial nerve injuries. Rare cases of familial hemifacial spasm have been reported, but most cases are sporadic and idiopathic.

Most cases of idiopathic hemifacial spasm begin in the fifth or sixth decades of life. Hemifacial spasm is seldom found in children or adolescents. Pediatric hemifacial spasm may result from an underlying intracranial tumor. Hemifacial spasm must be differentiated from facial dystonia, blepharospasm, facial myokymia ("bag of worms"), facial tics, hemimasticastory spasm, tardive dyskinesia, oromandibular dystonia, epilepsia partialis continua, and psychogenic facial spasm (fixed lower lip deviation).

Relief of hemifacial spasm can be achieved through chemodenervation with botulinum toxin injection or with microvascular decompression. 3D-TOF MRA may identify the vascular compression at the exit zone of the facial nerve and assist in preoperative planning. MR cisternography is valuable in identifying the blood vessels and nerve bundles in the cerebellopontine cistern. Gabapentin, carbamazepine, clonazepam, and phenytoin may be considered for the few patients with hemifacial spasm who fail chemodenervation and may not be appropriate candidates for microvascular decompression.

SELECTED REFERENCES

Brazis PW, Masdeu JC, Biller J. *Localization in clinical neurology*, 6th ed. Philadelphia: Lippincott Williams & Wilkins, Wolters Kluwer Health, 2011.

Campos-Benitez M, Kaufmann AM. Neurovascular compression findings in hemifacial spasm. *J Neurosurg* 2008;109(3):416–420.

Samii M, Gunther T, Iaconetta G, et al. Microvascular decompression to treat hemifacial spasm: long-term results for a consecutive series of 143 patients. *Neurosurgery* 2002;50:712–718.

Wang A, Jankovic J. Hemifacial spasm: clinical correlates and treatments. *Muscle Nerve* 1998;21: 1740–1747.

SEE QUESTION: 152, 312

CASE **65**

TIC DISORDER

- To discuss the clinical classification of tics.
- To review the spectrum of clinical disorders associated with tics.
- To briefly review the clinical characteristics and management of Tourette syndrome.

A 38-year-old man had throat clearing and blinking in childhood, evolving into head shaking and shoulder twitches in adulthood. He did not seek medical attention until about 10 years earlier because of social embarrassment. Being in crowds reliably increased the frequency of his movements. He had no head or shoulder twitches during sleep. Taking hot baths also reduced the intensity and frequency of his movements.

Our patient had a long history of brief, intermittent, stereotyped, purposeless, and irregularly repetitive clonic movements consistent with a motor tic disorder. He also had a history of generalized anxiety disorder. The motor tics initially became noticeable in grade school with persistent throat clearing and blinking. In middle and high school, these symptoms worsened, and at the time of this consultation, they had evolved into rapid head shaking and shoulder shrugging. The throat clearing abated. He had no grunting or barking. He described the period before the tics as characterized by an initial buildup of tension, relieved transiently by the tics.

He worked night shifts at his job, but he preferred to work at home as he felt less anxious. Although the absence of other workers at night helped with his anxiety, the thought of pending or incomplete work made him extremely nervous. He also used to sit in the back of movie theaters and at church, as he felt embarrassed about his symptoms. He had neither ritualistic thoughts surrounding the tics nor intrusive, uncontrollable, or recurrent thoughts. He had no compulsive behaviors. Other than throat clearing, he never had phonic tics.

His anxiety symptoms included worrying constantly, having different thoughts about a large range of daily issues, problems with concentration, and feeling panicky and overwhelmed at times, sometimes in anticipation of his own movements. He had been placed on haloperidol, but this caused incoordination and thus was discontinued. He also received carbamazepine, baclofen, and valproic acid with no benefit. He had some modest control of the tics with clonazepam. Cranial computed tomography (CT) and electroencephalography (EEG) were normal.

On examination, he had good insight into his illness. There were no hallucinations or delusions. There was no psychomotor agitation or retardation. Thoughts were well organized, logical, and goal oriented. The patient had simple motor tics, about three to four per minute, on average. The tics involved head twisting and jerking and shoulder shrugging, left greater than right. He had no coprolalia, echolalia, hiccoughs, or other vocal disturbances.

His fund of general knowledge was average for his age and reading was low average. Speech was fluent without dysarthria or aphasia. Digit span was normal. Visual motor scanning speed was intact. Novel problem solving was largely normal. Immediate recall was average. Learning with rehearsal was low normal. Long-term recall was average. Visual confrontation naming was normal. Constructional praxis was intact. The Personality Assessment Inventory was primarily remarkable for mild symptoms of anxiety. The remainder of his neurological examination was unremarkable.

Our diagnosis was motor tic disorder and generalized anxiety disorder. The onset of his symptoms under the age of 21 years with evolution of the type and distribution of tics made Tourette syndrome (TS) the most likely etiology for his motor tics.

Tics are characterized by brief, rapid, usually stereotyped, purposeless, irregularly repetitive, and predominantly clonic hyperkinetic movements involving one or more muscular groups. Tics may consist of simple motor movements (e.g., eye blinking, nose twitch, shoulder shrug, and head jerking), complex motor movements (e.g., head shaking, and skipping), simple phonic sounds (e.g., throat clearing, grunting, barking), or complex vocalizations (e.g., coprolalia, echolalia, palilalia, and hiccoughs).

Tics may present suddenly or gradually and may have spontaneous remissions. Besides temporary suppressibility, premonitory urge, and stereotypic appearance, tics may be exacerbated with stress, excitement, boredom, and fatigue. Tics have been clinically classified as (a) simple motor tics (clonic, dystonic, or tonic), (b) complex motor tics (seemingly purposeful or seemingly nonpurposeful), (c) simple phonic tics, (d) complex phonic tics, and (e) compulsive tics. There is also a transient tic syndrome of childhood, where the tics may occur for no longer than 12 consecutive months.

Secondary tics, to be considered when tics appear after the age of 20 years, may result from drugs (L-dopa, neuroleptics, methylphenidate, carbamazepine, phenytoin, phenobarbital, and lamotrigine) or striatal disorders (e.g., chorea–acanthocytosis, Huntington disease, Sydenham chorea, Wilson disease, primary dystonia, encephalitis lethargica, posttraumatic, poststroke, and carbon monoxide poisoning), frontotemporal dementias, and Creutzfeldt-Jakob disease. Childhood tic disorders have been associated with group A β-hemolytic streptococcal infections and termed PANDAS (pediatric autoimmune neuropsychiatric disorders associated with streptococcus), but this construct has remained the subject of long and ongoing debate.

TS is the most common involuntary movement disorder of childhood (4:1 male-to-female ratio) of onset before 21 years. Besides the motor and vocal/phonic tics, there often are coexistent behavioral disorders, especially attention deficit hyperactivity disorder (ADHD) and obsessive–compulsive disorder (OCD). The diagnosis is made when multiple waxing-and-waning motor and one or more phonic tics have been present for more than 1 year and the location, number, frequency, type, complexity, and/or severity of tics have changed over time. Inheritance of TS may involve autosomal dominant, bilinear, or polygenic mechanisms.

Coprolalia, one of the hallmark features of TS, may also occur with Lesch-Nyhan syndrome, postencephalitic parkinsonism, chorea–acanthocytosis, and other basal ganglia disorders. Treatment may be challenging. Given the high frequency of psychiatric comorbidity and marked severity and pervasiveness of tics, their complete elimination may not be the primary goal of therapy. Timely and accurate diagnosis and education of the patient and family are essential elements of effective management. A large variety of pharmacologic agents are now available to treat patients with tics, including neuroleptics, dopamine-depleting drugs (tetrabenazine, and reserpine), clonidine, guanfacine, clonazepam, trazodone, verapamil, deprenyl, pergolide, nicotine, and botulinum toxin injections (for dystonic tics). Plasma exchange and intravenous immunoglobulin have been used with variable success in children with infection-triggered tic disorder and obsessive–compulsive disorder.

SELECTED REFERENCES

Biller J, Ed. *Practical neurology*, 4th ed. Philadelphia: Lippincott Williams & Wilkins, Wolters Kluwer Health, 2012.

Brazis PW, Masdeu JC, Biller J. *Localization in clinical neurology*, 6th ed. Philadelphia: Lippincott Williams & Wilkins, Wolters Kluwer Health, 2011.

Espay AJ, Biller J. *Concise neurology*. Philadelphia: Lippincott Williams & Wilkins, Wolters Kluwer Health, 2011.

Perlmutter SJ, Leitman SF, Garvey MA, et al. Therapeutic plasma exchange and intravenous immunoglobulin for obsessive-compulsive disorder and tic disorders in childhood. *Lancet* 1999;354: 1137–1138.

Shapiro AK, Shapiro ES, Young JG, et al., eds. *Gilles de la Tourette syndrome*, 2nd ed. New York: Raven Press, 1988.

SEE QUESTIONS: 44, 189, 313

CASE **66**

HEMIDYSTONIA (SARCOIDOSIS)

OBJECTIVES

■ To discuss lesion localization in cases of hemidystonia.
■ To briefly review the major neurological manifestations of sarcoidosis.

VIGNETTE

This 34-year-old man was diagnosed with sarcoidosis through a lymph node biopsy 1 year earlier. He presented to the neurology clinic after rapid onset of abnormal movements of the left arm. Over time, the movements spread to the left side of his neck and face and to a lesser extent his trunk and left leg.

CASE SUMMARY

Our patient had biopsy-proven sarcoidosis. He presented with a mixed hyperkinetic movement disorder, hemidystonia and athetosis (also referred to as "slow chorea" or "mobile" dystonia). Most patients with unilateral hyperkinetic disorders have neuroimaging evidence of contralateral basal ganglia lesions. Hemidystonia most often complicates contralateral lesions in the globus pallidus. Hemichoreoathetosis tend to result from contralateral lesions of the anteroventral portion of the caudate, as demonstrated in our patient. Leaning or falling to one side while sitting, standing, or walking may result from contralateral pallidal–putaminal lesions. Our patient had combined lesions in the globus pallidus and caudate, expressing as a combination of dystonia and choreoathetosis.

Hyperkinetic disorders may be caused by abnormal excitatory input from the thalamus to the premotor cortex due to lesions either of the thalamus itself or of the striatum projecting by way of the globus pallidus to the thalamus, or the globus pallidus itself. Lesions associated with dystonic spasms or myoclonic dystonia tend to localize in the striatopallidal complex or thalamus contralateral to the dystonia. Paroxysmal hemidystonia may also occur with contralateral midbrain lesions. The most common cause of hemidystonia is stroke. In many patients the hemidystonia is preceded by hemiparesis, which often resolves as the hemidystonia develops. Other causes of hemidystonia include head trauma, perinatal injury, encephalitis, vascular malformations, porencephalic cysts, thalamotomy, and a variety of neurodegenerative disorders.

Sarcoidosis is a chronic multisystem granulomatous disease characterized by a noncaseating granulomatous reaction of unknown origin. Sarcoidosis most frequently involves the lymph nodes and lungs and occurs most commonly among young adults. Sarcoidosis is more common in women, and in the United States, African-Americans are more commonly affected than whites. Involvement of the nervous system accounts for 5% to 15% of cases. The clinical course is highly variable, with occasional exacerbations and spontaneous remissions.

Major neurological manifestations of sarcoidosis include cranial neuropathies (most commonly the facial nerve), encephalopathy, aseptic chronic or recurrent basilar meningitis, diabetes insipidus, brain mass, seizures, angiopathy, hydrocephalus, basal ganglia dysfunction, myelopathy, polyneuropathy, mononeuritis multiplex, and acute or chronic myopathy. The triad of parotitis, uveitis, and facial nerve palsy is known as Heerfordt syndrome. Hemidystonia due to CNS sarcoidosis is highly unusual.

SELECTED REFERENCES

Brazis PW, Masdeu JC, Biller J. *Localization in clinical neurology*, 6th ed. Philadelphia: Lippincott Williams & Wilkins, Wolters Kluwer Health, 2011.

Caviness JN, Knox CA. Hemidystonias occurring in a patient with sarcoidosis. *Mov Disord* 1996;11(3): 340–341.

Chuang C, Fahn S, Frucht SJ. The natural history and treatment of acquired hemidystonia: report of 33 cases and review of the literature. *J Neurol Neurosurg Psychiatry* 2002;72:59–67.

Fahn S, Bressman S, Marsden CD. Classification of dystonia. *Adv Neurol* 1998;78:1–10.

Stern BJ, Krumholz A, Johns C, et al. Sarcoidosis and its neurological manifestations. *Arch Neurol* 1985;42:909–917.

SEE QUESTIONS: 190, 204, 234, 240

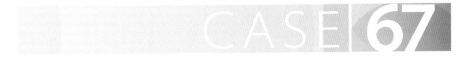

ACUTE DYSTONIC REACTION

OBJECTIVES

- To illustrate a neurologic complication of a dopamine receptor blocking agent.
- To review management guidelines of neuroleptic-induced acute dystonic reactions.

VIGNETTE

This 41-year-old woman had systemic lupus erythematosus and a prior branch retinal vein occlusion of the right eye. She also had a history of what was labeled as "allergic reaction" to prochlorperazine (Compazine) following abdominal surgery.

CASE SUMMARY

Our patient suffered an acute dystonic reaction induced by prochlorperazine. Neurologic complications of dopamine receptor blocking agents (neuroleptics) can occur within days, such as in acute dystonic reactions, acute akathisia, and neuroleptic malignant syndrome, or may occur after several months or years of exposure, such as in neuroleptic-induced parkinsonism (sometimes yielding a "rabbit syndrome," or perinasal tremor) and tardive dyskinesia. Acute dystonic reaction is an often dramatic and potentially life-threatening complication of neuroleptic treatment. Although traditionally antipsychotics are the neuroleptics considered as the typical offending agents, there is a growing prevalence of nonantipsychotic neuroleptics, particularly those used for nausea and cough (Table 67.1).

Acute dystonic reactions most commonly involve the muscles of the face, tongue, jaw, neck, or throat. Jaw-opening dystonia, in particular, is a common presentation, as demonstrated in second video. Most characteristic features include oculogyric crisis, trismus, and opisthotonic posturing. Pure truncal flexion (camptocormia) and the Pisa syndrome may occur as an acute dystonic reaction. A rarely reported extrapyramidal reaction is acute laryngeal dystonia (laryngospasm), a potentially life-threatening disorder, which may cause asphyxia.

Risk factors for acute dystonic reactions include young age, male gender (particularly African-American and Asian-American), and use of high-potency neuroleptics (e.g., haloperidol, and fluphenazine). Prior cocaine exposure increases the risk of acute dystonic reaction by 40-fold. Parenteral administration of benztropine (Cogentin) or diphenhydramine (Benadryl) are the most effective medications in the majority of cases, but

---

TABLE 67.1 NONANTIPSYCHOTIC NEUROLEPTIC DRUGS

For Nausea	For Depression
1. Phenothiazines, thiethylperazine [Torecan]	6. Tricyclic amoxapine [Asendin]
2. Prochlorperazine [Compazine]	7. Perphenazine/amitriptyline [Triavil]
3. Substituted benzamides, metoclopramide [Reglan], sulpiride, tiapride, and clebopride	
For Cough	**For Tourette Syndrome**
4. Promethazine [Phenergan]	8. Pimozide [Orap]
For Menopausal Flushes	**For Hypertension**
5. Veralipride	9. Calcium channel blockers flunarizine and cinnarizine

In bold, commonly used brand names of neuroleptics associated with acute dystonic reaction and other motor complications.

prophylactic use of oral anticholinergics should be continued as outpatient therapy for 48 to 72 hours. Intravenous administration of anticholinergics usually relieves symptoms within 2 to 3 minutes, whereas intramuscular administration requires approximately 15 to 30 minutes for symptom relief. Geriatric patients generally require lower doses of anticholinergic drugs. Phencyclidine (PCP) exposure should be suspected in cases of acute dystonic reactions failing to respond to diphenhydramine.

▶ **Case 67, Video 2 (Part 1):** This 66-year-old woman with chronic renal failure was given scheduled daily promethazine (Phenergan) for nausea. After 10 days of exposure, she developed confusion and jaw-opening dystonia.

▶ **Case 67, Video 3 (Part 2):** Complete resolution of her jaw-opening dystonia is documented after two 25-mg doses of diphenhydramine (Benadryl) were administered.

SELECTED REFERENCES

Brazis PW, Masdeu JC, Biller J. *Localization in clinical neurology*, 6th ed. Philadelphia: Lippincott Williams & Wilkins, Wolters Kluwer Health, 2011.

Espay AJ, Biller J. *Concise neurology*. Philadelphia: Lippincott Williams & Wilkins, Wolters Kluwer Health, 2011.

Fahn S, Bressman S, Marsden CD. Classification of dystonia. *Adv Neurol* 1998;78:1–10.

Koek RJ, Pi EH. Acute laryngeal dystonic reactions to neuroleptics. *Psychosomatics* 1990;31:236–237.

Piecuch S, Thomas U, Shah BR. Acute dystonic reactions that fail to respond to diphenhydramine: think of PCP. *J Emerg Med* 2000;18:379–381.

SEE QUESTIONS: 108, 204, 314, 315

CASE **68**

ATAXIA DUE TO BILATERAL PICA INFARCTIONS

◖| **OBJECTIVES** |◗

- ■ To highlight the cardinal features of cerebellar dysfunction.
- ■ To review the arterial supply of the cerebellum.
- ■ To discuss the clinical presentation and management of large cerebellar infarcts.

◖| **VIGNETTE** |◗

This 47-year-old man had a right cerebellar hemispherectomy secondary to a large cerebellar stroke (bilateral posterior inferior cerebellar artery [PICA] infarcts, right greater than left).

◖| **CASE SUMMARY** |◗

Our patient was a previously healthy 47-year-old man who had sudden-onset dyspnea, nausea, diaphoresis, disequilibrium, and dysarthria. These events occurred in association with an acute myocardial infarction. A 2D echocardiogram showed a left ventricular ejection fraction of 55% and no intracardiac thrombi. Magnetic resonance imaging (MRI) of the brain showed bilateral PICA territory infarctions. A cerebral angiogram demonstrated an occluded right vertebral artery and near occlusion of the left vertebral artery. During the angiographic procedure, he experienced neurologic decline with disconjugate gaze and bradycardia.

Hospital course was complicated by obstructive hydrocephalus requiring placement of a drain and subsequent resection of cerebellar necrotic tissue. He also developed heparin-induced thrombocytopenia and was treated with plasmapheresis and lepirudin, a direct thrombin inhibitor. Since hospital discharge, he had no recurrent transient ischemic attacks (TIAs) or strokes. He was rendered wheelchair bound and unable to walk due to marked ataxia. Follow-up magnetic resonance angiography (MRA) showed complete recanalization of the vertebral arteries. The underlying cause of his vascular events was determined to be polycythemia vera.

Cardinal features of cerebellar dysfunction involve disturbances in motor control, muscle tone regulation, and coordination of skilled movements. To coordinate means to adjust the rate, range, force, and sequence of willed muscular contractions. As shown in the video, salient neurologic findings were gait and limb ataxia, dysmetria on finger-to-nose and heel–knee–shin testing, dysdiadochokinesia, and impaired checking response. Speech was scanning and slurred. He also had a wide-based stance and gait.

Ischemic strokes account for more than 85% of all strokes, whereas intracerebral hemorrhage and subarachnoid hemorrhage account for the remainder. The TOAST classification categorizes ischemic strokes into five subtypes: (1) large artery atherosclerotic, (2) cardioembolism, (3) small vessel occlusion, (4) stroke of other determined etiology, and (5) stroke of undetermined etiology.

The arterial blood supply of the cerebellum derives from the posterior inferior cerebellar artery (PICA), the anterior inferior cerebellar artery (AICA), and the superior cerebellar artery (SCA). PICA branches from the vertebral artery, whereas AICA and SCA branch from the basilar artery. PICA encircles the medulla to supply the lateral medulla. The distal portions of PICA bifurcate into a medial trunk that supplies the vermis and the adjacent cerebellar hemisphere and a lateral trunk that supplies the cortical surface of the tonsil and cerebellar hemisphere. AICA supplies the lateral tegmentum of the lower two-thirds of the pons and the ventrolateral cerebellum. The internal auditory artery arises from AICA and supplies the facial and auditory nerves. SCA supplies the superolateral cerebellar hemispheres, the superior cerebellar peduncle, the dentate nucleus, and part of the middle cerebellar peduncle.

Cerebellar infarctions usually result from thrombotic or embolic occlusion of a long circumferential cerebellar vessel and can be caused by a variety of disorders. Cerebellar arterial occlusions often result from cardioembolism, embolism from a vertebral artery plaque, or local arterial thrombosis. The infarctions may be limited to the cerebellum or may involve the brainstem or other structures. Four types of cerebellar infarction are recognized corresponding to the arterial territories of (a) PICA, (b) AICA, (c) SCA, and (d) the cortical watershed and deep cerebellar white matter border-zone infarcts.

Cerebellar infarction typically presents with severe vertigo, nausea, vomiting, and ataxia. Loss of balance and difficulty maintaining posture, standing, and walking should suggest the presence of cerebellar disease. With large or bilateral cerebellar infarcts, the increased space-occupying effect of an edematous cerebellum may compress the aqueduct of Sylvius or the fourth ventricle, causing acute obstructive hydrocephalus, or may compress the brainstem, resulting in a decreased level of alertness, horizontal gaze palsy, skewed deviation, pinpoint pupils, decreased corneal reflexes, and/or paralysis of upward gaze. With a cerebellar pressure cone, there is downward displacement of the cerebellar tonsils through the foramen magnum, resulting in neck stiffness, cardiac and respiratory rhythm disturbances, apnea, and death. With upward transtentorial herniation, there is upward displacement of the superior aspect of the cerebellar hemisphere through the edge of the tentorial incisura, resulting in midbrain compression. Clinical manifestations of upward cerebellar herniation include lethargy, coma, paralysis of upward gaze, midposition and unreactive pupils, and abnormal extensor posturing.

Patients with cerebellar infarctions should be admitted to a neuroscience intensive care unit or dedicated stroke unit. Large space-occupying edematous cerebellar infarcts tend to involve the territory of PICA, SCA, or both. Emergency suboccipital craniotomy in clinically deteriorating patients or those who fail to improve, or ventriculostomy if clinical deterioration is due to obstruction hydrocephalus, is often required.

SELECTED REFERENCES

Adams HP Jr, Bendixen BH, Kapelle LJ, et al. Classification of subtype of acute ischemic stroke. Definition for use in a multicenter clinical trial. TOAST. Trial of ORG 10172 in acute stroke treatment. *Stroke* 1993;24:35–41.

Brazis PW, Masdeu JC, Biller J. *Localization in clinical neurology,* 6th ed. Philadelphia: Lippincott Williams & Wilkins, Wolters Kluwer Health, 2011.

Jauss M, Krieger D, Horning C, et al.; for the GASCIS Study Centers. Surgical and medical management of patients with massive cerebellar infarctions: result of the German-Austrian cerebellar infarction study. *J Neurol* 1999;249:257–264.

Love BB, Biller J. Neurovascular system. In: Goetz CG, ed. *Textbook of clinical neurology,* 2nd ed. Philadelphia: WB Saunders, 2003.

SEE QUESTIONS: 19, 92, 143, 183

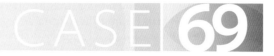

CASE 69

FRIEDREICH ATAXIA

OBJECTIVES

- To present an example of Friedreich ataxia.
- To discuss the differential diagnosis of Friedreich ataxia.
- To summarize current management strategies for Friedreich ataxia.

VIGNETTE

This 24-year-old woman dates the onset of her problems to about 6 years ago, when she first noted balance problems, with progressive difficulty walking straight but no falls. Physical therapy exercises were helpful, though stress at college made symptoms worse. More recently, she noted that her eyes tended to jerk away when trying to focus and her speech was hesitant and slowed. Of note, when she closes her eyes, she may feel transiently imbalanced (one of her early symptoms was to hold on to the shower wall when showering because she would perceive a tendency to fall when closing her eyes while shampooing). At the age of 11 years (sixth grade), she developed progressively worsening scoliosis, which was treated with spinal fusion at the age of 14. She had normal developmental milestones and had been a straight-A student.

CASE SUMMARY

Our patient had ataxia with scoliosis of onset in early teens, associated with areflexia and mild Romberg sign in the absence of cognitive impairment. These findings were most consistent with Friedreich ataxia, supported by atrophy of the cervical cord on MRI and confirmed by an expansion in the frataxin gene in both alleles (956 and 433 repeats). Despite the magnitude of the repeat expansion, there was no measurable proprioceptive impairment (except indirectly through a mild Romberg sign) and no cardiovascular or glycemic control symptoms, though periodic monitoring for these disease-associated complications was warranted.

The diagnosis of Friedreich ataxia (FRDA), in its classic form, requires the onset of ataxia or scoliosis before age 20, along with rapid subsequent appearance of areflexia, extensor plantar response, position and vibration loss, and other skeletal deformities (pes cavus), in the absence of ophthalmoplegia and dementia. Pes cavus or scoliosis in parents should suggest an autosomal dominant ataxia, such as Charcot-Marie-Tooth (CMT). The ataxia of FRDA is, however, more sensory than cerebellar and should be included in the differential diagnosis of other sensory ataxias, such as vitamin E deficiency, vitamin B_{12} deficiency, and nitrous oxide myeloneuropathy (Table 69.1).

FRDA is caused by an unstable GAA repeat within the first intron of the *frataxin* (*FXN*) gene on chromosome 9q13. Affected persons have from 81 to over 1,000 repeats in both their alleles (homozygous expansion). When the expansion is heterozygous, the other allele must have a point mutation. Hypertrophic cardiomyopathy and diabetes mellitus develop when

TABLE 69.1 (NONCEREBELLAR) SENSORY ATAXIAS

Localization	Classification	Etiologies
Posterior column	Myelopathies	**Friedreich ataxia** **Metabolic** (vitamin B_{12} deficiency,[a] folate deficiency,[a] vitamin E deficiency,[a] copper deficiency,[a] POLG1 mutation) **Toxic** (nitrous oxide myeloneuropathy,[a] clioquinol [antiprotozoal hydroxyquinoline], cassava ingestion) **Infectious** (HIV and HTLV myelopathies, tabes dorsalis) compressive/vascular myelopathy
Sensory ganglia	Sensory neuronopathies or ganglionopathies	**Metabolic** (thiamine [B_1] deficiency[b]) **Paraneoplastic** (subacute sensory neuronopathy due to anti-Hu and anti-CV2/CRMP5 antibodies) **Autoimmune** (Sjögren syndrome, Miller-Fisher syndrome, and Bickerstaff brainstem encephalitis) **Drugs** (cisplatin, pyridoxine [B_6] intoxication) **Inherited** disorders with degeneration of dorsal root ganglion cells
Peripheral nerves	Immune-mediated *demyelinating neuropathies—polyra-diculopathies*	Ataxic variant of Guillain-Barré syndrome: Miller-Fisher syndrome (anti-GQ1b) sensory ataxic neuropathy (anti-GD1b) anti-MAG neuropathy

[a]Vitamins B_{12} and E, folate, and copper deficiencies as well as nitrous oxide intoxication may present with a picture reflecting myeloneuropathy or subacute combined degeneration of the spinal cord (pyramidal, cerebellar, and neuropathic signs). Folate supplementation alone improves the anemia and peripheral neuropathy of B_{12} deficiency but not any CNS manifestations. Vitamin E deficiency is similar to Friedreich ataxia plus retinopathy.

[b]CNS manifestations of thiamine deficiency include Wernicke encephalopathy and optic neuropathy. Other manifestations include axonal peripheral neuropathy (*dry beriberi*), in severe cases mimicking the axonal type of Guillain-Barré syndrome, and high-output heart failure (wet beriberi).

MAG, myelin-associated glycoprotein.

From Espay, Lang. *Common movement disorders pitfalls: case-based teaching*. New York: Cambridge University Press, 2012, with permission.

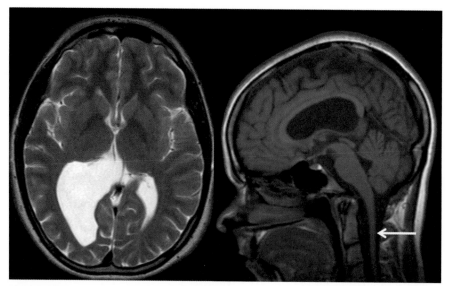

Figure 69.1   Axial T2-weighted (**left**) and midsagittal T1-weighted brain MRI demonstrating nonspecific, likely incidental, congenital colpocephaly of the posterior horn of the right lateral ventricle and disease-associated thinning of the cervical spinal cord (*arrow*), an imaging hallmark of Friedreich ataxia. There typically is no cerebellar atrophy.

GAA repeats exceed 500. Brain MRI shows atrophy of the upper cervical cord with nearly normal cerebellum (Fig. 69.1). Another ataxic disorder characterized by cervical cord atrophy is adult-onset Alexander disease, whereby palatal tremor is often part of the clinical picture.

Development of diabetes mellitus and cardiomyopathy in patients with FRDA should be monitored at regular intervals. Treatment can prevent or delay a number of related complications, including strokes and myocardial infarction. Orthopedic problems such as foot deformities and scoliosis can be treated with braces or surgery. Physical therapy may prolong use of the arms and legs and speech therapy improve enunciation and articulation.

▶ **Case 69, Video 2:**   Presence of early postural swaying from proprioceptive impairment (early Romberg sign) is demonstrated. This suggests that the ataxia is at least in part sensory in nature. Scoliosis is also demonstrated.

SELECTED REFERENCES

Biller J, ed. *Practical neurology*, 4th ed. Philadelphia: Lippincott Williams & Wilkins, Wolters Kluwer Health, 2012.

Espay AJ, Biller J. *Concise neurology*. Philadelphia: Lippincott Williams & Wilkins, Wolters Kluwer Health, 2011.

Espay AJ, Lang AE. *Common movement disorders pitfalls: case-based teaching*. New York: Cambridge University Press, 2012.

SEE QUESTIONS: 305, 306, 307

CASE **70**

CEREBELLAR ATAXIA

- To review the clinical presentation of midline cerebellar dysfunction.
- To outline the differential diagnosis of acquired progressive cerebellar degeneration and summarize the appropriate laboratory evaluation.

VIGNETTE

Seven years earlier, this 75-year-old woman was just about to descend some concrete steps when she hesitated because of poor balance. Since then, she felt increasing need to hold onto the rails or walls for support. Sometimes, she made sure that both feet were on one step at the same time, but in doing so, she still felt she was rocking back and forth.

CASE SUMMARY

 This 75-year-old woman had a 7-year history of slowly progressive ataxia, mild sensory loss, and downbeat nystagmus. Finger-to-nose testing showed a very mild symmetric endpoint tremor, left greater than right, but no overt dysmetria. Heel–shin testing was mildly abnormal bilaterally. Rapid alternating movements were decreased bilaterally. Sensory examination showed decreased sensation to pinprick in both hands and feet. She had a wide-based stance, could not stand unassisted, and had to use a walker to ambulate.

Identification of the type of cerebellar syndrome could predict a probable etiology. Four cerebellar syndromes are recognized: hemispheric syndrome, rostral vermis syndrome, caudal vermis syndrome, and pancerebellar syndrome. The cerebellar hemisphere syndrome (ipsilateral appendicular greater than truncal ataxia) often results from acute ischemic or hemorrhagic vascular events, trauma, neoplasms, or abscess. The rostral vermis syndrome (truncal ataxia with wide-based stance and gait but relatively minor or no dysmetria on heel-to-shin testing) results from alcoholism or nutritional deficiencies. The caudal vermis syndrome (truncal ataxia with staggering but rarely wide-based gait and little if any limb ataxia) often results from a midline cerebellar neoplasm such as medulloblastoma, ependymoma, or astrocytoma. The pancerebellar syndrome usually results from vitamin deficiencies (e.g., vitamin E), toxic/metabolic disorders, and demyelinating, immune-mediated, paraneoplastic, or hereditary (autosomal recessive, autosomal dominant, or X-linked ataxias) or nonhereditary degenerative ataxias (e.g., multiple system atrophy [MSA], cerebellar type). Besides the spectrum of hereditary cerebellar ataxias, other inheritable genetic or metabolic causes include abetalipoproteinemia, ataxia telangiectasia, adrenoleukodystrophy, ataxia with Co-Q deficiency, late-onset G_{M2} gangliosidoses, mitochondrial diseases, sialidosis, maple syrup urine disease, organic acidurias, cerebrotendinous xanthomatosis (CTX), Refsum disease, Wilson disease, and Niemann-Pick type C.

Acquired causes of progressive ataxia include among others paraneoplastic cerebellar degeneration. Among women with subacute progressive ataxia, a thorough search for

TABLE 70.1 **SELECTED CEREBELLAR ATAXIAS BASED ON TEMPORAL PROFILE**

Acute Ataxias	Subacute Ataxias	Rapidly Progressive	Chronic Ataxias
Alcohol poisoning Stroke	Thiamine deficiency Miller-Fisher syndrome Multiple sclerosis Parainfectious cerebellitis Autoimmune	Paraneoplastic cerebellar degeneration Creutzfeldt-Jakob disease SREAT Anti-GAD–associated ataxia	Spinocerebellar ataxias Friedreich ataxia MSA-C (formerly sOPCA) Nutritional (vit E/B$_{12}$ def) Toxins (toluene, mercury) Iatrogenic (phenytoin)

MSA, multiple system atrophy, cerebellar variant; sOPCA, sporadic olivopontocerebellar atrophy; SREAT, steroid-responsive encephalopathy with antithyroid antibodies, previously referred to as Hashimoto encephalopathy; GAD, glutamic acid decarboxylase.

ovarian cancer is essential. Anti-Yo (anti–Purkinje cell) antibodies are typically present in the serum of such patients. Less commonly, patients with malignancy develop cerebellar ataxia associated with anti-Hu, anti-Ri, anti-Ta, or anti-Ma antibodies. Ethanol toxicity should be considered as should thiamine deficiency. Elderly patients are occasionally prone to poor diets, especially those who live alone. Thiamine deficiency should be considered in any patient presenting with unexplained ataxia.

Multiple sclerosis, posterior fossa tumors, and vascular disease, such as Chiari malformation, are relatively easy to diagnose based on clinical presentation and MRI. Hypothyroidism is a rare cause of cerebellar ataxia, as is B$_{12}$ deficiency. Toxins other than alcohol include phenytoin, chemotherapy, solvents such as toluene, and mercury intoxication. Prior disorders such as Creutzfeldt-Jakob disease (CJD) should be considered. Immune-mediated cerebellar degeneration (other than paraneoplastic) includes a form seen with anti–glutamic acid decarboxylase (anti-GAD) antibodies and gluten ataxia (neurologic celiac disease) associated with antigliadin and antiendomysial antibodies. The temporal profile is helpful in guiding the type of cerebellar ataxia that needs to be investigated (Table 70.1).

Our patient's MRI showed atrophy of the anterosuperior vermis. She had negative anti-Hu antibodies and negative anti–Purkinje cell antibodies. Immunoelectrophoresis, very long chain fatty acids (VLCFAs), phytanic acid, and ammonia were normal. Porphyrin screen was unremarkable. Plasma cholestanol was normal. Thyroid-stimulating hormone (TSH) and vitamin E were normal. SCA ataxia screen was normal, including normal testing for Friedreich ataxia as well as dentatorubral-pallidoluysian atrophy (DRPLA). Serum B$_{12}$ levels were below normal, and B$_{12}$ replacement was initiated.

SELECTED REFERENCES

Biller J, Gruener G, Brazis P. *DeMyer's the neurologic examination. A programmed text*, 6th ed. New York: McGraw-Hill Medical, 2011.

Posner J, Dalmau JO. Paraneoplastic syndromes of the nervous system. *Clin Chem Lab Med* 2000;38: 117–122.

Selim M, Drachman DA. Ataxia associated with Hashimoto's disease: progressive non-familial adult onset cerebellar degeneration with autoimmune thyroiditis. *J Neurol Neurosurg Psychiatry* 2001;71(Jul): 81–87.

Verino S, Lennon VA. New Purkinje cell antibody (PCA-2): marker of lung cancer-related neurological autoimmunity. *Ann Neurol* 2000;47:297–305.

SEE QUESTIONS: 42, 85, 143, 241, 316, 317

HEREDITARY ATAXIA

. . . .

OBJECTIVES

- To review clinical features of hereditary cerebellar ataxia.
- To outline distinctive clinical features of common spinocerebellar ataxia (SCA) subtypes.

VIGNETTE

A 31-year-old woman had a progressive history of gait and limb incoordination and head tremor.

CASE SUMMARY

Our patient had a 4-year history of progressive ataxia beginning in her early 20s. Family history was remarkable, suggesting a dominant pattern of inheritance (with age of onset in the 20s). Her most prominent features were diplopia, sensory loss, and tremor. Frequent headaches complicated her clinical course. Neurologic examination demonstrated prominent dysarthria, left esotropia, and marked head and hand tremors. Muscle stretch reflexes were hypoactive. Gait was wide based and ataxic.

Our patient appeared to have a hereditary cerebellar ataxia. Investigation of these patients requires appropriate use of clinical algorithms based on mode of inheritance and MRI patterns of atrophy (Fig. 71.1).

SCA 1 begins with isolated gait ataxia, but over time patients develop severe dysarthria and dysphagia. Ophthalmoparesis, spasticity, and choreoathetosis are common associated manifestations. Most patients become wheelchair bound within 15 years of ataxia onset. SCA 3 (Machado-Joseph disease) is the most common dominantly inherited ataxia worldwide. The clinical picture varies, but usually involves progressive ataxia along with abnormalities of eye movements, speech, and swallowing. Onset is typically in the 30s or 40s, but occasionally patients present in the 60s. Most patients develop supranuclear ophthalmoparesis. Facial myokymia (resembling fasciculations) is also common. SCA 2 is more common than SCA 3 in individuals of Asian ancestry. Patients typically develop slow saccades with eventual gaze paresis due to marked pontine atrophy (see second video).

Peripheral neuropathy, dystonia, parkinsonism, and motor neuron disease may occur. SCAs 2, 3, and 6 are among the more common of the dominantly inherited ataxias. SCA 6 typically presents as a "pure" cerebellar ataxia with a very slower progression. Patients may have mild sensory loss. SCA 7 is associated with retinal degeneration. Interpretation of SCA 8 results is more problematic as some individuals have a very large SCA 8 expansion but do not develop the disease. SCA 10 often described in Mexican families is accompanied by seizures (second most common after SCA 2). SCA 12 is associated with prominent early tremors of the arms and head and is common in India. SCA 17 presents in midlife, and the ataxia tends to be associated with cognitive decline and a variety of movement disorders, including dystonia and chorea.

In patients with a dominant family history, the yield of current genetic testing is still less than 50% in identifying a specific defect. All genetic testing for commercially

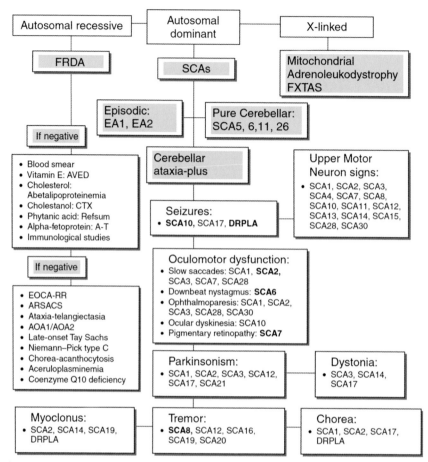

Figure 71.1   Proposed Algorithm for the Rational Investigation of Cerebellar Ataxias Based on Mode of Inheritance, Clinical Features, and MRI Pattern of Atrophy. (From Espay AJ, Biller J. *Concise neurology.* Philadelphia: Lippincott Williams & Wilkins, Wolters Kluwer Health, 2011, with permission.)

available SCAs were negative in our patient. New genetic causes of SCAs are identified every year.

An alternative diagnosis to SCA would be a mitochondrial disorder. MR spectroscopy (MRS) of the brain looking for lactate peaks, serum lactate, and pyruvate; mitochondrial DNA studies; and muscle biopsy may provide laboratory evidence in support of a mitochondrial disorder. These studies have been normal in our patient as well.

▶ **Case 71, Video 2:** Patient with genetically confirmed SCA 2, demonstrating the typical slowed saccades of this disorder. The last part of the video segment shows the marked wide-based gait ataxia.

SELECTED REFERENCES

Espay A, Biller J. *Concise neurology*. Philadelphia: Lippincott Williams & Wilkins, Wolters Kluwer Health, 2011.
Di Donato S, Gellera C, Mariotti C. The complex clinical and genetic classification of inherited ataxias. II. Autosomal recessive ataxias. *Neurol Sci* 2001;22:219–228.
The inherited ataxias. In: Conneally M, ed. *Neurogenetics.* Philadelphia: Continuum, 2000:73–99.
Paulson H, Ammache Z. Ataxia and hereditary disorders. *Neurol Clin* 2001;19:759–782.
Subramony SH, Vig PJ, McDaniel DO. Dominantly inherited ataxias. *Semin Neurol* 1999;19:419–425.

SEE QUESTIONS: 27, 85, 143, 241, 318

CASE 72

SPINOCEREBELLAR ATAXIA TYPE 3

OBJECTIVES

- To review the clinical features of spinocerebellar ataxia type 2 (SCA 3).
- To outline the features most helpful in distinguishing this form of ataxia from other SCAs.

VIGNETTE

This 61-year-old nurse admitted to have been "always been somewhat clumsy" with the eyes closed. For about a decade, she has felt she could fall when she was taking a shower with the eyes closed. She could just as easily walk into walls. She started to stagger, and some even thought she was drunk. About 8 years ago, she had fallen frequently enough to warrant the use of a walker. She continued to work as a nurse but in the computer support division. More recently, her hand dexterity became compromised. She noted an incipient tremor in both hands when trying to unlock a door or when holding a spoon or fork by her mouth, forcing the use of both hands to stabilize. Speech became somewhat garbled. Her tongue felt thick and she reported some choking episodes. She also has noted occasional horizontal double vision. Her father, paternal uncle, and paternal aunt have had difficulty with walking and balance. She feels her daughter is also clumsy.

CASE SUMMARY

Our patient had a long history of slowly progressive truncal and appendicular ataxia associated with peripheral neuropathy, areflexia, and upgaze impairment, in the absence of cognitive impairment (Montreal Cognitive Assessment = 29/30) in the setting of a heavy family history of ataxia. The history and findings were most consistent with a form of spinocerebellar ataxia. The ophthalmoparesis and the "bulging eyes" appearance suggested SCA 3, which was indeed confirmed through a CAG repeat expansion on *ataxin3* (14q32) of 64 repeats in one allele (normal, 12 to 44). Brain MRI showed atrophy of the cerebellar hemispheres without involvement of the pons, olives, or cervical cord.

SCA 3, also known as Machado-Joseph disease, is an autosomal dominant cerebellar ataxia due to CAG repeat expansions in *ataxin3*. The CAG repeat length determines age at disease onset, severity of the clinical phenotype, and rate of progression. Patients with SCA 3 may have among the latest onset and slowest progression of any of the SCAs, with or without ophthalmoparesis. Unlike the dystonia–parkinsonism presentation associated with an earlier onset and larger repeat size, the older adult presentation is most often associated with ataxia and small repeat expansions. In these patients, there often are slow saccades, areflexia, diplopia, and "bulging eyes" (in part due to eyelid retraction), all of which were present in our case. An axonal, distal, symmetric, sensorimotor polyneuropathy may be severe enough to independently contribute to the ataxia and prompt a sensation of imbalance when eyes were closed. Fasciculations and facial myokymia have also been documented in these patients.

Clinically, SCA 3 has been divided into four clinical types: type 1, dystonia and spasticity (earlier onset, more severe course with progressive nuclear ophthalmoplegia, especially affecting the abducens nucleus); type 2, spasticity and cerebellar ataxia (most common phenotype); type 3 (our patient's), cerebellar ataxia and peripheral neuropathy with amyotrophic changes (ophthalmoplegia is supranuclear—rather than nuclear—and may also express with a limitation in upward gaze and convergence); and type 4, levodopa-responsive parkinsonism and peripheral neuropathy. Importantly, cognitive impairment is not a feature of SCA 3.

▌ **Case 72, Video 2:** Same patient with genetically proven SCA 3 discusses a diagnostically important feature: her "bulging" eyes.

SELECTED REFERENCES

Coutinho P, Andrade C. Autosomal dominant system degeneration in Portuguese families of the Azores Islands: a new genetic disorder involving cerebellar, pyramidal, extrapyramidal and spinal cord motor functions. *Neurology* 1978;28(7):703–709.

Espay A, Biller J. *Concise neurology*. Philadelphia: Lippincott Williams & Wilkins, Wolters Kluwer Health, 2011.

Paulson H, Ammache Z. Ataxia and hereditary disorders. *Neurol Clin* 2001;19:759–782.

van Gaalen J, van de Warrenburg BP. Republished: a practical approach to late-onset cerebellar ataxia: putting the disorder with lack of order into order. *Postgrad Med J* 2012;88(1041):407–417.

SEE QUESTIONS: 319, 320, 321

CASE 73

MULTIPLE SYSTEM ATROPHY, CEREBELLAR TYPE

OBJECTIVES

- To review the clinical features of multiple system atrophy, cerebellar type (MSA-C).
- To outline the features most helpful in distinguishing this disorder from other forms of MSA.

VIGNETTE

This 63-year-old man was evaluated for a 3-year history of progressive unsteadiness when walking and clumsiness with fine motor tasks. A year prior to that, he had an episode of sudden-onset vertigo associated with nausea and vomiting, which resolved without recurrence. After 2 years of unsteadiness, he started to fall, with increasing frequency of at least once per month, mostly sideways, especially when steps were "not landing evenly on the ground." He resorted to using a cane to minimize the frequency of falls. His speech had become somewhat slurred, and he was choking to liquids, especially hot ones, but not to solids. He had some urinary urgency and increasing episodes of urinary incontinence. He noted some light-headedness upon standing up or bending forward. Hepatitis C was recently diagnosed. His brother, maternal cousin, and one of his sister's daughters had childhood-onset mental retardation.

CASE SUMMARY

Our patient had progressive truncal greater than appendicular ataxia in the absence of oculomotor impairment (other than hypermetric saccades), peripheral neuropathy, pyramidal dysfunction, or overt cognitive impairment (Montreal Cognitive Assessment = 26/30). The phenotype was that of a pure cerebellar ataxia with mild parkinsonism. Associated dysphagia, mild neurogenic bladder, and early orthostatic hypotension reflected concurrent dysautonomia. The presumptive diagnosis was multiple system atrophy, cerebellar type (MSA-C), which was supported by an olivopontocerebellar pattern of atrophy on brain MRI (Fig. 73.1).

Two other conditions were suggested by the vignette given the past history of hepatitis C and family history of children with mental retardation: acquired hepatolenticular degeneration and fragile X tremor–ataxia syndrome, respectively. However, the diagnosis of hepatitis C was recent and there was no liver cirrhosis. Also, the family history did not follow the X-linked inheritance of fragile X syndrome, whereby only boys should be affected. Importantly, both of these disorders include tremor in their phenotype, whereas MSA-C is classically a tremorless ataxic disorder. Also, a paraneoplastic disorder could be considered but a 3-year course seemed excessively long for this entity.

MSA is an oligodendrogliopathy that can be categorized into two main subtypes: MSA-C (cerebellar) and MSA-P (parkinsonian). In Asian countries, particularly Taiwan, MSA-C is more common than MSA-P, while MSA-P is more common elsewhere in the

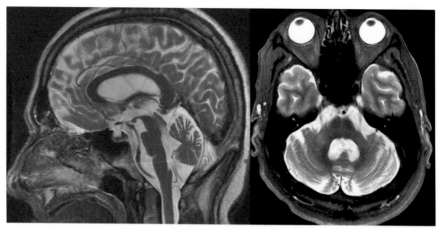

Figure 73.1   Midsagittal and axial T2-weighted brain MRI showing moderate atrophy in the medulla, cerebellum, and pons ("olivopontocerebellar" distribution of regional atrophy). The pontine atrophy yielded a "hot cross bun" appearance.

world. In MSA-C, truncal and appendicular ataxia are typically followed by dysarthria, tremor, and parkinsonian or other extrapyramidal symptoms. Sporadic olivopontocerebellar atrophy (OPCA), due to atrophy of the brainstem and cerebellum, most often implies MSA-C.

There is no disease-specific treatment for MSA-C. Management of orthostatic hypotension includes liberalizing salt intake, use of elastic stocking, and head elevation at night. Pharmacologic interventions include fludrocortisone (Florinef, 0.1 to 0.3 mg per day) and midodrine (ProAmatine, 15 to 30 mg per day). The latter may cause piloerection, scalp pruritus, urinary retention, and supine hypertension.

SELECTED REFERENCES

Espay A, Biller J. *Concise neurology*. Philadelphia: Lippincott Williams & Wilkins, Wolters Kluwer Health, 2011.

Gilman S, Wenning GK, Low PA, et al. Second consensus statement on the diagnosis of multiple system atrophy. *Neurology* 2008;71:670–676.

van Gaalen J, van de Warrenburg BP. Republished: a practical approach to late-onset cerebellar ataxia: putting the disorder with lack of order into order. *Postgrad Med J* 2012;88(1041):407–417.

SEE QUESTIONS: 322, 323

CASE 74

LIPID STORAGE ATAXIA: NIEMANN-PICK TYPE C

OBJECTIVES

■ To review the clinical features of Niemann-Pick C.
■ To outline the differential diagnosis of the various forms of ataxia whose features may overlap with those of Niemann-Pick C.

(Case courtesy of Dr. Donald Gilbert, University of Cincinnati)

VIGNETTE

This 15-year-old girl, previously healthy and of normal early development, had progressive deterioration of gait and coordination normal motor and language development. At the age of 5 years, she started having difficulty with early-reading skills. After age 7 years, she developed hand tremor, balance problems with tripping, clumsiness, and difficulty moving her eyes quickly (needed to move her head to compensate). After the age of 9 years, she has developed generalized tonic–clonic seizures, with poor control with a growing regimen of antiepileptics and further decline in gait, coordination, school performance, and behavior.

CASE SUMMARY

Our patient had a progressive ataxia beginning in her early childhood. Family history of neurological disease was negative for three generations but a distant cousin died in early adulthood due to progressive neurologic disease. Her general examination, including chest and abdomen, was normal. Her neurologic examination demonstrated slightly brisk reflexes with normal sensation. An important feature on examination was the greatly reduced range of vertical and, to a lesser extent, horizontal saccades, which was overcome with oculocephalic maneuvers, consistent with supranuclear gaze palsy.

The combination of cerebellar ataxia and supranuclear vertical gaze palsy, in the context of seizures and progressive cognitive decline is typical of Niemann-Pick type C (NPC). Some patients may have hepatosplenomegaly, as it is common in the neurovisceral infantile form. Marked cerebellar and, variably, callosal atrophy can be documented by neuroimaging (Fig. 74.1). Liver and bone marrow biopsy will demonstrate foamy (lipid-laden) cells or "sea-blue histiocytes." In our patient, the diagnosis was confirmed by the identification of two NPC1 mutations by NPC1 gene sequence analysis: a heterozygous deletion of two nucleotides in exon 3, c.251_252delAA, and a heterozygous C to G change at nucleotide 3019 in exon 20, c.3019C>G, predicting a substitution of proline to alanine at residue 1007, p.P1007A.

The demonstration of supranuclear vertical gaze palsy on examination conveniently reduced the potential diagnostic considerations of ataxia to only a handful of disorders: NPC, Tay-Sachs disease, Gaucher disease, CTX, and spinocerebellar ataxias type 3 and 7

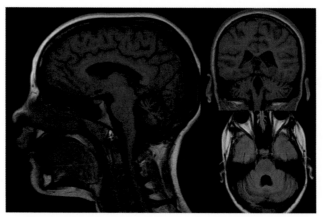

Figure 74.1 Brain MRI demonstrating marked cerebellar atrophy and thinning of the corpus callosum, two typical features in NPC.

(SCA 3 and SCA 7). The association with seizures and dementia is more typical of NPC than of any of any of the other disorders listed here.

NPC can present in infancy, adolescence, or adulthood with a core set of clinical features including ataxia, dementia, dysarthria, and vertical supranuclear ophthalmoplegia, followed by seizures, corticospinal features, and dysphagia with disease progression. Variable systemic features include hepatosplenomegaly. Variable neurologic features include dystonia and choreoathetosis. NPC is an autosomal recessive neurovisceral disorder of lipid storage occurring in 1 of 100,000 live births, biochemically and phenotypically distinct from Niemann-Pick diseases types A and B, which result from deficiency of lysosomal sphingomyelinase. Most cases are caused by abnormalities in the NPC1 gene on 18q, which codes for the lysosomal NPC1 protein. The less common NPC2 variant is caused by mutations in the NPC2 gene on 14q, whose product resides in the Golgi apparatus and late endosomes. Impairment in these proteins results in endosomal accumulation of cholesterol, some glycolipids, and selected gangliosides, causing axonal spheroid formation, particularly of the cerebellum, and hypomyelination with eventual demyelination of white matter tracts, especially of the corpus callosum, with hippocampal and cortical regions affected later.

Management is based on symptomatic therapy for seizures and some of the associated movement disorders, such as dystonia, nocturnal sedatives to improve sleep hygiene, and physical therapy to maintain mobility as long as possible. Carrier testing for at-risk relatives and prenatal testing for pregnancies at increased risk are possible when the two disease-causing mutations have been identified in the family.

SELECTED REFERENCES

Espay A, Biller J. *Concise neurology*. Philadelphia: Lippincott Williams & Wilkins, Wolters Kluwer Health, 2011.

Patterson M. Niemann-Pick Disease Type C. 2000 Jan 26 [Updated 2008 Jul 22]. In: Pagon RA, Bird TD, Dolan CR, et al., eds. *GeneReviews™ [Internet]*. Seattle (WA): University of Washington, 1993. Available from: http://www.ncbi.nlm.nih.gov/books/NBK1296/

Paulson H, Ammache Z. Ataxia and hereditary disorders. *Neurol Clin* 2001;19:759–782.

SEE QUESTIONS: 324, 325, 326

SECTION 7

DEMYELINATING DISORDERS

CASE 75

BILATERAL INTERNUCLEAR OPHTHALMOPLEGIA SECONDARY TO MULTIPLE SCLEROSIS

OBJECTIVES

- To briefly discuss multiple sclerosis.
- To highlight the main features of internuclear ophthalmoplegia (INO).

VIGNETTE

This 44-year-old woman had a history of neurologic symptoms dating back to her early teenage years. In her early 20s, she had an acute onset of vertigo, lower extremity weakness, and fatigue followed by progressive balance difficulties and urinary incontinence.

CASE SUMMARY

Our patient had intermittent symptoms, most notably fatigue, dizziness, leg weakness, poor balance, urinary impairment, and ocular dismotility for several years. Examination was notable for bilateral INO and a spastic and ataxic gait. She was diagnosed with multiple sclerosis (MS).

MS is a chronic demyelinating disease of the central nervous system (CNS) resulting in injury to the myelin sheaths, oligodendrocytes, and eventually axons. The clinical diagnosis of MS requires two temporally dissociated attacks of demyelination referable to two anatomically separate white matter pathways of the brain or spinal cord. Such definition can be met at the initial clinical event if magnetic resonance imaging (MRI) lesions are sufficient proof for dissemination in space and time, according to the McDonald criteria (2001). The clinical profile of MS can be classified as relapsing–remitting (RRMS 85%), progressive relapsing (PRMS), secondary progressive (SPMS), and primary progressive (PPMS). Most common symptoms at onset of MS are visual, oculomotor dysmotility, sensory disturbances, or incoordination. Approximately 20% of patients with MS present with optic neuritis (ON) as the first demyelinating event. Traditionally, MS has been diagnosed on the basis of clinical findings and supporting evidence from ancillary investigations such as MRI of the brain, and cerebrospinal fluid (CSF) analysis. However, CSF is no longer routine in the investigation of MS, although it remains useful when MRI is either nondiagnostic or not available.

In MS, the CSF cell count may be normal or show a modest increase in mononuclear leukocytes. The total CSF protein concentration is normal in two-thirds of patients or may show mild elevation in the other third. CSF immunoglobulin levels are typically elevated. The CSF IgG may be increased. The IgG index ([CSF IgG/serum IgG]/[CSF albumin/serum albumin]) is used to demonstrate an increased amount of IgG present in the CSF compared to serum. It is often greater than 0.7 in patients with MS. CSF protein electrophoresis frequently demonstrates the presence of oligoclonal bands (OCBs). OCBs may be present in 80% to 90% of patients. The presence of myelin basic protein (MBP), thought to correlate with active demyelination, is a nonspecific finding.

TABLE 75.1   SELECTED OCULOMOTOR BRAINSTEM SYNDROMES

Oculomotor Syndrome	Features	Localization
INO	Ipsilateral adduction paresis with contralateral abducting nystagmus	Ipsilateral MLF
Bilateral INO	Bilateral adduction weakness with exotropia and preserved convergence	Bilateral MLF
One-and-a-half syndrome	Ipsilateral INO plus horizontal gaze palsy (only contralateral eye abduction is preserved)	Ipsilateral CN VI/PPRF nucleus and adjacent MLF
Vertical saccade impairment	Impaired downward saccades	Ipsilateral riMLF lesions
Parinaud syndrome	Supranuclear vertical (upward) gaze palsy, light-near dissociation, convergence–retraction nystagmus, eyelid retraction (Collier sign)	Posterior commissure (dorsal midbrain)
Horizontal gaze palsy	Nuclear horizontal gaze palsy (away from affected pons)	Ipsilateral abducens nucleus
Ocular bobbing	Repetitive rapid conjugate downward eye movements with slow return to primary position	Central pons
Skew deviation	Acquired vertical eye misalignment and head tilt toward lower eye	Lesion anywhere in the brainstem affecting the connections between the vestibular and oculomotor nuclei

INO, internuclear ophthalmoplegia; MLF, medial longitudinal fasciculus; PPRF, paramedian pontine reticular formation.

In order to understand the ocular dysmotility shown by our patient, a basic understanding of applied neuroanatomy is required. The brainstem neurons responsible for conjugate horizontal saccadic eye movements are located in the paramedian pontine reticular formation (PPRF) and interneurons of the abducens nucleus. When gazing to the left, the left lateral rectus (abducens nerve) and the right medial rectus (oculomotor nerve) must activate synchronously. Axons of the abducens interneurons cross to the contralateral side in the lower pons and ascend in the medial longitudinal fasciculus (MLF) to the contralateral oculomotor nucleus. INO is characterized by impaired horizontal eye movements with impaired adduction of the affected eye and abduction nystagmus of the contralateral eye. The adduction weakness results from disruption of signals carried by the MLF destined for the oculomotor nucleus. An INO is named by the side of the lesion. Thus, a right INO results in impaired adduction of the right eye. An INO may or may not affect convergence, previously known as Cogan posterior INO and Cogan anterior INO, respectively. Unilateral or bilateral INOs in young adults most often result from MS.

The more common oculomotor syndromes arising from brainstem lesions are listed in Table 75.1.

SELECTED REFERENCES

Biller J, ed. *Practical neurology*, 4th ed. Philadelphia: Lippincott Williams & Wilkins, Wolters Kluwer Health, 2012.

Brazis PW, Masdeu JC, Biller J, eds. *Localization in clinical neurology*, 6th ed. Philadelphia: Lippincott Williams & Wilkins, Wolters Kluwer Health, 2011.

Espay A, Biller J. *Concise neurology*. Philadelphia: Lippincott Williams & Wilkins, Wolters Kluwer Health, 2011.

SEE QUESTIONS: 2, 28, 51, 62, 63, 111, 150, 168, 177, 180, 191, 193, 208, 209, 245

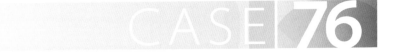

NYSTAGMUS/ATAXIA SECONDARY TO RELAPSING–REMITTING MULTIPLE SCLEROSIS

OBJECTIVES

- To discuss relapsing–remitting multiple sclerosis (MS).
- To discuss the treatment of MS.

VIGNETTE

A 27-year-old African-American woman had several episodes of neurologic deficits. The first event consisted of marked fatigue, decreased vision, and gait unsteadiness. The second event was characterized by decreased vision in both eyes. The third and fourth episodes were again characterized by impaired vision and disequilibrium.

CASE SUMMARY

This 27-year-old woman has had several episodes of neurologic dysfunction resulting in fatigue, blurred vision, and gait unsteadiness. Examination was notable for gaze-evoked nystagmus and an unsteady gait. Magnetic resonance imaging (MRI) showed increased T2 signal hyperintensities involving the left pons, and bilateral periventricular white matter. She was diagnosed with relapsing–remitting MS.

MS is a chronic demyelinating disease of the central nervous system (CNS) resulting in injury to the myelin sheaths, oligodendrocytes, and eventually axons. The clinical diagnosis of MS requires two temporally dissociated attacks of demyelination referable to two anatomically separate white matter pathways of the brain or spinal cord. The McDonald criteria for diagnosis of MS (Table 76.1) have resulted in earlier diagnosis of MS with a high degree of both specificity and sensitivity.

MS can affect any area of the CNS. Relapsing–remitting MS is the most common form of MS. Neurologic dysfunction may increase over days or weeks, then plateaus, and subsequently resolves over days or weeks. Initially, patients recover normal functioning after these attacks. MRI of the brain is the most helpful and sensitive neuroimaging tool to diagnose MS. MRI typically demonstrate multiple, often ovoid areas of increased T2 or fluid-attenuated inversion recovery (FLAIR) signal abnormalities in the periventricular

---

TABLE 76.1 McDONALD CRITERIA FOR DIAGNOSIS OF MS

1. Two or more attacks with objective clinical evidence of two or more clinical lesions is enough to make a diagnosis of MS
2. Two or more clinical attacks:
   a. But only one clearly defined lesion on clinical examination
   b. Fulfillment of additional criteria of dissemination on space may be evidenced by
      1. New MRI lesion
      2. Combination of an MRI lesion plus positive CSF findings or another clinical attack at a new site
3. Isolated clinical attack occurs; criteria for MS may be met if there are two or more lesions with evidence of dissemination in time by either
   a. New lesion by MRI or
   b. Second clinical attack
4. Clinically isolated syndrome with only one objective lesion PLUS can make a diagnosis of MS with
   a. Dissemination in space demonstrated by second MRI lesion with positive CSF findings
   b. Dissemination in time if demonstrated by
      1. MRI or
      2. Second clinical attack
5. Insidious progression of disease can lead to a diagnosis of MS:
   a. If disease has progressed for at least 1 y
   b. Two of the following three conditions are met:
      1. Positive brain MRI findings
      2. Positive spinal cord MRI findings (given more weight than previously)
      3. Positive CSF findings

CSF, cerebrospinal fluid.

white matter. These periventricular lesions may be confluent. Other typical MRI findings include involvement of the corpus callosum and involvement of U-fibers adjacent to cerebral cortex. Lesions may demonstrate gadolinium enhancement.

Management of acute MS exacerbations consists of intravenously administered methylprednisolone over 3 to 5 days in order to hasten recovery. A number of disease-modifying therapies have been proven to alter the course of relapsing–remitting MS. These medications include interferon beta (IFN-β) [IFN-β-1a] (Avonex, Rebif), IFN-β-1b (Betaseron), and glatiramer acetate (Copaxone). Mitoxantrone (Novantrone), a chemotherapeutic agent, has been shown to be helpful in worsening relapsing–remitting MS, but its use as a second-line agent is limited by cardiac toxicity. Fingolimod (Gilenya) and Teriflunomide (Aubagio) are oral therapies recently shown to reduce the frequency of MS exacerbations.

A number of other medications are used for symptomatic control of spasticity, fatigue, depression, urinary dysfunction, and neurogenic pain.

SELECTED REFERENCES

Biller J, ed. *Practical neurology*, 4th ed. Philadelphia: Lippincott Williams & Wilkins, Wolters Kluwer Health, 2012.

Bitsch A, Brück W. MRI—pathological correlates in MS. *Int MS J* 2001;8(3):89–95.

Mattson DH. Alphabet soup: a personal, evolving, mostly evidence-based and logical, sequential approach to the "ABCNR" drugs in multiple sclerosis. *Semin Neurol* 2002;22(1):17–25.

Pohlman CH, Reingold SC, Edan et al. Diagnostic criteria for multiple sclerosis: 2005 revisions to the "McDonald criteria." *Ann Neurol* 2005;58(6):840–846.

SEE QUESTIONS: 28, 51, 111, 150, 168, 177, 180, 191, 193, 208, 209, 245, 257

CASE 77

MULTIPLE SCLEROSIS (PONTINE LESION)

OBJECTIVES

- To discuss the clinical manifestations of a pontine lesion.
- To discuss ancillary tests used to diagnose multiple sclerosis (MS).

VIGNETTE

A 35-year-old man was admitted for evaluation of right and left hemibody numbness, incoordination, diplopia, and right-sided facial weakness.

CASE SUMMARY

This 35-year-old man was admitted with bilateral numbness, incoordination, diplopia, and right facial weakness. On examination he had paralysis of conjugate gaze to the right, right upper and lower facial muscle weakness, left hemiparesis leading to gross dysmetria on finger-to-nose and heel-to-shin testing, and an ataxic wide-based gait (ataxic hemiparesis). Magnetic resonance imaging (MRI) demonstrated a focus of high signal intensity in the pons at the level of the middle cerebellar peduncle (brachium pontis) and smaller areas of high signal intensity involving the subcortical white matter of both hemispheres. He was diagnosed with MS.

This combination of deficits has been referred to as the dorsal pontine syndrome and also as Foville syndrome (among those with meningovascular syphilis): ipsilateral gaze palsy and peripheral facial palsy with contralateral face-sparing hemiparesis. The gaze palsy (deviation of the eyes away from the side of the lesion, not overcome by oculocephalic maneuvers) is due to a lesion in the abducens nucleus, which coordinates the action of both eyes to produce horizontal gaze. The facial palsy is nuclear and fascicular, thus affecting the upper and lower face. On attempting to close the eye on the affected side, the right eyeball deviated up and slightly outward. Known as Bell phenomenon, this is due to relaxation of the inferior rectus and contraction of the superior rectus. The Bell phenomenon is a normal response that becomes apparent due to weakness of ipsilateral eyelid closure. However, it may be absent in about 10% of normal people. Although MRI showed smaller areas of high signal intensity in the subcortical white matter of both hemispheres, the right pontine lesion accounted for most of his clinical findings.

MS is diagnosed on the basis of clinical findings and supporting evidence from ancillary investigations, such as MRI of the brain, and exclusion of alternative diagnosis. Spinal cord or optic nerve imaging may be indicated in selected cases. Approximately 20% of patients with MS present with optic neuritis (ON) as the first demyelinating event, while about 40% of patients experience ON at some other point during the course of the disease. Spinal cord involvement has a predilection for the dorsolateral cervical spinal cord. The previously described McDonald criteria (Table 76.1) have been further revised.

Evoked responses evaluate the integrity of central and peripheral nervous system pathways and may be helpful in selected instances. Visual evoked responses (VER) may show conduction defects in the central visual pathways. The major positive deflection at the latency of approximately 100 ms (the P100 response) is the most useful clinically and may assist in the detection of a clinically "silent" lesion in a patient suspected of having MS. Somatosensory evoked potentials (SSEPs) and brainstem auditory evoked potentials (BAEPs) may show defects in the somatosensory and auditory pathways, respectively. However, SSEPs and BAEPs are no longer of major diagnostic utility in patients with MS.

SELECTED REFERENCES

Biller J, ed. *Practical neurology*, 4th ed. Philadelphia: Lippincott Williams & Wilkins, Wolters Kluwer Health, 2012.

Brazis PW, Masdeu JC, Biller J, eds. *Localization in clinical neurology*, 6th ed. Philadelphia: Lippincott Williams & Wilkins, Wolters Kluwer Health, 2011.

Polman CH, Reingold SC, Banwell B, et al. Diagnostic criteria for multiple sclerosis: 2010 revisions of the McDonald criteria. *Ann Neurol* 2011;69:292–302.

SEE QUESTIONS: 28, 51, 111, 150, 152, 168, 180, 191, 193, 208, 209, 245

CASE 78

SPASTIC GAIT/DYSARTHRIA DUE TO PRIMARY PROGRESSIVE MULTIPLE SCLEROSIS

OBJECTIVES

■ To discuss primary progressive multiple sclerosis (MS).
■ To discuss the treatment of primary progressive MS.

VIGNETTE

This 65-year-old man presented with a 4-year history of left-leg stiffness and weakness. He complained that his left foot will "slap" when walking. A lumbar laminectomy had not improved his symptoms. Recently, his wife noted his speech was slurred.

CASE SUMMARY

This 65-year-old man had a 4-year history of progressive lower extremity weakness and stiffness, and more recently he had slurred speech. Examination was remarkable for spasticity in both legs, a weak left leg, a left Babinski sign, and a spastic gait. He was diagnosed with primary progressive MS.

Most patients with MS have a relapsing course of the disease, but about 1 in 10 people do not. Progressive forms of MS include primary progressive (PPMS), secondary progressive (SPMS), and progressive relapsing (PRMS). Primary progressive MS (PPMS) occurs in approximately 10% to 15% of patients with MS. PPMS is characterized by steady disease progression from onset with no overt exacerbations or remissions. Occasional plateaus and temporary minor improvements are allowed. By far the most common clinical presentation is a progressive myelopathy often with spastic paraparesis. A small minority of patients present with a progressive cerebellar syndrome. Among patients with PPMS, magnetic resonance imaging (MRI) of the brain and spinal cord show few gadolinium enhancing lesions. PPMS is associated with less inflammation and more neurodegenerative pathology. Because of its slowly progressive nature, other disorders to entertain in the differential diagnosis of a 65-year-old man with spastic paraparesis are primary lateral sclerosis and hereditary spastic paraparesis, both of which can be complicated with dysarthria and dysphagia.

PPMS is more refractory to treatment than any of the other forms of MS. None of the currently available immunomodulatory therapies (interferon β-1a, interferon β-1b, glatiramer acetate and mitoxantrone) have been shown to be definitively helpful and have not been approved by the U.S. Food and Drug Administration (FDA) to treat PPMS.

A number of medications can be considered in PPMS including short courses of high-dose intravenous methylprednisolone, methotrexate, cyclophosphamide, cladribine, azathioprine, and intravenous gamma globulin. Unfortunately, none of these strategies have been proven to be of sustained benefit in these patients, and moreover, they carry the potential for considerable side effects.

SELECTED REFERENCES

Biller J, ed. *Practical neurology*, 4th ed. Philadelphia: Lippincott Williams & Wilkins, Wolters Kluwer Health, 2012.

Mattson DH. Alphabet soup: a personal, evolving, mostly evidence-based and logical, sequential approach to the "ABCNR" drugs in multiple sclerosis. *Semin Neurol* 2002;22(March):17–25.

McDonnell GV, Hawkins SA. Primary progressive multiple sclerosis: increasing clarity but many unanswered questions. *J Neurol Sci* 2002;199:1–15.

Polman CH, Reingold SC, Banwell B, et al. Diagnostic criteria for multiple sclerosis: 2010 revisions of the McDonald criteria. *Ann Neurol* 2011;69:292–302.

Thompson AJ, Polman CH, Miller DH, et al. Primary progressive multiple sclerosis. *Brain* 1997;120:1085–1096.

SEE QUESTIONS: 111, 150, 168, 191, 193, 208, 209, 245

SECTION 8

NEURO-OPHTHALMOLOGY

CASE 79

HORNER SYNDROME IN PATIENT WITH WALLENBERG SYNDROME

OBJECTIVE

- To review the neuro-ophthalmological manifestations of vertebrobasilar dissections.

VIGNETTE

A 39-year-old woman had sudden onset of severe left posterior neck pain, left face numbness, and left-sided incoordination. She veered to the left, vomited on numerous occasions, and had drooping of her left eyelid. Subsequently, she noted impaired heat perception on the right hemibody and dysesthesias of the right leg. She had no vertigo, diplopia, dysarthria, tinnitus, hearing loss, or hiccups. She had had no prior spinal manipulations or neck injuries.

CASE SUMMARY

Our patient had a classic history of a lateral medullary (Wallenberg) syndrome. She had a left vertebral artery dissection. In addition to her residual dysesthetic sensory symptomatology, she had a preganglionic left Horner syndrome due to involvement of the hypothalamospinal pathway at the dorsolateral brainstem tegmentum. A Horner syndrome results from underactivity of the oculosympathetic pathway and is characterized by miosis, partial eyelid ptosis, and at times facial anhidrosis. The anisocoria is more pronounced in darkness, a typical feature of Horner compared to other forms of anisocoria (Fig. 79.1). The affected pupil dilates more slowly than the normal pupil (dilation lag). Other neuro-ophthalmological manifestations of vertebrobasilar dissections include diplopia, nystagmus, oscillopsia, ocular misalignment, skew deviation, ocular motor nerve palsies (CN III, IV, and VI), lateral gaze palsy, internuclear ophthalmoplegia, and homonymous visual field defects.

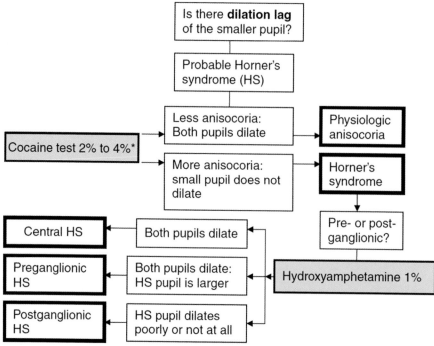

Figure 79.1 Diagnostic Algorithm When Anisocoria Is Greater in Dim Light (Smaller Pupil Abnormal). *Apraclonidine (0.5% to 1%) is an alternative to cocaine. (From Espay AJ, Biller J. *Concise neurology*. Philadelphia: Lippincott Williams & Wilkins, Wolters Kluwer Health, 2011, with permission.)

The lateral medullary syndrome is due to occlusion of the intracranial vertebral artery or less commonly its prebasilar offshoot, the posterior inferior cerebellar artery (PICA). Horner syndrome can also occur within the context of anterior or carotid circulation stroke, in which case it is always postganglionic. Indeed, an acute and painful Horner syndrome should be considered due to an acute internal carotid artery dissection until proven otherwise. Hydroxyamphetamine 1% given after cocaine or apraclonidine can help distinguish a preganglionic (both pupils dilate, with the affected pupil becoming larger) versus a postganglionic Horner syndrome (the affected pupil dilates poorly or none) (Fig. 79.1).

SELECTED REFERENCES

Espay AJ, Biller J. *Concise neurology*. Philadelphia: Lippincott Williams & Wilkins, Wolters Kluwer Health, 2011.

Love BB, Biller J. Neurovascular system. In: Goetz G, ed. *Textbook of clinical neurology*. Philadelphia: WB Saunders, 2003:395–424.

Love BB, Biller J. Stroke in young adults. In: Samuels MA, Keske SF, eds. *Office practice of neurology*, 2nd ed. New York: Churchill Livingstone, 2003:337–358.

SEE QUESTIONS: 59, 113, 114

CASE 80

ADIE TONIC PUPIL/ROSS SYNDROME

OBJECTIVES

- To demonstrate a tonic pupil (Adie tonic pupil).
- To show testing for light-near dissociation.
- To review pharmacological testing for patients with a tonic pupil.
- To review manifestations of Holmes-Adie and Ross syndromes.

VIGNETTE

A 49-year-old man had frequent episodes of heat exhaustion and excessive sweating involving the left lower quadrant of his back, associated with lack of sweating on his forehead, axilla, hands, and feet. He also had difficulty focusing with his left eye.

CASE SUMMARY

Our patient had episodes of heat exhaustion associated with hyperhidrosis and segmental anhidrosis. He also had problems with accommodation of his left eye. Examination was remarkable for anisocoria (left pupil larger than right pupil) with absent reaction to light but with a slow constriction to prolonged near effort (light-near dissociation). Redilation after constriction (not shown) was slow and tonic. The patellar and ankle reflexes were absent.

Our patient had a tonic pupil. Tonic pupils result from damage to the ciliary ganglion or the short ciliary nerves, as part of a widespread autonomic neuropathy, or in otherwise healthy individuals (Adie tonic pupil syndrome). Unlike Horner syndrome, Adie syndrome creates an anisocoria greater in bright light because the magnitude of the deficit is magnified when only the unaffected contralateral pupil reacts to light. In general, lack of light response in a large pupil can be due to either Adie syndrome or an old third cranial nerve palsy if unilateral, or a dorsal midbrain syndrome due to a mesencephalic tectal tumor or neurosyphilis (Argyll Robertson pupil) (Fig. 80.1). However, Adie syndrome may be unilateral or bilateral (it tends to become bilateral at a rate of about 4% per year) and may be associated with depressed or absent patellar and ankle reflexes, in which case it is referred to as Holmes-Adie syndrome. Ross syndrome applies to the combination of a tonic pupil, hypo- or areflexia, and progressive segmental hypohidrosis with compensatory hyperhidrosis.

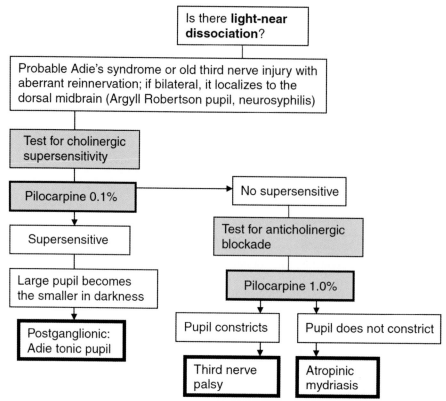

Figure 80.1   Diagnostic Algorithm When Anisocoria Is Greater in Bright Light (Larger Pupil Abnormal). Mechanical anisocoria where pupilloconstriction is subnormal in the abnormal, larger pupil, may be seen in angle-closure glaucoma, trauma, infection, inflammation (prior uveitis), iris tumor or mass (iris melanoma), and laser treatment. (From Espay AJ, Biller J. *Concise neurology.* Philadelphia: Lippincott Williams & Wilkins, Wolters Kluwer Health, 2011, with permission.)

SELECTED REFERENCES

Corbett JJ. The bedside and office neuro-ophthalmology examination. *Semin Neurol* 2003;23(1):63–76.

Espay AJ, Biller J. *Concise neurology.* Philadelphia: Lippincott Williams & Wilkins, Wolters Kluwer Health, 2011.

Thompson HS, Miller NR. Disorders of pupillary function, accommodation, and lacrimation. In: Miller NR, Newman NJ, eds. *Walsh and Hoyt's clinical neuro-ophthalmology,* 5th ed. Baltimore: Williams & Wilkins, 1998:1016–1018.

Weller M, Wilhelm H, Sommer N, et al. Tonic pupil, areflexia, and segmental anhidrosis. Two cases of Ross syndrome and review of the literature. *J Neurol* 1992;239:231–234.

SEE QUESTIONS: 113, 114, 135

CASE 81

NONARTERITIC ANTERIOR ISCHEMIC OPTIC NEUROPATHY

OBJECTIVES

- To list the most common symptom of nonarteritic anterior ischemic optic neuropathy (NA-AION).
- To recognize the most common signs and causes of NA-AION.
- To describe the most common visual field abnormalities observed in NA-AION.

VIGNETTE

A 44-year-old woman awoke with a scotoma involving the superior visual field of the oculus dexter (OD). On examination, visual acuity was 20/30 OD and 20/20 oculus sinister (OS). She had right optic disc swelling and a partial superior altitudinal visual field defect of the OD. Erythrocyte sedimentation rate (ESR) and C-reactive protein (CRP) were normal.

CASE SUMMARY

Our patient experienced painless visual loss of her right eye (OD). She had no systemic symptoms such as anorexia, weight loss, jaw claudication, headaches, or scalp tenderness. She took one tablet of sumatriptan, as she thought she had a migrainous aura. Examination was remarkable for decreased visual acuity of the OD, right optic disc edema, and right relative afferent pupillary defect (RAPD). Magnetic resonance imaging (MRI) of the brain and orbits was normal. Magnetic resonance angiography (MRA) of the intracranial vessels showed narrowing of the right proximal (A1) segment of the anterior cerebral artery (ACA). Catheter cerebral arteriography showed an occluded supraclinoid right inferior cerebellar artery (ICA) after the origin of the ophthalmic artery. There was also an occluded right P2 segment with a hypoplastic right P1 segment of the posterior cerebral artery (PCA). ESR, CRP, and plasma homocysteine were normal. She was heterozygous for the methylenetetrahydrofolate reductase (MTHFR) C677T gene mutation.

Our patient had an anterior ischemic optic neuropathy (AION). Ischemic optic neuropathy may affect the anterior part of the optic nerve (AION) or a segment of the posterior aspect of the optic nerve (posterior ischemic optic neuropathy or PION). AION may be arteritic (A-AION) or non-arteritic (NA-AION). PION may be arteritic (A-PION), nonarteritic (NA-PION), or surgical/postoperative.

NA-AION is characterized by acute painless monocular visual loss. Visual impairment ranges from a central scotoma to complete monocular visual loss. Examination may show poor visual acuity on the affected eye, although visual acuity may be normal. There is a swollen or edematous optic disc often associated with flame hemorrhages or cotton wool spots around the disc and a relative afferent pupillary defect (RAPD). A combination of a relative inferior altitudinal visual field defect with an absolute inferior nasal defect is the most commonly observed visual field pattern in NA-AION.

AION results from occlusion of the posterior ciliary arteries. Nocturnal arterial hypotension is a frequent precipitant of NA-AION. NA-AION seldom results from ICA steno-occlusive disease. NA-AION may be associated with arterial hypertension, diabetes mellitus, migraines, dyslipidemia, collagen vascular disease, thrombophilic states including the antiphospholipid antibody syndrome (APAS), nocturnal arterial hypotension, profound acute blood loss, or following cataract extraction. NA-AION has also been reported in association with the use of phosphodiesterase-5 inhibitors. A small cup-to-disc ratio ("disc at risk") is now considered to be secondary contributing factor.

Giant cell arteritis is the most common cause of arteritic AION. A-AION results in more severe visual loss than NA-AION. Severity of visual field defects is also more marked in cases of A-AION, and the optic disc swelling has a chalky white appearance.

Our patient was diagnosed as having an NA-AION and was treated with aspirin, verapamil, and a combination of folic acid, pyridoxine, and cobalamin. She was advised to avoid sympathomimetic or vasoconstrictive drugs. Optic nerve sheath decompression is not indicated in patients with NA-AION.

SELECTED REFERENCES

Brouzas D, Charakidas A, Andrioti E, et al. Non-arteritic anterior ischemic optic neuropathy associated with coexistent factor V Leiden and methylenetetrahydrofolate reductase mutations. *Neuro-Ophthalmology* 2001;26:201–204.

Hayreh SS. Erectile dysfunction drugs and non-arteritic anterior ischemic optic neuropathy: is there a cause and effect relationship? *J Neuroophthalmol* 2005; 25: 295–298.

Hayreh SS. Ischemic optic neuropathy. *Prog Retin Eye Res* 2009;28:34–62.

The Ischemic Optic Neuropathy Decompression Trial Research Group. Optic nerve decompression for non-arteritic ischemic optic neuropathy (NAION) is not effective and may be harmful. *JAMA* 1995;273:625–632.

Lee AG, Brazis PW. *Clinical pathways in neuro-ophthalmology. An evidence-based approach.* New York: Thieme, 1998.

SEE QUESTIONS: 43, 44, 45, 90, 112, 147, 196, 223, 256

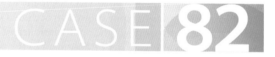

POSTOPERATIVE ACUTE LEFT CN III PALSY

OBJECTIVES

- To demonstrate characteristic findings of a third cranial nerve palsy.
- To describe the phenomenology of aberrant regeneration of the third cranial nerve.

VIGNETTE

Following surgery of an intracranial mass lesion, a 60-year-old woman complained of a droopy left eyelid and diplopia.

Our patient had a recent craniotomy for an intracranial mass. On examination, she had complete left eyelid ptosis. Upon lifting her drooped eyelid, she had exotropia (lateral deviation) and hypotropia (downward deviation) of the left eye. She also had anisocoria; the left pupil measured 5 mm in diameter, and the right pupil measured 2 mm in diameter. There was no constriction directly or consensually of the left pupil. She had impaired adduction (medial rectus muscle), supraduction (superior rectus and inferior oblique muscles), and infraduction (inferior rectus muscle) of the left eye. On attempted adduction of the left eye, there was normal depression and intorsion (superior oblique muscle). She had full abduction of the left eye (lateral rectus muscle). Range of eye movements of the right eye was completely normal.

Normal contraction of the medial rectus muscle produces adduction (inward turning), whereas abduction (outward turning) is driven by the lateral rectus muscle. The superior and inferior recti muscles are best evaluated on abduction. Elevation in abduction is caused by the superior rectus muscle. Depression of the globe in abduction is caused by the inferior rectus muscle. The oblique muscles are best evaluated on adduction. Elevation of the eye on adduction is caused by the inferior oblique muscle. Depression of the globe in adduction is caused by the superior oblique.

Why could she not open her left eye? With a third cranial nerve lesion, eye opening is impaired. The levator palpebrae superioris, innervated by the third nerve, plays the major role in eyelid opening. On the other hand, with a cranial nerve VII lesion, eyelid closure (orbicularis oculi) is impaired, and the palpebral fissure is wider. Why did she have anisocoria? Two iris muscles regulate pupil size. The sphincter (pupilloconstrictor) is innervated by the parasympathetic system, and the dilator (pupillodilator) is innervated by the sympathetic system. As a result of parasympathetic dysfunction, there was unrestrained activity of the sympathetic pupillodilator and the left pupil became larger and unreactive to light.

In summary, our patient had a left third cranial nerve (CN III) palsy characterized by complete eyelid ptosis, pupillary dilation, impaired pupillary reaction to light, and impaired adduction, supraduction, and infraduction. The third nerve innervates the levator palpebrae superioris; the superior, inferior, and medial recti; the inferior oblique muscles; and the pupillary constrictors (sphincter pupillae muscle and ciliary muscles). Lesions can affect the third nerve in the midbrain (nucleus or fascicular portion), in the subarachnoid space, in the cavernous sinus, at the superior orbital fissure, or in the orbit.

The oculomotor nuclear complex is located in the midbrain, rostral to the level of the nucleus of cranial nerve IV. The fascicular portion of the third nerve travels ventrally traversing the red nucleus and exits anteriorly, medial to the cerebral peduncles. In the subarachnoid space, each third nerve passes between the posterior cerebral and superior cerebellar arteries. At the internal carotid-posterior communicating artery junction, aneurysms may cause a complete CN III palsy. The third nerve then enters the lateral wall of the cavernous sinus. The fourth cranial nerve and the first division of the trigeminal nerve (V1) also lie along the lateral wall of the cavernous sinus, whereas the sixth cranial nerve and the oculosympathetic fibers lie more medially. Once it reaches the superior orbital fissure, the third nerve divides into a superior division that innervates the levator palpebrae muscles and the superior rectus and an inferior division that innervates the medial and inferior recti, the inferior oblique, and the presynaptic parasympathetic outflow to the ciliary ganglion.

Magnetic resonance imaging (MRI) with gadolinium demonstrated a large left cavernous sinus/sphenoid wing mass that proved to be a meningioma. Cranial nerves III, IV,

VI, and V1 and the ophthalmic division of cranial nerve V (V1) sympathetic/parasympathetic connections are present in the cavernous sinus. Blood supply to the cavernous cranial nerves arises from the inferolateral trunk of the internal carotid artery (ICA) and, in some cases, from the accessory meningeal artery. Sympathetic fibers extend along the intradural ICA, whereas the parasympathetic fibers and ganglion cells are associated with the cavernous ICA. Lesions affecting the third nerve in the cavernous sinus may be painless or painful. They may occur in isolation or may often compromise cranial nerves four (CN IV), six (CN VI), and the ophthalmic division of cranial nerve five (V1).

Compressive lesions of the third nerve in the cavernous sinus may spare the pupil. Conversely, a third nerve palsy associated with a small pupil (Horner syndrome) due to oculosympathetic compromise virtually localizes the lesion to the cavernous sinus. Another clue of a cavernous sinus localization for a third nerve palsy is the concurrent presence of trochlear palsy (superior oblique weakness), but its testing is difficult because testing requires adduction, which cannot be performed. Instead, the patient should be instructed to abduct the eye and then look down. If the trochlear nerve is intact, there will be intorsion.

Features of primary aberrant regeneration also help localize the lesion to the cavernous sinus and exclude a primary vasculopathic injury such as a diabetic third nerve palsy. Signs of aberrant regeneration of the third cranial nerve include the following: retraction and elevation of the lid on downward gaze (pseudo–Graefe sign); elevation of the involved lid on attempted adduction of the eye (gaze lid dyskinesis); retraction of the globe on attempted vertical eye movements; adduction of the involved eye on attempted elevation or depression; lack of pupillary reactivity to light, but adequate response when the medial rectus muscle, inferior rectus muscle, or elevators of the eye are activated (pseudo–Argyll Robertson pupil); delayed onset abduction defect; and lagophthalmos.

Aberrant regeneration of the third nerve usually follows injury from intracavernous aneurysms, following aneurysm surgery, or trauma. Aberrant regeneration of the third cranial nerve has also been reported in cases of ophthalmoplegic migraine, a β-lipoproteinemia, and in cases of idiopathic oculomotor nerve palsies.

Differential diagnosis of cavernous sinus lesions also includes intracavernous aneurysms, carotid-cavernous fistulas, pituitary adenoma, pituitary apoplexy, metastases, schwannomas, infections such as mucormycosis or aspergillosis, and idiopathic granulomatous inflammation of the cavernous sinus (Tolosa-Hunt syndrome).

SELECTED REFERENCES

Brazis PW, Masdeu JC, Biller J. *Localization in clinical neurology*, 6th ed. Philadelphia: Lippincott Williams & Wilkins, Wolters Kluwer Health, 2011.

Carrasco JR, Savino PJ, Bilyk JR. Primary aberrant oculomotor nerve regeneration from a posterior communicating artery aneurysm. *Arch Ophthalmol* 2002;120:663–665.

Rush JA, Younge BR. Paralysis of cranial nerves III, IV, and VI. *Arch Ophthalmol* 1981;99(1):76–79.

Tytle TL, Punukollu PK. Carotid cavernous fistula. In: Biller J ed. *Seminars in cerebrovascular diseases and stroke*. Philadelphia: WB Saunders, 2001;1:83–111.

SEE QUESTIONS: 113, 114, 142, 194, 195, 196, 197, 229, 235

CASE 83

PROGRESSIVE LEFT CN III PALSY SECONDARY TO CAVERNOUS SINUS MASS LESION

OBJECTIVES

■ To demonstrate the characteristic pattern of a third nerve palsy.
■ To discuss differential diagnosis of cavernous sinus mass lesions.

VIGNETTE

A 38-year-old man had a 6-year history of painless progressive left eyelid drooping, impaired near vision, and horizontal diplopia.

CASE SUMMARY

Our patient had a 6-year history of progressive painless left upper eyelid ptosis and binocular horizontal diplopia, worse on gaze to the right. He also noticed a larger left pupil and had blurred vision of his left eye when looking at near objects.

On examination, visual acuity was 20/20 on the right eye (OD) and 20/25 on the left eye (OS). Confrontation visual fields were normal. On funduscopy, the appearance of the discs, maculae, vessels, and periphery was normal. On center gaze, there was a slight exotropia (lateral deviation) and hypotropia (downward deviation) of the left eye. The range of eye movements was normal on the right eye. There was left upper eyelid ptosis.

He had inability to fully adduct his left eye. With the left eye abducted, he had weakness of elevation and depression of that eye. On attempted adduction of the left eye, there was restricted elevation but normal depression and intorsion. He had full abduction of the left eye. The right pupil measured 2 mm in diameter, and the left measured 4 mm. There was no apparent constriction directly or consensually of the left pupil. Corneal sensation was normal. There was no hypesthesia of the left forehead or cheek.

Our patient had a left third nerve (CN III) palsy characterized by eyelid ptosis, pupillary dilation, impaired pupillary reaction to light, and limitation of adduction (medial rectus muscle), supraduction (superior rectus and inferior oblique muscles), and infraduction (inferior rectus muscle). The third nerve innervates the levator palpebrae superioris; the superior, inferior, and medial recti; the inferior oblique muscles; and the pupillary constrictors (sphincter pupillae muscle and ciliary muscles). Lesions can affect the third nerve in the midbrain (nucleus or fascicular portion), in the subarachnoid space, in the cavernous sinus, at the superior orbital fissure, or in the orbit.

Magnetic resonance imaging (MRI) with gadolinium showed a left cavernous sinus/medial sphenoid wing mass. Lesions affecting the third nerve in the cavernous sinus may be painless or painful. They may occur in isolation or may compromise the trochlear (CN IV), abducens (CN VI), and the ophthalmic division of the trigeminal cranial nerve (V1). Compressive lesions of the oculomotor nerve in the cavernous sinus may spare the pupil.

Conversely, a third nerve palsy associated with a small pupil (Horner syndrome) due to oculosympathetic compromise virtually localizes the lesion to the cavernous sinus. Features of primary aberrant regeneration also help localize the lesion to the cavernous sinus.

Our patient had a left frontotemporal orbitozygomatic craniotomy with subtotal resection of a left cavernous sinus meningioma. Meningiomas account for approximately 15% to 20% of intracranial tumors. Meningiomas are slow-growing tumors and are the most common extraaxial tumors. Meningiomas arise from arachnoid cells and are more common in women than in men. Most meningiomas are supratentorial. Frequent locations are parasagittal along the falx cerebri and laterally over the cerebral convexity. Other important locations are the olfactory groove, sphenoid wing, juxtasellar region, tentorium, posterior fossa (petrosal), foramen magnum, and clivus. Occasionally, meningiomas are intraventricular. Spinal meningiomas account for approximately 10% of all meningiomas and predominate in the thoracic spine.

Differential diagnosis of cavernous sinus lesions also includes intracavernous aneurysms, carotid-cavernous fistulas, pituitary adenoma, pituitary apoplexy, metastases, schwannomas, infections such as mucormycosis or aspergillosis, and idiopathic granulomatous inflammation of the cavernous sinus (Tolosa-Hunt syndrome). Most patients with ischemic (vasculopathic) third nerve palsies have pupillary sparing and recover within 8 to 12 weeks.

SELECTED REFERENCES

Ayerbe J, Lobato RD, de la Cruz J, et al. Risk factors predicting recurrence in patients operated on for intracranial meningioma. A multivariate analysis. *Acta Neurochir (Wien)* 1999;141:921–932.

Biller J, ed. *Practical neurology*, 4th ed. Philadelphia: Lippincott Williams & Wilkins, Wolters Kluwer Health, 2012.

Brazis PW, Masdeu JC, Biller J. *Localization in clinical neurology*, 6th ed. Philadelphia: Lippincott Williams & Wilkins, Wolters Kluwer Health, 2011.

Rush JA, Younge BR. Paralysis of cranial nerves III, IV, and VI. *Arch Ophthalmol* 1981;99(1):76–79.

SEE QUESTIONS: 13, 113, 114, 142, 194, 195, 196, 197

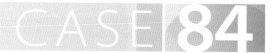

ABDUCENS PALSY

OBJECTIVES

- To describe diagnostic criteria of an abducens (CN VI) palsy.
- To review the topographical locations accounting for CN VI palsy.
- To describe potential causes of CN VI palsy.

VIGNETTE

An 82-year-old man with arterial hypertension and hyperlipidemia was referred for evaluation of headaches and horizontal diplopia.

CASE SUMMARY

 Our patient had a history of horizontal nonpositional headaches and sudden onset of binocular diplopia. He had a more pronounced horizontal separation of the images when looking at a distance. There was no associated scalp or occipital tenderness, eyelid ptosis, or history of thyroid disease. There was no diurnal variation of the diplopia and no fatigability. There was no history of diabetes, sore shoulders or hips, anorexia, weight loss, fever, or jaw claudication. On examination, he had impaired abduction (lateral rectus muscle) of the right eye and nasal deviation (esotropia) of the right eye in center gaze. There was no proptosis, chemosis, or lid swelling. He had no evidence of eyelid ptosis, papilledema, or a Horner syndrome. The remainder of his neurologic examination was unremarkable.

Magnetic resonance imaging (MRI) of the brain showed changes compatible with small vessel ischemic disease. There were no brainstem acute ischemic changes on diffusion-weighted MRI. Magnetic resonance angiography (MRA) showed minimal tortuosity of the vertebrobasilar system, but no dolichoectasia, aneurysms, or vascular abnormalities. MRI of the orbits was unremarkable.

Our patient had an isolated abducens (CN VI) palsy. There was no evidence of ipsilateral gaze palsy as seen with lesions involving the abducens nucleus. The abducens nucleus is located in the dorsal lower aspect of the pons. The abducens nerve exits ventrally at the level of the horizontal sulcus between the pons and medulla and courses anterolaterally passing over the petrous apex to enter the lateral wall of the cavernous sinus. Along with the oculomotor nerve (CN III) and trochlear nerve (CN IV), the CN VI nerve enters the orbit through the superior orbital fissure to innervate the lateral rectus muscle.

Movement of the eye nasally is termed adduction; temporal movement is termed abduction. Elevation and depression of the eye are termed supraduction and infraduction, respectively. Intorsion refers to nasal rotation of the 12 o'clock position on the vertical meridian; extorsion is temporal rotation of the 12 o'clock position on the vertical meridian. The abducens nerve supplies the lateral rectus muscle. The lateral rectus muscle has only horizontal actions and is the primary abductor of the eye.

A sixth nerve palsy may result from nuclear, fascicular, subarachnoid, cavernous, or orbital lesions. Etiologies of sixth nerve palsies are myriad including ischemic and hemorrhagic disorders; aneurysms or other vascular anomalies; demyelinating, neoplastic, metabolic, traumatic, and inflammatory/infectious disorders; hydrocephalus; raised intracranial pressure; or cerebrospinal fluid (CSF) hypotension. However, despite extensive investigations, the etiology of a sixth nerve palsy remains undetermined in a considerable number of adults and children.

As in our patient, the most common etiologic factor of a sixth nerve palsy in older adults is microvascular occlusion of the abducens nerve, also known as a vasculopathic sixth nerve palsy. Most vasculopathic sixth nerve palsies recover over a period of 3 to 6 months. Isolated sixth nerve palsies have also been described with pontine strokes. Our patient had a complete resolution of symptoms in 3 months.

SELECTED REFERENCES

Biller J, ed. *Practical neurology,* 4th ed. Philadelphia: Lippincott Williams & Wilkins, Wolters Kluwer Health, 2012.

Brazis PW, Masdeu JC, Biller J. *Localization in clinical neurology,* 6th ed. Philadelphia: Lippincott Williams & Wilkins, Wolters Kluwer Health, 2011.

Fukutake T, Hirayama K. Isolated abducens nerve palsy from pontine infarction in a diabetic patient. *Neurology* 1992;42:226.

Rush JA, Younge BR. Paralysis of cranial nerves III, IV, and VI. *Arch Ophthalmol* 1981;99(1):76–79.

SEE QUESTIONS: 215, 235

CASE 85

CHRONIC PROGRESSIVE EXTERNAL OPHTHALMOPLEGIA

OBJECTIVES

- To discuss the clinical features of chronic progressive external ophthalmoplegia (CPEO).
- To review inheritance patterns of CPEO.
- To discuss the differential diagnosis of CPEO with myasthenia gravis.

VIGNETTE

At the age of 23, this 48-year-old woman complained of diplopia. Thereafter, she had a history of stepwise bilateral impairment of eye movements. On examination, VA was 20/30 OD, pinhole increased the acuity to 20/20; 20/100 OS, pinhole increased the acuity to 20/40. Visual fields were full. Funduscopy was normal, without pigmentary retinopathy. Pupils were 4 and 4.5 mm in diameter with normal reaction to light. There was no relative afferent pupillary defect (RAPD). Ocular motility is shown in the video.

CASE SUMMARY

At the age of 23, our patient had diplopia due to abduction weakness of the right eye. This was preceded by a 2-week history of a sharp needlelike pain behind that eye. Thereafter, she had a history of stepwise bilateral impairment of eye movements. About 8 years prior to this assessment, she noted severe ptosis of the left upper lid. Because of the marked ophthalmoplegia of the right eye and tonic deviation downward of that eye, she had strabismus surgery to elevate the globe. She continued to suffer from intermittent headaches.

Subsequently, she noted bowel incontinence and occasional dizziness, probably related to head movements and her severe eye movement impairment. She also had occasional dull bitemporal headaches and had more difficulty with nocturnal vision. She had no skeletal muscle weakness, hearing loss, seizures, incoordination, diabetes, or other endocrinopathy. She had no diurnal variability of her left eyelid ptosis or dry eyes.

On examination, she was of normal stature. There was a slight chin-up head position and complete left upper lid ptosis. There was no exophthalmos. Visual acuity was 20/30-1 in the OD; pinhole increased acuity to 20/20. Visual acuity in the OS was 20/100; pinhole increased acuity to 20/40. Confrontation visual fields were full. On color vision examination, she identified 11 out of 15 plates with each eye. Funduscopy showed normal appearance of the discs, vessels, and periphery. There was a slight enhancement of the pigmentation in the macula, but no definite sign of pigmentary retinopathy. Ocular motility showed marked restriction of range of movements in every direction of gaze, with lack of horizontal movements and slowed saccades on the minimal residual vertical gaze. Oculocephalic and Bell eye movements were absent. Remainder of the neurologic examination was unremarkable.

Our patient had extensive unrevealing evaluations, including magnetic resonance imaging (MRI) of the orbits and brain, cerebrospinal fluid (CSF) analyses, edrophonium (Tensilon) test, thyroid function tests, and blood tests for mitochondrial disorders. Serum lactic acid and pyruvic acid were normal. An electroretinogram was performed for photopic and scotopic reactions; the results were normal. Repetitive stimulation studies and single-fiber electromyography (EMG) were unremarkable in many occasions. Chest computed tomography (CT) was normal. Biopsy of the left vastus lateralis muscle showed moderate perifascicular atrophy, mild angulated muscle fibers, and increased fat in the muscle fibers, findings that were not conclusive. There were no ragged-red fibers on Gomori trichrome stain. Southern blot analysis of the skeletal muscle mitochondrial DNA was normal.

She also had a biopsy of two of her extraocular muscles that were fibrotic in nature. Acetylcholine receptor antibodies, except for only one occasion that yielded a positive result, were not detectable. Antistriational (skeletal) antibodies and anti-MuSK antibodies were not detectable. Electrocardiogram (EKG) did not show any conduction abnormality. Trials of coenzyme Q (CoQ10), vitamin E, menadione (vitamin K$_3$), riboflavin, carnitine, corticosteroids, cholinesterase inhibitors (Mestinon), mycophenolate mofetil, and intravenous immunoglobulin therapy were unsuccessful.

Our patient probably had an unusual presentation of chronic progressive external ophthalmoplegia (CPEO). CPEO encompasses different conditions characterized by slowly progressive paralysis of the external ocular muscles combined with ptosis. Patients typically have bilateral and symmetrical ophthalmoparesis and ptosis. The ciliary and iris muscles are not involved. Due to the symmetric restriction of eye movements, unlike myasthenia gravis, patients seldom complain of diplopia. Cases have been described with ophthalmoplegia but no ptosis, or with unilateral or asymmetric ptosis.

CPEO may occur in isolation or may be associated with a constellation of ophthalmologic, neurologic, or systemic features. If the ophthalmoplegia appears before age 20 and is accompanied by atypical retinitis pigmentosa (salt and pepper pattern), along with a cerebellar ataxia, cardiac conduction defects, and elevated CSF protein (greater than 100 mg/dL), the condition is known as Kearns-Sayre syndrome (KSS). Other abnormalities often seen in KSS include short stature, hearing loss, vestibular dysfunction, pendular nystagmus, Babinski sign, delayed puberty, and various other endocrine disorders. It is important to note, however, that up to 10% of patients with CPEO due to KSS have no ragged-red fibers on muscle biopsy, and the causative large mtDNA deletion often escapes detection by PCR (which is used for virtually all of the mitochondrial diseases). Southern blot is recommended for suspected CPEO/KSS cases.

The extraocular muscles are primarily involved in many mitochondrial diseases. CPEO is considered the most frequent manifestation in mitochondrial encephalomyopathies. In addition to the preferential involvement of the ocular and cranial musculature, mitochondrial encephalomyopathies are often associated with dysfunction in other organ systems. Some mitochondrial disorders are associated with prominent vascular headaches. Mitochondrial encephalomyopathies are a complex group of disorders resulting from mtDNA mutations. Most cases occur sporadically.

Familial cases have been described. Modes of inheritance include maternal transmission associated with mitochondrial point mutations, autosomal recessive inheritance, and autosomal dominant inheritance. Differentiation of CPEO from other neurogenic, neuromuscular junction or myogenic disorders may be difficult. In the case of our patient, the extreme asymmetry characterizing the onset of the ophthalmoplegia as seen in the lid ptosis of the left was unusual. The history of stepwise progressive loss of eye movements and the presence of diplopia were unusual as well.

However, by history, careful evaluation for other causes of ophthalmoplegia had been negative. A major concern for an atypical presentation of myasthenia gravis motivated the therapeutic trials of Mestinon, corticosteroids, mycophenolate mofetil, and intravenous immunoglobulins. Her greater difficulty with vision at night was probably related to impaired ability to use visual clues for orientation and balance as there was no overt retinopathy. She did notice dizziness on rapid eye movements of the head, which was probably due to the absence of effective vestibular ocular movements.

SELECTED REFERENCES

DiMauro S, Hirano M, Schon EA. Mitochondrial encephalomyopathies: therapeutic approaches. *Neurol Sci* 2000;21:5901–5908.

Lee AG, Brazis PW. Chronic progressive external ophthalmoplegia. *Curr Neurol Neurosci Rep* 2002;2: 413–417.

Sahashi K, Yoneda M, Ohno K, et al. Functional characterisation of mitochondrial tRNA (Tyr) mutation (5877—>GA) associated with familial chronic progressive external ophthalmoplegia. *J Med Genet* 2001;38:703–705.

Shrama NK, Gujrati M, Kumar J, et al. Chronic asymmetric progressive external ophthalmoplegia with right facial weakness: a unique presentation of mitochondrial myopathy. *J Neurol Neurosurg Psychiatry* 2002;73(1):95.

SEE QUESTIONS: 2, 231

CASE **86**

RIGHT HOMONYMOUS HEMIANOPSIA DUE TO PCA INFARCT

OBJECTIVES

- To review the neuro-ophthalmological manifestations of posterior cerebral artery (PCA) territory infarcts.
- To discuss the differential diagnosis of PCA infarcts in patients with a history of migraines.
- To summarize the main neurological manifestations associated with the antiphospholipid antibody syndrome (APAS), the etiology of the PCA infarct.
- To caution against the premature diagnosis of migrainous cerebral infarction.

VIGNETTE

A 34-year-old woman with history of migraines without aura had sudden onset of loss of peripheral vision of her right visual field. She also experienced a brief episode of horizontal diplopia and bifrontal headaches. She did not have nausea, vomiting, photophobia, phonophobia, or osmophobia.

CASE SUMMARY

Our patient had an isolated congruous right homonymous hemianopia due to an occlusion of cortical branches of the left posterior cerebral artery (PCA). A unilateral PCA infarction often results in contralateral homonymous hemianopia with macular sparing. The extracranial vertebral arteries were unremarkable. Magnetic resonance angiography (MRA) showed an occluded P2 segment with no visualization of the calcarine artery, parietooccipital artery, and posterior temporal artery. Further investigations failed to demonstrate a possible cardiac source of embolism. As shown by the MRA, she had no evidence of proximal vertebrobasilar steno-occlusive disease nor evidence of intrinsic atheromatous disease of the PCA. She did not smoke cigarettes and was not on oral contraceptives. Although she had a history of migraine headaches, and cerebral infarctions complicating migraine mostly involve the PCA distribution, she was found to have persistent elevations of antiphospholipid antibodies titer. Her infarction was ultimately attributed to a prothrombotic state due to a primary APAS.

The PCAs arise from the distal basilar artery in most (70%) patients. Occasionally (20%), one or rarely both PCAs arise from the internal carotid artery (ICA) from a large posterior communicating artery (PComA). In 10% of the patients, the PCAs have a mixed origin. The PCAs are divided into four segments: P1 from the distal basilar artery to the PComA, P2 after the PComA, and the P3 and P4 segments which refer to the distal segments with cortical branches. The PCAs and their branches supply the mamillary bodies, thalami, and medial and basal temporal lobes, including the hippocampi. Manifestations of PCA territory infarctions are variable, depending on site of occlusion and availability of collaterals. Occlusion of the precommunal P1 segment causes midbrain, thalamic, and hemispheric infarction.

Occlusion of the PCA in the proximal segment before branching in the thalamogeniculate pedicle causes lateral thalamic and hemispheral symptoms. Occlusions also may affect a single PCA branch, primarily the calcarine artery, or cause a large hemispheric infarction of the PCA territory. Unilateral infarctions in the distribution of hemispheral branches of the PCA may produce a contralateral homonymous hemianopsia caused by infarction of the striate cortex, optic radiations, or lateral geniculate body.

If the infarction does not reach the occipital pole, there is partial or complete macular sparing. The visual field defect may be limited to a quadrantanopsia. A superior homonymous visual field defect results from infarction of the striate cortex inferior to the calcarine fissure or the inferior optic radiations in the temporo-occipital lobes. An inferior homonymous quadrantanopia results from infarction of the striate cortex superior to the calcarine fissure or the superior optic radiations in the parietooccipital lobes. Patients with unilateral homonymous hemianopsia due to occipital lobe lesions exhibit a normal optokinetic response.

More complex visual changes may also occur with PCA territory infarctions, including formed or unformed visual hallucinations, visual and color agnosias, or prosopagnosia. The syndrome of alexia without agraphia is discussed in cases 27 and 50.

APAS may be primary or secondary. Primary APAS is an immune-mediated coagulopathy, the etiology of which remains unknown. Secondary APAS can occur within the context of several diseases such as systemic lupus erythematosus, rheumatoid arthritis, Sjögren syndrome, Sneddon syndrome (livedo reticularis and ischemic cerebrovascular disease), malignancies, syphilis, acute and chronic infections including AIDS, and inflammatory bowel disease; administration of certain drugs; liver transplantation; early onset severe preeclampsia; and also in individuals without demonstrable underlying disorder. Ischemic stroke is the most common arterial thrombotic event in APAS.

Neurologic involvement associated with antiphospholipid antibodies includes ischemic strokes, transient ischemic attacks (TIAs), ocular ischemia, migrainous-like events, cerebral venous thrombosis, dementia (with or without Sneddon syndrome), acute ischemic encephalopathy, transient global amnesia, seizures, chorea, transverse myelopathy, and Guillain-Barré syndrome.

The best therapeutic strategy for preventing strokes in patients who have APAS remains unclear. In patients who have stroke and APAS, aspirin is as effective as moderate-intensity warfarin for preventing recurrent cerebral events. Our patient received warfarin.

Migrainous infarction is a rare event, considering the high prevalence of migraine in the general population. Criteria for migrainous infarction according to HIS-II require one or more aura symptoms lasting more than an hour associated with neuroimaging confirmation of ischemic infarction with history of migraine with aura, a concurrent attack typical of previous attacks except for duration of the neurological deficits, and exclusion of other causes of infarction. Migraine, particularly migraine with aura, may increase the risk of ischemic stroke in young women, especially if they also have other risk factors such as smoking and use of oral contraceptives.

SELECTED REFERENCES

Caplan LR. *Posterior circulation disease. Clinical findings, diagnosis, and management.* Boston: Blackwell Science, 1996.

Cuadrado MJ, Hughes GRV. Antiphospholipid (Hughes) syndrome. *Rheum Dis Clin North Am* 2001;27:507–524.

Headache classification subcommittee of the International Headache Society. The International Classification of Headache Disorders: 2nd Edition. *Cephalalgia.* 2004;24(Suppl 1):9–160.

Levine SR, Welch KMA. The spectrum of neurologic disease associated with antiphospholipid antibodies. Lupus anticoagulants and anticardiolipin antibodies. *Arch Neurol* 1987;44:876–883.

Tzourio C, Tehindrazanarivelo A, Iglesias S, et al. Case-control study of migraine and risk of ischemic stroke in young women. *Br Med J* 1995;310:830–833.

SEE QUESTIONS: 29, 47, 48, 52, 54, 90, 147, 167, 223

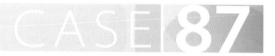

UPBEAT NYSTAGMUS: WERNICKE ENCEPHALOPATHY

OBJECTIVES

- To describe a case of upbeat nystagmus and associated manifestations.
- To discuss the relatively small differential diagnosis of upbeat nystagmus.
- To discuss the treatment strategy for Wernicke encephalopathy.
- To caution against the delayed diagnosis of Wernicke encephalopathy.

VIGNETTE

This 33-year-old woman was admitted to the psychiatry ward with a combination of abnormal behaviors ("little girl" speech, screaming, and amnesia) and what was referred as "bizarre" ataxia. She had had intractable vomiting for approximately 3 weeks prior to her admission, reportedly triggered by a remorseful confession to her husband of an extramarital affair. She complained of feeling that "the ground is moving."

CASE SUMMARY

 Our patient had a combination of unusual features, which were suggestive of a psychogenic etiology to the admitting physician. Of her symptoms, however, the "moving ground" was the most important because it led to the careful oculomotor characterization, which disclosed upbeat nystagmus. She also had a wide-based gait that in no way showed the "bizarre" features it had been attributed, which justified a delayed neurologic evaluation as outpatient after discharge, preventing prompt diagnosis and initiation of therapy.

The patient had the classic triad of ataxia, anterograde amnesia, and ophthalmologic impairment that characterizes Wernicke encephalopathy, triggered by thiamine (B_1) depletion due to protracted vomiting. A brain MRI obtained almost 1 month showed only mild signal abnormality in the medial thalami (Fig. 87.1), given presumably a partial restoration of the nutritional deficiency since the cessation of vomiting. The patient

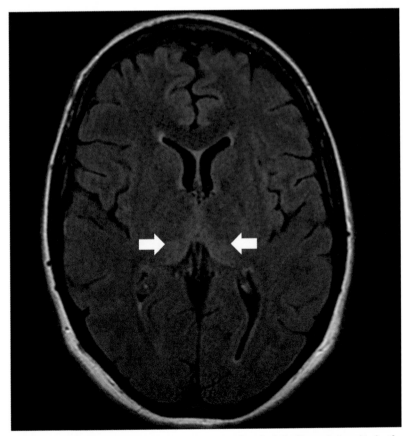

Figure 87.1 **FLAIR Axial Brain MRI Demonstrating Subtle Hyperintensity in the Dorsomedial Thalami (*Arrows*).**

underwent B_1 replacement, first intravenously (500 mg) followed by oral supplementation, which resolved the oscillopsia (with corresponding normalization of eye movements) but only partially improved her gait, possibly because of the delay in the initiation of treatment.

Upbeat nystagmus is associated with a relatively short number of disorders, which includes Wernicke encephalopathy as well as other lesions affecting paramedian region of the medulla and, less commonly, pons and midbrain. Arsenic poisoning is also a cause of upbeat nystagmus and may present with clinical picture similar to that of Wernicke encephalopathy. A "top of the basilar" syndrome due to occlusion of posterior thalamo-perforating arteries could also be entertained in the setting of an abrupt onset of a "confusional state" associated with symmetric lesions in the paramedian thalami.

The upbeat nystagmus of Wernicke encephalopathy should be present in primary position (not just evoked exclusively on upgaze) and may be suppressed or converted to downbeat nystagmus on convergence. Associated or alternative oculomotor deficits reported in Wernicke encephalopathy are restriction of gaze range and eyelid ptosis.

Established or presumptive Wernicke encephalopathy is treated with high-potency vitamin B complex. This includes a minimum of thiamine 100 mg IV for 3 days followed by daily B complex with B_1 250 mg for 5 days or until clinical improvement ceases. Parenteral thiamine replacement improves ocular abnormalities within hours to a few days, whereas confusion and ataxia have slower improvement rates. The amnestic syndrome may not recover in roughly 25% of patients, with higher rates when treatment is delayed.

SELECTED REFERENCES

Abouaf L, Vighetto A, Magnin E, et al. Primary position upbeat nystagmus in Wernicke's encephalopathy. *Eur Neurol* 2011;65(3):160–163.

Biller J, ed. *Practical neurology*, 4th ed. Philadelphia: Lippincott Williams & Wilkins, Wolters Kluwer Health, 2012.

Espay AJ, Biller J. *Concise neurology*. Philadelphia: Lippincott Williams & Wilkins, Wolters Kluwer Health, 2011

Espay AJ, Lang AE. *Common movement disorders pitfalls: case-based teaching.* New York: Cambridge University Press, 2012.

SEE QUESTIONS: 328, 329, 330, 331

SECTION 9

NEUROINFECTIOUS DISEASES

CASE 88

HERPES ZOSTER (POSTHERPETIC NEURALGIA)

OBJECTIVES

- To review the most frequent neurologic complications associated with varicella-zoster virus (VZV) infections.
- To review the clinical presentation and management of uncomplicated herpes zoster.

VIGNETTE

A 63-year-old man had left-sided chest pain and a skin rash.

CASE SUMMARY

VZV causes chickenpox (varicella) and shingles. Following initial infection, usually as varicella in childhood, VZV, one of the herpes family of viruses, remains dormant in the dorsal spinal root ganglion neurons and the fifth cranial nerve (CN V) ganglion neurons. Upon reactivation, a spectrum of clinical manifestations may occur including herpes zoster (shingles), postherpetic neuralgia, cranial neuropathies, Ramsay Hunt syndrome (geniculate neuralgia, nervus intermedius neuralgia, or herpes zoster oticus), cerebellar ataxia, myelitis, radiculitis, brachial plexus neuritis, motor neuropathies, encephalitis, thrombotic cerebral vasculopathy, keratitis, and so forth. Once herpes zoster rash resolves, many patients continue to suffer from pain persisting longer than 1 to 3 months (postherpetic neuralgia).

Our patient had a typical painful dermatomal rash associated with reactivation of VZV infection. The gradual onset of unilateral dermatomal paresthesias may precede the onset of pain. Dermatomal pain is the most common symptom of herpes zoster and may antedate the cutaneous eruption by days to weeks. After a prodromal illness, erythematous macules and papules appear and progress to vesicles. They then begin to crust and resolve. The crusts usually resolve within 2 to 3 weeks. Patients may experience pain and sensory loss in the distribution of the rash.

The incidence of herpes zoster increases with advancing age, doubling approximately in each decade after the age of 50 years. Motor weakness, especially in cervical and lumbar radicular distributions, may be overlooked. Herpes zoster typically affects a single dermatome, most commonly a thoracic dermatome. The dermatomes most commonly involved are T5 and T6. However, multiple contiguous or noncontiguous dermatomes may be involved. The ophthalmic division of the fifth cranial nerve (CN V) is the most frequently affected cranial nerve. Rarely, VZV reactivation can occur without cutaneous vesicles ("zoster sine herpete").

For typical zoster in an immunocompetent patient, nonopioid analgesics and local anesthetic creams have been used. Antiviral agents within 24 hours (acyclovir, famciclovir, and valacyclovir) after the onset of rash decreases the duration and severity of pain associated with the rash. Some studies have shown the potential benefit of prednisone (if no contraindications) in preventing postherpetic neuralgia.

SELECTED REFERENCES

Kost RG, Starus SE. Postherpetic neuralgia-pathogenesis, treatment, and prevention. *N Engl J Med* 1996;335:32–42.

Mahalingam R, Wellish MC, Dueland AN, et al. Localization of herpes simplex virus and varicella zoster virus DNA in human ganglia. *Ann Neurol* 1992;31:444–448.

Stankus SJ, Dlugopolski M, Packer D. Management of herpes zoster (shingles) and postherpetic neuralgia. *Am Fam Physician* 2000;61(8):2437–2444.

SEE QUESTIONS: 157, 158, 165

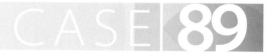

RECURRENT ASEPTIC MENINGITIS

OBJECTIVES

- To define aseptic meningitis.
- To list the common causes of aseptic meningitis.
- To briefly discuss Mollaret meningitis.

VIGNETTE

A 34-year-old African-American woman was admitted with new-onset bilateral frontal headaches, posterior neck pain, vomiting, photophobia, generalized weakness, and numbness in face, arms, and legs. She had no fever and denied ill contacts, recent foreign travel, skin lesions, or upper respiratory symptoms. On examination, blood pressure was 137/74 mm Hg, heart rate was 92 beats/min, respirations were 18 breaths/min, and temperature was 97.1°F.

CASE SUMMARY

Our patient had three recurrent episodes of headaches, posterior neck pain and stiffness, nausea, vomiting, and fever. Examination showed limited flexion of the neck. She did not have a Brudzinski sign (the patient did not exhibit flexion of her knees and hips when passive flexion of her neck was attempted in the supine position). Cerebrospinal fluid (CSF) studies at three points over the span of 3 years demonstrated a lymphocytic pleocytosis with normal glucose level, minimal elevation of protein content, and negative Gram stain, a profile compatible with the diagnosis of aseptic meningitis (Table 89.1). We concluded that our patient had three episodes of recurrent self-limited aseptic meningitis, probably representing Mollaret meningitis.

Aseptic meningitis is a diagnosis given to patients with clinical and laboratory evidence of meningeal inflammation with negative routine bacterial cultures. The clinical presentation often includes headache (100%), fever (93%), neck stiffness, nausea, vomiting, and confusion. Signs of meningeal irritation include Brudzinski sign and Kernig sign. A positive Kernig sign is present when extension of the knee in a patient lying supine with the hips flexed 90 degrees elicits pain or resistance in the lower back or posterior thigh. CSF generally demonstrates lymphomononuclear pleocytosis (fewer than 500 cells), moderately elevated protein content, and normal glucose and lactate levels.

The term *aseptic meningitis* is often used to describe a viral meningitis, but there are multiple infectious and noninfectious causes. Infectious conditions may be viral or nonviral. Viral disorders causing aseptic meningitis syndrome include the following: enterovirus, herpes simplex virus (HSV) 1 and 2, varicella-zoster virus, adenovirus, Epstein-Barr virus, lymphocytic choriomeningitis virus, human immunodeficiency virus, arbovirus, and influenza virus types A and B. Enteroviruses are the most common cause of viral aseptic meningitis. Bacterial disorders causing aseptic meningitis syndrome include the following: partially treated bacterial meningitis, parameningeal infections, infective endocarditis, *Mycoplasma pneumoniae*, *Mycobacterium tuberculosis*, Ehrlichiosis, *Borrelia burgdorferi*, *Treponema pallidum*, *Brucella* sp., and *Leptospira* sp.

Fungal disorders causing aseptic meningitis syndrome include *Cryptococcus neoformans*, *Histoplasma capsulatum*, *Coccidioides immitis*, and *Blastomyces dermatitidis*. Parasitic disorders causing the aseptic meningitis syndrome include *Toxoplasma gondii* and *Taenia solium*.

Noninfectious causes of the aseptic meningitis syndrome include certain drugs and systemic diseases. Most drug-induced cases are due to nonsteroidal antiinflammatory drugs (NSAIDs); antimicrobials such as trimethoprim–sulfamethoxazole, metronidazole, and cephalosporins; intravenous immunoglobulin (IVIG); OKT$_3$ antibodies; intrathecal agents; and vaccinations. NSAIDs probably account for most of the drug-related cases. Systemic diseases causing the aseptic meningitis syndrome include the following:

TABLE 89.1   RECURRENT ASEPTIC MENINGITIS

Year	CSF WBC (% Lymphocytes)	CSF RBC	CSF Protein	CSF Glucose (Serum Glucose)
First year	15 (99%)	3	69	52
Second year	501 (97%)	72	Not recorded	Not recorded
Fourth year	160 (97%)	4	54	54 (90)

CSF, cerebrospinal fluid; WBC, white blood count; RBC, red blood count.

sarcoidosis, systemic lupus erythematosus, Wegener granulomatosis, central nervous system (CNS) vasculitis, Behçet disease, Vogt-Koyanagi and Harada syndromes, leptomeningeal cancer, posttransplantation lymphoproliferative disorder, and others.

Mollaret meningitis is a condition where recurrent episodes of fever are associated with an aseptic meningitis syndrome. CSF findings may show large fragile "endothelial" cells, mild hypoglycorrhachia, and a mild increase in the gamma globulin content. The episodes are typically self-limited. No definitive cause has been noted although HSV-2, and less frequently HSV-1, is thought to be the etiology in many cases. This would make acyclovir a reasonable treatment option in patients with Mollaret meningitis.

SELECTED REFERENCES

Hermans PE, Goldstein NP, Wellman WE. Mollaret's meningitis and differential diagnosis of recurrent meningitis: report of case, with review of the literature. *Am J Med* 1972;52(1):128–140.

Jolles S, Sewell WA, Leighton C. Drug-induced aseptic meningitis: diagnosis and management. *Drug Saf* 2000;22(3):215–226.

Moris G, Garcia-Monco JC. The challenge of drug-induced aseptic meningitis. *Arch Intern Med* 1999; 159(11):1185–1194.

Nowak DA, Boehmer R. A retrospective clinical, laboratory and outcome analysis in 43 cases of acute aseptic meningitis. *Eur J Neurol* 2003;10(3):271–280.

Roos K. Viral meningitis and aseptic meningitis. In: Roos K, ed. *Central nervous system infectious diseases and therapy.* New York: Marcel Dekker Inc, 1997:127–139.

SEE QUESTIONS: 137, 151, 153, 154, 155, 163, 165

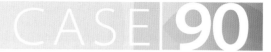

POSTENCEPHALITIC PARKINSONISM

OBJECTIVES

- To define postencephalitic parkinsonism.
- To list the common causes of postencephalitic parkinsonism.
- To list the most common neurotropic viruses associated with basal ganglia lesions.

VIGNETTE

This 35-year-old woman with history of hypertension, pancreatitis, and idiopathic renal disease developed decreased verbal output, sleepiness, and disorientation within a few days from renal transplantation. She evolved into a state of akinetic-rigid mutism with apraxia of eyelid opening reaching a peak 3 months after recovering from her encephalopathy. She had had a static course thereafter, remaining unresponsive to levodopa and other dopaminergic therapies.

CASE SUMMARY

Although our patient was unable to articulate words, she had adequate comprehension of instructions and normal orobuccolingual praxis. She was markedly parkinsonian, virtually akinetic with severe gait and postural impairment. Other deficits included apraxia of eyelid opening, square-wave jerks, inability to initiate horizontal saccades (which themselves were normal) without blinking, and glabellar reflex. Her handwriting was severely micrographic. By the time of her last examination, 2 years after her triggering encephalopathy, she exhibited a moonlike facies from chronic prednisone treatment and an orthopedic cast in both feet placed following tendonectomy to alleviate excessive bilateral plantar flexion.

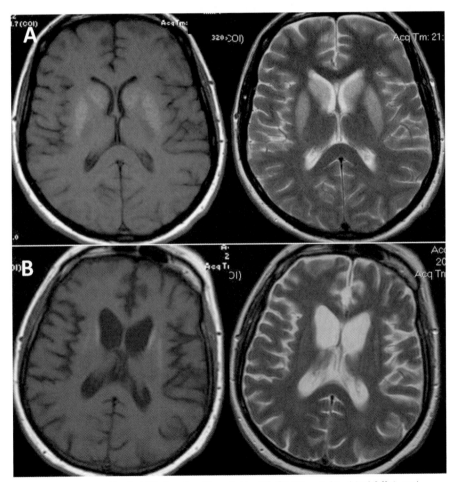

Figure 90.1   Axial brain MRI showing T1-weighted (**left**), T2-weighted (**middle**), and fluid-attenuated inversion recovery (FLAIR) sequences at 1 week (**A**) and 12 months (**B**) after symptom onset showing hyperintensity of the caudate nuclei, putamen, and external portion of the globus pallidum bilaterally with progressive atrophy of these deep nuclei over time. Ventricular enlargement results from striatal volume loss.

During the initial encephalopathic state, her cerebrospinal fluid (CSF) showed 32 white blood cells (100% lymphocytes) with normal protein (47 mg/dL) and glucose (68 mg/dL).Serial levels of FK506 (tacrolimus), which she received for rejection prophylaxis, were within therapeutic range. Her brain magnetic resonance imaging (MRI) demonstrated striatal hyperintensity with progressive atrophy, suggestive of striatal necrosis (Fig. 90.1). Epstein-Barr virus (EBV) DNA was detected by PCR (1.5×10^2 copies/mL).

Postencephalitic parkinsonism (PEP) was known as a complication of encephalitis lethargica related to the influenza epidemic of 1917 to 1927, described by Constantin von Economo and popularized in the movie *Awakenings*. PEP cases continue to emerge outside of epidemic settings after infections with neurotropic viruses, such as Japanese B encephalitis, St. Louis encephalitis, Eastern equine encephalitis, Coxsackie B3 and B4, and West Nile Virus. Parkinsonism develops months or even years after the acute encephalitic illness. Other deficits in PEP patients may include dysarthria and palilalia, cervical and facial dystonia (particularly blepharospasm and jaw opening dystonia), motor tics, and obsessive–compulsive disorder. Compared to old survivors of the influenza of von Econo-mo's, modern cases of PEP tend to have a shorter latency to the onset of parkinsonism and less common occurrence of oculogyric crises (which are more commonly an idiosyncratic reaction to the use of metoclopramide and phenothiazine neuroleptics).

Our case of EBV-induced encephalitis lethargic-like PEP presentation may have been more severe due to her post–renal transplantation status, which rendered her immuno-compromised. When PEP is due to viruses that affect the substantia nigra but relatively spare the putamen (St. Louis encephalitis and Coxsackie B3 and B4), response to levodopa tends to be more rewarding.

SELECTED REFERENCES

Biller J, ed. *Practical neurology*, 4th ed. Philadelphia: Lippincott Williams & Wilkins, Wolters Kluwer Health, 2012.

Dale RC, Church AJ, Surtees RAH, et al. Encephalitis lethargica syndrome: 20 new cases and evidence of basal ganglia autoimmunity. *Brain* 2004;127;21–33.

Dimova PS, Bojinova V, Georgiev D, et al. Acute reversible parkinsonism in Epstein-Barr virus-related encephalitis lethargica-like illness. *Mov Disord* 2006;21:564–566.

Espay AJ, Henderson KK. Post-encephalitic parkinsonism and basal ganglia necrosis due to Epstein-Barr virus infection. *Neurology* 2011;76(17):1529–1530.

SEE QUESTIONS: 332, 333, 334

CASE 91

CREUTZFELDT-JAKOB DISEASE

OBJECTIVES

- To describe a case of Creutzfeldt-Jakob disease (CJD).
- To define the Heidenhain variant of CJD.
- To highlight an example of the posterior or sensory variant of the alien limb syndrome.
- To generate a differential diagnosis of rapidly progressing dementias.

This 65-year-old right-handed woman was admitted to the hospital because of progressive confusion. She had been apparently healthy until about 2 months prior to admission, when she disclosed to her husband that "people were growing funny, long noses" and that "everyone on TV looked like cartoons." By the time of our evaluation, 3 months into her illness, she was globally aphasic, exhibited an alien limb syndrome, and had increased sound-sensitive startle.

 This patient had a rapidly progressive encephalopathy, heralded by the development of metamorphopsias (distortions of visual images, in this case expressed as "funny, long noses" she noted in people), followed by cortical blindness, and eventually aphasia, apraxia, a left dystonic and levitating arm, and ultimately (not shown) intermittent myoclonus. The protein 14-3-3 was elevated in cerebrospinal fluid (CSF). Her brain magnetic resonance imaging (MRI) showed a cortical ribbon in the parietooccipital region (Fig. 91.1). These features suggested the posterior or Heidenhain variant of CJD. The patient died 4 months after the onset of symptoms, 1 month after the video was recorded.

Our patient demonstrated the posterior or sensory variant of the alien hand syndrome, which is manifested by withdrawal or avoidance of the nondominant hand. This form of alien syndrome, unlike the frontal and callosal forms, is due to lesions in the nondominant parietotemporal area and may co-occur with hemianesthesia, hemianopia, and ultimately anosognosia. The presence of a left alien limb syndrome is more often associated with CJD than with any other form of corticobasal syndrome and may be its presenting feature. This feature, along with the rapidly progressive cortical blindness associated with restricted diffusion in the parietooccipital gyri as detected by MRI, was typical of CJD,

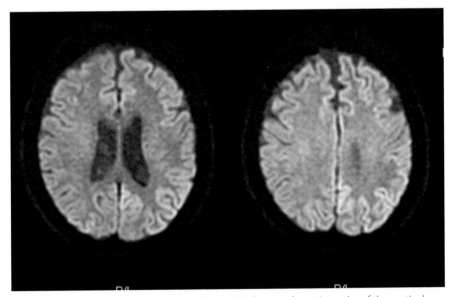

Figure 91.1   Axial diffusion-weighted brain MRI showing hyperintensity of the cortical ribbon in the parietooccipital cortex, left greater than right.

presenting as a rapidly progressive corticobasal syndrome. Cases of cortical blindness with predominant occipital lobe involvement have been referred to as the Heidenhain variant of CJD.

CJD is a rapidly progressive dementia with myoclonus, cerebellar ataxia, and cortical blindness. Although spontaneous myoclonus is a classic manifestation, it may not be present early on, or only be apparent as stimulus-sensitive myoclonus or pathologic startle. Progression to akinetic mutism and death may occur in 2 to 3 months, with 70% of patients dying within 6 months from symptom onset. Raised CSF 14-3-3 protein, neuronal-specific enolase, and S-100 are helpful but nonspecific findings. The electroencephalography (EEG) may show pseudoperiodic sharp wave discharges in approximately 70% of cases. Atypical forms of CJD may have a prolonged clinical course (greater than 2 years) or an ataxic rather than cognitive presentation.

Besides CJD, other disorders of potentially rapid progression that should be considered in the differential diagnosis include some forms of Alzheimer disease, dementia with Lewy bodies, frontotemporal dementias associated with motor neuron disease, adult ceroid lipofuscinosis (Kufs disease), AIDS–dementia complex, paraneoplastic encephalopathies, steroid-responsive autoimmune encephalitis (aka, Hashimoto encephalopathy), and some toxic/iatrogenic encephalopathies such as mercury and bismuth toxicity.

SELECTED REFERENCES

Biller J, ed. *Practical neurology*, 4th ed. Philadelphia: Lippincott Williams & Wilkins, Wolters Kluwer Health, 2012.

Espay AJ, Biller J. *Concise neurology*. Philadelphia: Lippincott Williams & Wilkins, Wolters Kluwer Health, 2011.

Fogel B, Wu M, Kremen S, et al. Creutzfeldt-Jakob disease presenting with alien limb sign. *Mov Disord* 2006;21(7):1040–1042.

Kropp S, Schulz-Schaeffer WJ, et al. The Heidenhain variant of Creutzfeldt-Jakob disease. *Arch Neurol* 1999;56(1):55–61.

SEE QUESTIONS: 335, 336, 337

SECTION 10

NEUROOTOLOGY

CASE 92

VERTIGO/IMBALANCE SECONDARY TO ISOLATED VERMIAN INFARCTION

OBJECTIVES

- To highlight possible pitfalls in the diagnosis of acute isolated severe vertigo.
- To review the clinical presentation of the acute isolated vestibular syndrome.
- To describe vascular and nonvascular causes of the central vestibular syndrome.

VIGNETTE

A 62-year-old man had a sudden onset of dizziness, vertigo, imbalance, and blurred vision after suddenly turning his head to the right. This was followed by nausea and diaphoresis. The episode lasted for 12 hours.

CASE SUMMARY

 Our patient had acute onset of vertigo and imbalance upon suddenly turning in bed with his head to the right side. The episode lasted 12 hours. He also had nausea and diaphoresis. He had no prior upper respiratory infection or flulike illness and did not complain of auricular pain, hearing loss, tinnitus, aural fullness, emesis, headaches, diplopia, dysarthria, facial paresthesias, extremity weakness, clumsiness, or numbness. He had no lateropulsion. He did not have orthostatic hypotension or evidence of a vesicular rash in the external auditory canal and concha. There was no history of motion intolerance during car, boat, or air travel. He was initially diagnosed as having presyncope versus syncope, and extensive cardiac investigations were unremarkable.

Balance involves the overlapping function of the visual, proprioceptive, and vestibular systems. Vertigo is defined as an illusion of movement either of self or the environment. Our patient had an acute vestibular syndrome characterized by severe vertigo, nausea, and postural instability. As Neurology was not consulted at the time of presentation, we cannot comment as to the possible presence of spontaneous nystagmus. When an acute vestibular syndrome evolves over days in an otherwise healthy patient, it is often attributed to a viral vestibular neuritis (vestibular neuronitis). If there is associated hearing loss, it is often attributed to a neurolabyrinthitis.

Vestibular neuritis refers to a disorder of the vestibular system without associated hearing loss, characterized by sudden attacks of severe vertigo, nausea, vomiting, and abnormal vestibular function on caloric testing in otherwise healthy patients. An upper respiratory infection often precedes this condition. The vertigo usually resolves within a week. Viral labyrinthitis is characterized by acute onset of severe and often incapacitating vertigo and hearing loss, frequently associated with nausea and vomiting. The vertigo usually resolves over several days to weeks. Bacterial labyrinthitis is rare in the postantibiotic era.

Benign paroxysmal positional vertigo (BPPV), probably the most common cause of vertigo, is characterized by sudden vertigo lasting less than 1 minute that occurs when the individual is trying to sit up suddenly, rolling over in bed, or tilting the head backward. Classic BBPV involves the posterior semicircular canal. Cervical vertigo (a controversial entity) is associated with head extension and attributed to vascular compression of the vertebral arteries. As shown by the magnetic resonance imaging (MRI) studies, our patient had central vertigo due to a small caudal vermian infarction.

Vascular causes of the central vestibular syndrome include vertebrobasilar transient ischemic attacks, labyrinthine stroke, lateral medullary (Wallenberg) syndrome, migraine-associated vertigo, basilar artery migraine (Bickerstaff), subclavian steal syndrome, and cerebellar infarction and hemorrhage. Nonvascular causes of central vertigo include cerebellar, brainstem, and temporal lobe tumors; central nervous system (CNS) infections, multiple sclerosis, Chiari malformation, Wernicke encephalopathy, trauma, focal seizures, and familial episodic ataxia syndromes.

Emergency room physicians should have a low threshold for obtaining a neurological consultation in patients who present with isolated vertigo or with vertigo, imbalance, and nausea and who also have risk factors for cerebrovascular disease. As many as 25% of patients with cerebrovascular risk factors who present to an emergency room with isolated vertigo, nystagmus, and postural instability have an infarction involving the inferior cerebellum. Improved diagnostic capability has been demonstrated with a three-step bedside oculomotor examination (HINTS: head impulse–nystagmus–test of skew). This has been proposed as more sensitive for stroke diagnosis than early MRI in patients presenting with an acute vestibular syndrome (nausea often with vomiting, gait instability, head motion intolerance, and nystagmus). A normal horizontal head impulse test, an identifiable skew deviation (vertical ocular misalignment), or a direction-changing nystagmus in eccentric gaze provides 100% sensitivity and 96% specificity for the diagnosis of stroke compared to peripheral vestibulopathy (Table 92.1).

TABLE 92.1 CENTRAL VERSUS PERIPHERAL VERTIGO: THREE-STEP BEDSIDE OCULOMOTOR EXAMINATION

	Central Vertigo (Brainstem or Cerebellar Stroke)	Peripheral Vertigo (Acute Vestibulopathy)
Horizontal head impulse test[a]	Normal	Abnormal
Skew deviation[b]	Present	Absent
Nystagmus in eccentric gaze	Direction-changing nystagmus in eccentric gaze	Direction to same side regardless of gaze

[a]The horizontal head impulse test, a measure of vestibuloocular response (VOR), is measured by the head impulse test, whereby the examiner rapidly rotate the patient's head from lateral to midposition.
[b]Skew deviation represents vertical misalignment/strabismus, which may be apparent in primary gaze or on alternating eye covering.
The three-step approach was suggested by Kattah JC, Taekad AV, Wang DZ, et al. HINTS to diagnose stroke in the acute vestibular syndrome. Three-step bedside oculomotor examination more sensitive than early MRI diffusion-weighted-imaging. *Stroke* 2009;40:3504–3510.

SELECTED REFERENCES

Brazis PW, Masdeu JC, Biller J. *Localization in clinical neurology*, 6th ed. Philadelphia: Lippincott Williams & Wilkins, Wolters Kluwer Health, 2011.
Hotson JR, Baloh RW. Acute vestibular syndrome. *New Engl J Med* 1998;339:680–685.
Kattah JC, Taekad AV, Wang DZ, et al. HINTS to diagnose stroke in the acute vestibular syndrome. Three-step bedside oculomotor examination more sensitive than early MRI diffusion-weighted-imaging. *Stroke* 2009;40:3504–3510.
Norrving B, Magnusson M, Holtas S. Isolated acute vertigo in the elderly: vestibular or vascular disease? *Acta Neurol Scand* 1995;91:43–48.

SEE QUESTIONS: 19, 64, 65, 143

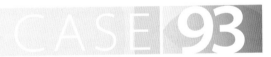

DEAFNESS/TINNITUS SECONDARY TO VESTIBULAR (ACOUSTIC) SCHWANNOMA

OBJECTIVES

■ To highlight the importance of a detailed evaluation of tinnitus and hearing loss.
■ To discuss the clinical manifestations of vestibular schwannomas.
■ To illustrate other etiologies of the cerebellopontine angle syndrome.
■ To analyze potential management strategies for vestibular schwannomas.

VIGNETTE

A 57-year-old man was evaluated because of a 3- to 4-month history of progressive unilateral right hearing loss and right ear tinnitus.

CASE SUMMARY

Our patient had progressive unilateral sensorineural hearing loss and subjective non-pulsatile tinnitus. Brain magnetic resonance imaging (MRI) demonstrated a small enhancing mass within the right internal auditory canal (IAC) consistent with a small right vestibular schwannoma. Vestibular schwannomas arise in the IAC in the cerebellopontine angle. Commonly but improperly called "acoustic neuromas," these tumors originate from the vestibular Schwann cells of CN VIII (cochleovestibular nerve) in the IAC at the glial–Schwann cell junction.

The tumor arises from the inferior or superior division of the vestibular nerve, but it typically causes symptoms due to mass effect on the adjacent cochlear nerve. In the IAC, the vestibular division of the cochleovestibular nerve courses in the posterior superior and inferior quadrants, and the cochlear division courses in the inferior–posterior quadrant. Besides vestibular schwannomas, other conditions causing the cerebellopontine angle syndrome include meningiomas, lipomas, cholesteatomas, arachnoid cysts, epidermoids, hemangiomas, vascular loops, vertebral dolichoectasia, arteriovenous malformations, and metastatic tumors.

Vestibular schwannomas are slow-growing benign tumors, accounting for approximately 10% of all intracranial tumors. The growth rate has been estimated to vary from 0.4 to 2.4 mm/year. Vestibular schwannomas are the most common cranial nerve schwannomas, followed by schwannomas of the trigeminal and facial nerves. Patients with vestibular schwannomas typically present with insidious cochlear nerve dysfunction, characterized by unilateral high-pitched tinnitus and progressive sensorineural hearing loss with early loss of speech discrimination. Rarely deafness may occur suddenly, most likely due to intratumoral hemorrhage or disruption of regional blood flow due to internal auditory artery occlusion.

Dizziness and a sense of imbalance or disequilibrium are more frequent complaints than vertigo. As the tumor grows, the internal auditory meatus progressively widens and complete ipsilateral deafness ensues. With medial tumor growth, neighboring cranial nerves are affected, and eventually brainstem and cerebellar compromise occur with very large tumors. Progressive tumoral enlargement may account for symptoms related to hydrocephalus or symptoms of increased intracranial pressure.

Dysfunction of neighboring cranial nerves varies according to the direction of tumoral growth. With anterior extension, the trigeminal nerve (CN V) and abducens nerve (CN VI) are compromised. With posteroinferior tumoral extension, the glossopharyngeal (CN IX), vagus (CN X), and spinal accessory (CN XI) may be involved. In either case, the facial nerve (CN VII) is usually involved. In patients presenting with *bilateral* vestibular schwannomas, neurofibromatosis type 2 should be suspected. MRI with gadolinium enhancement with specific IAC protocol is the preferred imaging modality to detect vestibular schwannomas. Vestibular schwannomas often demonstrate enhancement with gadolinium. Computed tomography (CT) with specific algorithms may also yield useful information. Pure tone and speech audiometry should be obtained. Auditory brainstem responses (ABRs) are abnormal in the majority of patients; the sensitivity is lowest among patients with small acoustic neuromas.

Management strategies include observation, surgery (retrosigmoid, middle fossa, and translabyrinthine approaches), and radiosurgery. Cerebellopontine angle mass lesions are usually surgically removed on an elective basis. The goal of surgery is to remove the tumor and preserve facial nerve function. Our patient was treated with stereotactic radiosurgery. Lesions smaller than 3 cm, particularly when there is no brainstem compression or in poor surgical risk patients, are often treated with stereotactic radiosurgery.

SELECTED REFERENCES

Biller J, ed. *Practical neurology*, 4th ed. Philadelphia: Lippincott Williams & Wilkins, Wolters Kluwer Health, 2012.

Brazis PW, Masdeu JC, Biller J. *Localization in clinical neurology*, 6th ed. Philadelphia: Lippincott Williams & Wilkins, Wolters Kluwer Health, 2011.

Hart RG, Davenport J. Diagnosis of acoustic neuroma. *Neurosurgery* 1991;9:450–463.

Myer SA, Post KD. Acoustic neuroma. In: Winn HR. *Youmans neurological surgery*, 6th ed., Vol 2. Philadelphia: Elsevier Saunders, 2011:Chapter 133, 1460–1475.

Samii M, Matthies C. Management of 1,000 vestibular schwannomas (acoustic neuromas): facial nerve preservation and restitution of function. *Neurosurgery* 1997;40:684–695.

SEE QUESTIONS: 38, 63, 64, 65, 166, 176, 197

CASE 94

VERTIGINOUS DIZZINESS

OBJECTIVES

- To review common causes of dizziness.
- To outline differential diagnosis of vertigo.
- To summarize management of Ménière disease and benign positional vertigo.

VIGNETTE

A 44-year-old man had recurrent dizziness and subjective sensation of profound environmental spin. He had occasional off and on high-pitched ringing in both ears. Past medical history was noteworthy for deep vein thrombosis of the lower extremity 11 years earlier following a limb fracture. Neurologic and neurootologic examinations were normal.

CASE SUMMARY

Our patient presented with a 1-year history of intermittent vertiginous dizziness. He had no hearing loss or ear fullness, but described an occasional high-pitched ringing in both ears. Magnetic resonance imaging (MRI) scan of the brain with and without contrast and additional extensive laboratory evaluation showed no apparent etiology for his vertigo.

The main categories of dizziness are vertigo, presyncopal dizziness (impending faint), disequilibrium (poor balance), and a *nonspecific* group. Vertigo is an illusion of spinning or motion, ranging from mild to severe. Peripheral vestibular afferents innervate the brainstem vestibular nuclei and project to the cerebellum, oculomotor nuclei, cerebral areas, and spinal cord. Otologic or peripheral vertigo may be present with pathology involving the labyrinth or the vestibular nerve and is often characterized by intense episodic vertigo, often leaving the patient immobile from the attack. There is often nausea, vomiting, tachycardia, and diaphoresis. In contrast, patients with presyncopal dizziness experience light-headedness, often postural, as if they might pass out. Causes of presyncopal dizziness include orthostatic hypotension, autonomic neuropathy, use of antihypertensive medications, vasovagal attacks, and cardiac arrhythmias.

Patients with disequilibrium often verbalize such descriptions as their "balance is off" or they have a "floating feeling." Common causes include medication side effects, brainstem or cerebellar dysfunction, deafferentation from cervical spondylosis or sensory neuropathy, and neurodegenerative disorders such as atypical parkinsonisms (progressive supranuclear palsy, and multiple system atrophy). The other group of patients with dizziness includes those who do not conform to the other three categories. Such patients often describe vague nonspecific symptoms and often have multiple somatic complaints.

Ménière disease is characterized by recurrent episodes of intense vertigo, tinnitus, hearing loss, and fullness in the head or ears. Ménière's may result from prior trauma, infection, or hereditary factors. In many instances, there is no clear trigger. Diagnosis is based on a detailed history and a structured examination. Ménière disease tends to be recurrent and increases with age; it is related to an accumulation of fluid/endolymph in the labyrinth. Preventative management includes a salt-restriction diet and potassium-sparing diuretics. Acute attacks are treated with meclizine, diazepam, or promethazine.

Benign paroxysmal positional vertigo (BPPV) is caused by debris in the semicircular canals (mostly posterior semicircular canal) leading to recurrent episodes lasting several hours to several days of intense positional vertigo. Patients do not experience deafness or tinnitus. Treatment includes an attempt to clear out the debris from the canal and into the vestibule (called the canalith repositioning maneuver or modified Epley maneuver). Repositioning is reported to work well in 70% to 80% of patients.

Acute labyrinthitis or vestibular neuronitis is a self-limited monophasic illness often seen in the setting of an upper respiratory infection. Vertigo from brainstem or cerebellar disease tends to be associated with other central nervous system (CNS) symptoms/signs and may be related to transient ischemic attacks (TIAs), strokes, multiple sclerosis, or neoplasms. Additional conditions to be considered among patients with chronic vertigo include syphilis, exposure to aminoglycoside antibiotics, and neurosarcoidosis.

Our patient's history of recurrent vertiginous dizziness and intermittent tinnitus would suggest an otologic or peripheral cause, most likely Ménière disease. The rather persistent and frequent occurrence of symptoms was somewhat unusual for early Ménière's. Although classic Ménière's is associated with hearing loss and subjective fullness, some patients may lack the complete tetrad of symptoms. The presence of tinnitus and absence of a striking positional trigger make benign positional vertigo less likely. The chronic nature of his symptoms is against the possible diagnosis of viral vestibular neuronitis or labyrinthitis. His improvement associated with corticosteroid therapy raises the question of a possible inflammatory process such as a viral or immune-mediated etiology.

SELECTED REFERENCES

Baloh RW. Clinical practice. Vestibular neuritis. *N Engl J Med* 2003;348:1027–1032.

Biller J, ed. *Practical neurology*, 6th ed. Philadelphia: Lippincott Williams & Wilkins, Wolters Kluwer Health, 2012.

Eggers SDZ, Zee DS. Evaluating the dizzy patient; bedside examination and laboratory assessment of the vestibular system. *Semin Neurol* 2003;23:47–58.

Epley JM. Human experience with canalith repositioning maneuvers. *Ann NY Acad Sci* 2001;942:179–191.

SEE QUESTIONS: 19, 64, 65, 338, 339

CASE 95

BENIGN PAROXYSMAL POSITIONAL VERTIGO

OBJECTIVES

- To review a classical presentation of benign paroxysmal positional vertigo (posterior semicircular canal).
- To illustrate the Dix-Hallpike maneuver for its diagnosis and Epley maneuver for its treatment.
- To describe the main clinical differences between central and peripheral forms of nystagmus.

VIGNETTE

This 71-year-old man, with well-controlled Parkinson disease, developed positional vertigo and minimal nausea whenever he changed the position of his head and, particularly, when looking up quickly. He was otherwise stable on levodopa treatment, at a dose of 200 mg q.i.d. with excellent function and only mild motor fluctuations, expressed as tremor reemergence toward the end of each dose cycle.

CASE SUMMARY

Our patient with well-controlled Parkinson disease presented with unrelated but classic right posterior semicircular canal variant of benign paroxysmal positional vertigo (BPPV), which was suggested by a history of positional vertigo appearing when in bed and turning or extending his head. The diagnosis of BPPV was confirmed with the Dix-Hallpike maneuver, which elicited nystagmus with a torsional component when rapidly extending the head toward the affected ear, which reproduced the intensity and severity of prior vertiginous episodes. The torsional nystagmus was "geotropic" and more prominent when the eye moved toward affected ear. This form of peripheral nystagmus has a latency of 3 to 20 seconds and exhibits fatigability with repeated testing.

BPPV is the most common cause of vertigo in the general population. It consists of sudden and short-lasting recurrent vertigo elicited by certain rotational movements of the head. It is caused by free-floating debris, typically calcium carbonate crystals (otoliths), that dislocate from the utriculus of the vestibular labyrinth and migrate to the more dependent semicircular canals, most often posterior. The otolith movement alters endolymphatic pressure and causes cupular deflection, triggering the spinning sensation that defines vertigo. Head trauma and labyrinthitis are considered risk factors for the development of BPPV, although they are documented in relatively few such patients. BPPV may be self-limited, but remissions can be induced at the bedside with the Epley maneuver, as illustrated in the video.

The Epley maneuver treats BPPV patients by relocating their free-floating debris from the posterior semicircular canal back into the vestibular labyrinth (Fig. 95.1). The maneuver may need to be repeated until the patient is asymptomatic. There is about 80% success rate after a single treatment. The patient is advised to remain upright for 24 hours following the Epley maneuver at the office in order to minimize the likelihood of debris remigration to the

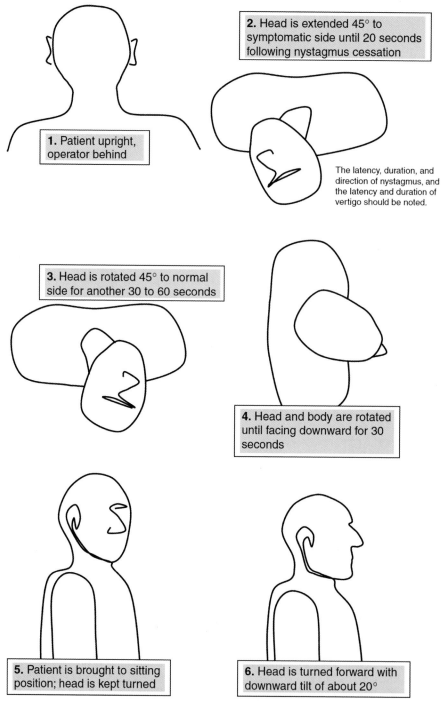

2. Head is extended 45° to symptomatic side until 20 seconds following nystagmus cessation

1. Patient upright, operator behind

The latency, duration, and direction of nystagmus, and the latency and duration of vertigo should be noted.

3. Head is rotated 45° to normal side for another 30 to 60 seconds

4. Head and body are rotated until facing downward for 30 seconds

5. Patient is brought to sitting position; head is kept turned

6. Head is turned forward with downward tilt of about 20°

Figure 95.1   Canalith Repositioning Maneuver (Epley). Positioning assumes left posterior semicircular canal affected. Reverse movements apply for right posterior semicircular canal. Note that the Dix-Hallpike test corresponds to the first two steps from Epley maneuver. (From Espay AJ, Biller J. *Concise neurology*. Philadelphia: Lippincott Williams & Wilkins, Wolters Kluwer Health, 2011, with permission.)

TABLE 95.1 DISTINGUISHING NYSTAGMUS OF CENTRAL VERSUS PERIPHERAL ORIGIN

	Peripheral Nystagmus	Central Nystagmus
Causes	Ménière, BPPV, vestibular neuritis, labyrinthitis	Lesions to the vestibulocerebellum (flocculus, nodulus, vermis)
Main features	Positional nystagmus has latency, adaptability, and *fatigability*	Positional nystagmus has no latency, no adaptability, and *no fatigability*
Directionality	Unidirectional (mixed horizontal/torsional[a]); fast phase opposite the affected labyrinth	Unidirectional or bidirectional; purely vertical (upbeating or downbeating),[b] torsional,[c] or horizontal[d]
Direction on eccentric gaze	Direction changes	Direction to same side regardless of gaze
Intensity	More pronounced in the side of the fast-beating component (away from vestibular lesion)	More pronounced toward side of gaze (e.g., left-beating in left gaze, upbeating in upgaze)
Effect of visual fixation	Nystagmus suppressed	Nystagmus not suppressed
Associated smooth pursuit	Intact	Broken in ipsilesional direction
Tinnitus or deafness	May be present	Absent

[a]Mixed horizontal/torsional nystagmus is typical for vestibular neuritis but can occur with central lesions.
[b]Pure vertical nystagmus is usually central but can occur with simultaneous lesions of both anterior or both posterior canals.
[c]Pure torsional nystagmus usually indicates a medullary lesion (syringobulbia and lateral medullary infarction) and may be part of the ocular tilt reaction (skew, torsion, and head tilt).
[d]Pure horizontal nystagmus is usually central but can occur with a single horizontal canal lesion.
Modified from Espay AJ, Biller J. *Concise neurology*. Philadelphia: Lippincott Williams & Wilkins, Wolters Kluwer Health, 2011, with permission.

posterior semicircular canal. When relapse develops, a second session is warranted. High-grade carotid stenosis and unstable heart disease are contraindications for this maneuver.

Nystagmus is a rhythmic oscillatory movement of the eyes that may be pendular (slow, and rare) or phasic (jerk nystagmus, and common). Jerk nystagmus is named after the direction of the fast, typically corrective eye movement. Nystagmus is seldom in and of itself symptomatic, representing a consequence rather than the underlying cause of vertigo. This consequence, however, when appropriately evaluated, can be of great value in determining whether the cause of the underlying vertigo is central or peripheral (Table 95.1).

SELECTED REFERENCES

Biller J, ed. *Practical neurology*, 6th ed. Philadelphia: Lippincott Williams & Wilkins, Wolters Kluwer Health, 2012.

Eggers SDZ, Zee DS. Evaluating the dizzy patient: bedside examination and laboratory assessment of the vestibular system. *Semin Neurol* 2003;23:47–58.

Epley JM. Human experience with canalith repositioning maneuvers. *Ann NY Acad Sci* 2001;942:179–191.

Espay AJ, Biller J. *Concise neurology*. Philadelphia: Lippincott Williams & Wilkins, Wolters Kluwer Health, 2011.

SEE QUESTIONS: 64, 338, 339

SECTION 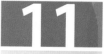 11

NUTRITIONAL/METABOLIC

CASE 96

WERNICKE ENCEPHALOPATHY SECONDARY TO HYPEREMESIS GRAVIDARUM

OBJECTIVES

- To review the clinical manifestations and differential diagnosis of Wernicke encephalopathy.
- To summarize the basic neuropathological findings of Wernicke encephalopathy.
- To list the most frequent conditions associated with Wernicke encephalopathy.
- To review management guidelines for Wernicke encephalopathy.

VIGNETTE

A 34-year-old woman was diagnosed with hyperemesis gravidarum. About 4 weeks after its onset, she started to complain of intermittent oscillopsia and dizziness. A month later, she had gallbladder surgery and induction of a stillborn child at 17 weeks of pregnancy.

CASE SUMMARY

 Our patient had intractable vomiting due to hyperemesis gravidarum resulting in Wernicke encephalopathy. Wernicke encephalopathy results from a deficiency in vitamin B_1 or thiamine. Because the body's reserves of thiamine are only 30 to 50 mg, they become depleted in approximately 4 to 6 weeks in the absence of thiamine intake. Global confusional state (greater than 60%), gait ataxia (50%), and a variety of ocular abnormalities (40%) are the hallmark of this disorder, although the occurrence of this triad in combination is unusual. Ocular findings most commonly encountered are vertical nystagmus, bilateral CN VI palsies, and conjugate gaze palsies, reflecting lesions of the vestibular nuclei, anterior and superior cerebellar vermis, abducens nuclei, and paramedian pontine reticular formation (PPRF).

Upgaze restriction reflecting compromise of the pretectum and periaqueductal gray is less common. Retinal hemorrhages and papilledema are rare. Pupillary abnormalities are present in less than 20% of patients. Vestibular paresis is uniformly present in the acute stage. The ataxia is predominantly cerebellar as a result of involvement of the superior cerebellar vermis and vestibular nuclei. Rarely, patients develop stupor, coma, or hypothermia.

Numerous conditions have been associated with Wernicke encephalopathy including chronic alcoholism, starvation, gastrointestinal tract malignancies, lymphoid–hemopoietic malignancies, anorexia nervosa, hunger strike, acquired immunodeficiency syndrome, pyloric stenosis, gastric stapling for morbid obesity, inappropriate parenteral nutrition, prolonged intravenous feeding, digitalis intoxication, chronic hemodialysis or long-standing peritoneal dialysis, drug treatment for obesity, thyrotoxicosis, and hyperemesis gravidarum.

In a review of 49 cases of Wernicke encephalopathy in pregnancy, the disorder manifested at a mean of 14 weeks of gestational age, when vomiting and feeding difficulties lasted just under 8 weeks.

Pathologically, there is evidence of bilateral symmetrical periventricular (third ventricle, aqueduct of Sylvius, and fourth ventricle) lesions in the brainstem and medial thalamus. The anterior cerebellar vermis is frequently involved, and atrophy of the mammillary bodies is seen in the majority of chronic cases. Affected structures show endothelial proliferation and the presence of microscopic petechial hemorrhages.

Diagnosis of Wernicke encephalopathy is facilitated by magnetic resonance imaging (MRI), which is more sensitive than computed tomography (CT) in detecting the acute periventricular and diencephalic lesions as demonstrated in our patient. Mirroring the pathological changes described above, typical findings are characterized by symmetric involvement of the medial thalami, mammillary bodies, and tectal plate. Differential diagnosis of patients presenting with confusion, ataxia, and oculomotor disturbances must include drug intoxication, posterior fossa strokes (particularly a "top of the basilar" stroke may affect most of the same structures listed above), subacute meningitides, subdural hematoma, and Leigh encephalomyelopathy. Management of Wernicke encephalopathy includes the administration of parenteral thiamine, bed rest, nutritional supplements, and the avoidance of glucose without thiamine. With thiamine administration, the nystagmus and abducens and conjugate palsies as well as the acute confusion are generally reversible; however, ataxia resolves completely in only approximately 40% of cases (see Case 87, "Upbeat Nystagmus").

In summary, Wernicke encephalopathy is a treatable disorder. Untreated, it carries a mortality of 10% to 20%. The major long-term complication is Korsakoff syndrome. Failure to diagnose Wernicke encephalopathy remains a serious concern. Numerous autopsy studies corroborate the rare occurrence of the full classical clinical triad.

SELECTED REFERENCES

Charness ME, Simon RP, Greenberg DA. Ethanol and the nervous system. *N Engl J Med* 1989;321:442–454.

Chiossi G, Neri I, Cavazzuti M. Hyperemesis gravidarum complicated by Wernicke encephalopathy: background, case report, and review of the literature. *Obstet Gynecol Surv* 2006;61(4):255–268.

Reuler JB, Girard DE, Cooney TG. Wernicke's encephalopathy. *N Engl J Med* 1985;312:1035–1038.

Zuccoli G, Pipitone N. Neuroimaging findings in acute Wernicke encephalopathy: review of the literature. *Am J Roentgenol* 2009;192(2):501–508.

SEE QUESTIONS: 166, 171, 328, 329, 330, 331

CASE 97

CEREBROTENDINOUS XANTHOMATOSIS

OBJECTIVES

- To review the main clinical features of cerebrotendinous xanthomatosis (CTX) in a patient free of neurological manifestations.
- To review some diagnostic pitfalls in the diagnosis of CTX.
- To review ancillary diagnostic criteria for CTX.
- To discuss management strategies of CTX.

VIGNETTE

A 53-year-old hypertensive woman had a history of multiple "lumps" involving her hands, knees, feet, and legs since age 9 and had "more than 400 surgeries" to remove these lesions. She also had three heart attacks and had a coronary artery bypass graft (CABG) 7 years earlier. She had no history of chronic diarrhea and had no neurologic complaints except for occasional blurry vision. She had three living brothers, eight living sisters, and two daughters. There was a history of heart disease in one brother (deceased). Two brothers had similar tender xanthomas.

On examination, her blood pressure was 138/72 mm Hg. She had bilateral carotid bruits and a grade II/VI systolic ejection murmur. There was a large pterygium nasally extending very close to the visual axis of the right eye and a dense arcus of both corneas. On funduscopic examination, the appearance of the discs, maculae, vessels, and periphery was normal. She had mild bilateral cataracts.

CASE SUMMARY

Our patient presented with pain around multiple xanthomatous lesions of the extremities. Initially she was diagnosed with neurofibromatosis, and subsequently she received the diagnosis of phytosterolemia. Examination showed numerous xanthomas present throughout her extremities. There were faint bilateral carotid bruits. Neurologic examination was normal. Carotid ultrasound showed 16% to 59% bilateral internal carotid artery stenosis.

Magnetic resonance imaging showed evidence of focal parietal atrophy but was otherwise unremarkable. Magnetic resonance spectroscopy (MRS) showed a mild increase in the *N*-acetylaspartate peak along with mild increased choline and lipid peaks. Serum cholesterol was 186, and serum cholestanol was elevated at 1.57 mg/dL (normal 0.2 ± 0.2 mg/dL). Urine was positive for tetrahydroxy, pentahydroxy, and hexahydroxy bile acid glucuronides, which are specific for sterol 27-hydroxylase deficiency. Cultured fibroblasts were checked for 27-sterol hydroxylase deficiency. The patient was switched from cholestyramine to colesevelam and started on chenodeoxycholic acid (CDCA).

CTX, van Bogaert disease, is a rare autosomal recessive lipid storage disorder caused by a mutation in the *CYP27A1* gene or chromosome 2q33, encoding the mitochondrial enzyme sterol 27-hydroxylase. The incidence of CTX has been estimated to be 3 to 5 per 100,000 people worldwide with an estimated prevalence of 1.9 per 100,000 in Caucasians of European ancestry. It typically presents as a slowly progressive ataxia in conjunction with tendinous xanthomas. Pyramidal, extrapyramidal (dystonia and parkinsonism), and cerebellar manifestations, along with dementia and seizures, are the predominant neurological manifestations. Other clinical features include myelopathy and polyneuropathy. The xanthomas may also be seen in the quadriceps, triceps, and fingers in addition to the Achilles tendons, or they may be absent. Thickening of the interatrial septum compatible with lipomatous hypertrophy has been described in a few patients with CTX. Elevated serum cholestanol and urine bile acid glucuronides help to confirm the diagnosis.

The primary treatment of CTX is with CDCA. HMG-CoA reductase inhibitors have also been used.

SELECTED REFERENCES

Federico A, Dotti MT. Cerebrotendinous xanthomatosis. *Neurology* 2001;57:1743.

Kuriyama M, Tokimura Y, Fujiyama J, et al. Treatment of cerebrotendinous xanthomatosis: effects of chenodeoxycholic acid, pravastatin, and combined use. *J Neurol Sci* 1994;125(Aug):22–28.

Lorincz MT, Rainier S, Thomas D, Fink JK. Cerebrotendinous xanthomatosis, possible higher prevalence than previously recognized. *Arch Neurol* 2005;62:1459.

Van Bogaert L, et al. *Une forme cérébrale de la cholestérinose généralise.* Paris, France: Mason et Cie, 1937.

SEE QUESTION: 251

SECTION 12

HEADACHES/PAIN

CASE 98

MIGRAINE HEADACHES/PREGNANCY

VIGNETTE

A 35-year-old woman, G2, P1, 36-week gestation, was evaluated for recurrent headaches.

CASE SUMMARY

This patient presented with headache during pregnancy. Patients with episodic headaches, throbbing or pounding in quality, associated visual aura, intolerance of light and noise, and nausea are typically diagnosed with migraine. Migraine headaches affect approximately 25% of women during childbearing years. The relationship between migraine and estrogens is well known, including the tendency for migraine to occur around menses, to be aggravated by contraceptive medication, to develop following removal of the ovaries, and to exacerbate or begin during pregnancy. Some women experience a reduction of migraine during and after menopause, whereas others begin to experience migraine in this setting. Similarly, pregnancy can be associated with a dramatic improvement in migraine for some women, especially those who have perimenstrual headaches. Approximately 60% to 70% of women have improvement in the frequency of migraines, mainly around the second and third trimesters. Conversely, approximately 10% of migraines start during pregnancy, while 4% to 8% of women experience worsening migraines during pregnancy.

Commonly migraine occurs early in the second trimester. Management of migraine in pregnancy is problematic as many of the standard drugs used for prevention and those used for acute management are relatively contraindicated. In general, acetaminophen is acceptable for PRN use in pregnancy. For more severe headaches, acetaminophen with codeine is used. Beta-blockers (propranolol), verapamil, valproate, and tricyclic antidepressants are avoided. Triptans and dihydroergotamine are best avoided as well. All triptans are considered to be pregnancy category C by the US Food and Drug Administration (US FDA). At times, headache severity and frequency require an open discussion between the patient, her neurologist, and her obstetrician to consider the risks and benefits of exposure to one of the drugs just named. Alternative therapies such as relaxation, biofeedback, acupuncture, and other nonpharmacologic interventions should be considered.

Serious causes of headache are important to consider when evaluating a pregnant patient, including intracranial venous or sinus thrombosis, idiopathic intracranial hypertension, stroke, tumor, severe preeclampsia, and subarachnoid or intracerebral hemorrhage. Intracerebral hemorrhage is 2.5 times more likely during pregnancy and 28 times more likely during the first 6 weeks postpartum. The risk of aneurysmal subarachnoid hemorrhage is greatest during the third trimester, whereas arteriovenous malformations may be slightly more likely to bleed in the second trimester.

SELECTED REFERENCES

Aube M. Migraine in pregnancy (review). *Neurology* 1999;53(4 Suppl 1):S26–S28.

Biller J, ed. *Practical neurology*, 4th ed. Philadelphia: Lippincott Williams & Wilkins, Wolters Kluwer Health, 2012.

Contag SA, Bushnell C. Contemporary management of migrainous disorders in pregnancy. *Curr Opin Obstet Gynecol* 2010;22:437–445.

Roos KL, ed. *Headache and pregnancy*. In: *Neurologic disorders and pregnancy*. Continuum, Philadelphia 2000:114–127.

SEE QUESTIONS: 90, 134, 145, 146, 147, 260

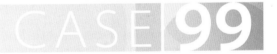

CASE 99

CLUSTER HEADACHES

OBJECTIVES

- To analyze characteristic clinical features of episodic cluster headache.
- To briefly review the current classification of the many varieties of cluster headache.
- To summarize management guidelines for episodic cluster headache.

VIGNETTE

A 28-year-old man was evaluated because of recurrent unilateral headaches.

CASE SUMMARY

Without any warning, our patient experienced a rather stereotypical syndrome characterized by recurrent brief attacks of severe unilateral pain centered around the left periorbital/retroorbital region, lasting 60 to 90 minutes. The pain was constant and more common nocturnal, awakening him from sleep. He had no gastrointestinal complaints. During attacks, he was restless, unable to lie flat, and constantly pacing.

There were ipsilateral autonomic signs related to sympathetic paresis and parasympathetic system overactivity such as conjunctival injection, lacrimation, rhinorrhea, and eyelid ptosis and miosis (as noted on his medical records). He had no manifestations of trigeminal nerve dysfunction. The attacks occurred with a frequency from once daily to once every other day, lasting for a few weeks to 2 months. There was a characteristic periodicity with pain-free intervals of many years. High-flow oxygen therapy was very effective in aborting an attack.

According to the International Headache Society (IHS), our patient fulfilled diagnostic criteria for episodic cluster headache. Cluster headache has been classified into (a) episodic, (b) chronic, (c) chronic paroxysmal hemicrania, and (d) cluster headache–like syndrome. Chronic cluster headaches have been further subdivided into primary chronic (chronic from onset) and secondary chronic (chronic cluster headache evolving from episodic cluster headache). Eighty percent of cluster sufferers have the episodic variety of cluster. Men are affected more than women (3 to 6:1 ratio). The exact prevalence of cluster headache is unknown but has been estimated to be at least 0.4% in men and 0.08% in women.

Periodicity is a main feature of episodic cluster headache, with the cluster period lasting 2 to 3 months, attributed to hypothalamic influences. Typical attacks often occur at the same time each day, awakening patients from sleep. There is no aura. Pain typically peaks in 10 to 15 minutes. Attacks usually last anywhere between 15 and 180 minutes and occur with a frequency from once every other day to eight times a day. Typical pain is described as excruciating, burning, or boring, but usually not throbbing. The pain is associated with symptoms and signs of cranial autonomic dysfunction including ipsilateral conjunctival injection and/or lacrimation, ipsilateral nasal congestion and/or rhinorrhea, and ipsilateral Horner syndrome. Cluster periods typically occur every 1 to 2 years.

Chronic cluster headache refers to typical cluster headaches whose cycle is longer than 6 months without remission or with remissions lasting less than 2 weeks. In chronic paroxysmal hemicrania, the attacks are considerably shorter (5 to 45 minutes) than in episodic cluster headache and also more frequent (7 to 22 per day).

Chronic paroxysmal hemicrania is more common among women. It consists of multiple (2 to 40 times), brief (2 to 45 minutes), unilateral, periorbital or temporal, daily painful attacks that persist unremittingly for years; and is highly responsive to indomethacin, to the extent that this response is part of the diagnostic criteria.

Symptomatic forms of cluster headache or cluster headache–like syndrome have been described in association with a variety of lesions, usually near the cavernous sinus, including tumors (e.g., parasellar meningiomas, pituitary adenomas, and nasopharyngeal carcinomas), vascular malformations, carotid and vertebral artery aneurysms, and giant cell arteritis, among others. Symptomatic clusterlike headaches should be suspected if there is a lack of periodicity to the patient's complaints, if there is residual background pain between pain clusters, if the neurologic examination is abnormal besides ptosis and miosis, or if traditional therapy is ineffective.

Management of episodic cluster headache may be symptomatic/abortive or prophylactic/preventive. Precise documentation of potential drug contraindications and potential drug interactions must be taken into consideration when selecting among the many available pharmacologic agents. The most effective symptomatic treatment of cluster headache is inhalation of high-flow concentrated oxygen, 6 to 8 L/min, by face mask, for no longer than 20 minutes. Other abortive strategies include intranasal administration of 4% lidocaine, subcutaneous sumatriptan, sublingual or inhaled ergotamine, and injectable dihydroergotamine (DHE 45 injection) preparations.

The prophylactic treatment of episodic cluster headaches includes verapamil, ergotamine, lithium carbonate, corticosteroids, valproic acid, gabapentin, baclofen, and topiramate. Verapamil is the most effective calcium channel blocker for cluster headache prophylaxis and the treatment of first choice. Combined therapy is often necessary and may be very effective. Refractory cluster headache patients have been treated with occipital nerve or hypothalamic neurostimulator. Patients should avoid alcohol.

SELECTED REFERENCES

Ashkenazi A, Schwedt T. Cluster headache and prophylactic therapy. *Headache* 2011;51:272–286.

Biller J, ed. *Practical neurology*, 4th ed. Philadelphia: Lippincott Williams & Wilkins, Wolters Kluwer Health, 2012.

Headache Classification Subcommittee of the International Headache Society. The international classification of headache disorders: 2nd edition. *Cephalalgia* 2004;24(Suppl 1):9–160.

Kudrow L. *Cluster headache: mechanisms and management.* London: Oxford University Press, 1980.

Kudrow L. The pathogenesis of cluster headache. *Curr Opin Neurol* 1994;7:278–282.

SEE QUESTIONS: 133, 134, 135, 136, 144, 145, 146, 147, 259

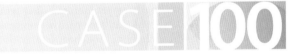

CSF HYPOTENSION SYNDROME

OBJECTIVES

- To analyze the characteristic clinical and neuroimaging features of spontaneous intracranial hypotension syndrome.
- To summarize management guidelines of the spontaneous intracranial hypotension syndrome.

VIGNETTE

A 49-year-old previously healthy woman was admitted for evaluation of new-onset headaches.

CASE SUMMARY

Without an apparent precipitating factor such as head trauma, back trauma, or lumbar puncture, our patient experienced an incapacitating positional headache. The headache was worse on assuming a sitting or standing position and was relieved when supine or prone. There had been no response to analgesics including codeine. She then developed horizontal binocular diplopia. She had no fever, neck stiffness, cerebrospinal fluid (CSF) rhinorrhea, or upper extremity radicular complaints. Eventually, a brain magnetic resonance imaging (MRI) showed diffuse thickening of the pachymeninges with diffuse, nonnodular intense enhancement with gadolinium. She was initially erroneously suspected of having meningitis. When a lumbar puncture (LP) was attempted, she was told she had a "dry tap" and was referred for further evaluation.

On initial examination, she was afebrile and only had mild limitation of abduction of the right eye. A radionuclide cisternogram showed asymmetric activity projecting in the right posterior lateral region of the cervical spine. A cervical computed tomography (CT) myelogram showed abnormal epidural collections of contrast focally at C2-3 anteriorly and C5-6 posterolaterally. There was also bilateral C7-T1 and T1-2 epidural contrast extending through the neural foramina and surrounding bilateral root sleeves and ganglia. These findings were more pronounced at C7-T1 on the left. After bed rest, administration of intravenous fluids, and two autologous epidural blood patches, she had marked recovery with complete resolution of her headaches and diplopia. Within 3 months, she became asymptomatic and returned to work full time.

Our patient had the cardinal features of spontaneous intracranial hypotension, a disorder most commonly observed among women, age 30 to 60, with underlying connective tissue disorders. The most common symptom of spontaneous intracranial hypotension is an orthostatic holocranial headache, similar to postdural puncture headaches. Relief of pain within a few minutes of lying flat is characteristic. Straining and coughing exacerbate the pain. Onset of headaches may be sudden or gradual. Patients may also complain of neck stiffness, neck or interscapular pain, nausea, vomiting, diplopia, visual blurring, photophobia, facial numbness, dysgeusia, decreased hearing, hyperacusis, tinnitus, dizziness, fainting when standing, or upper limb radicular symptoms.

Typical MRI features include diffuse pachymeningeal/dural enhancement following the administration of gadolinium, thought to represent engorgement of the dural vasculature. The ventricles may be slitlike. There may be evidence of caudal brain descent, manifested as herniation of the cerebellar tonsils ("secondary Chiari I malformation") and tight basilar cisterns. Subdural collections (hematomas and hygromas) have been described. Enlargement of the pituitary gland has been described.

By definition, the CSF pressure is low (60 mm H_2O or less) or unobtainable, and there is no history of previous dural puncture. However, some patients with spontaneous intracranial hypotension have normal CSF pressure; this suggests that CSF hypovolemia rather than hypotension may play a pathogenic role. The CSF composition is usually normal, but there may be slight elevation of the CSF protein elevation, a variable lymphocytic pleocytosis, and few red blood cells. A thorough investigation to test for CSF leaks along the neuraxis should be undertaken.

A CSF leak is documented in most, if not all, cases of spontaneous intracranial hypotension, usually at the level of the cervicothoracic junction or thoracic spine. MRI of the spine may demonstrate the level of the CSF leak or associated meningeal diverticula or dilated epidural veins in the high cervical region. CT myelography of the entire spine may be necessary. Management involves bed rest, oral or intravenous fluids, oral or intravenous caffeine therapy, analgesics, steroids, and the administration of autologous epidural blood patches or continuous epidural saline infusions. Many patients require repair of the CSF leak. MRI findings of meningeal enhancement decrease or disappear as clinical symptoms subside. Prognosis is generally favorable. Most patients can be cured after a correct diagnosis is made.

SELECTED REFERENCES

Bell WE, Joynt RJ, Sahs AL. Low spinal fluid pressure syndromes. *Neurology* 1961;10:512–521.

Mokri B, Piepgras DG, Miller GM. Syndrome of orthostatic headaches and diffuse pachymeningeal gadolinium enhancement. *Mayo Clin Proc* 1997;72:400–413.

Mokri B, Posner JB. Spontaneous intracranial hypotension. The broadening clinical and imaging spectrum of CSF leaks. *Neurology* 2000;55:1771–1772.

Pannullo SC, Reich JB, Krol G, et al. MRI changes in intracranial hypotension. *Neurology* 1993;43:919–926.

SEE QUESTIONS: 96, 97, 136, 137, 144, 145, 151, 154, 162, 258

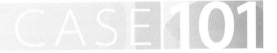

CASE 101

IDIOPATHIC INTRACRANIAL HYPERTENSION

OBJECTIVES

- To describe criteria for the diagnosis of idiopathic intracranial hypertension (IIH).
- To describe potential causes of IIH.
- To discuss the differential diagnosis of IIH.
- To review treatment guidelines for patients with IIH.

VIGNETTE

A 31-year-old woman was evaluated because of headaches.

CASE SUMMARY

 This young obese normotensive woman presented with a combination of long-standing headaches, visual scotomata, bilateral papilledema, and enlarged blind spots on visual field testing. She was not on contraceptives. Visual acuity was 20/20 OU. Remainder of her neurologic examination was unremarkable. She had a normal brain magnetic resonance imaging (MRI) and normal magnetic resonance venography (MRV). Having excluded hydrocephalus, an intracranial mass, or cerebral venous thrombosis as the etiology of the papilledema, she had a lumbar puncture (LP), which showed elevated opening pressure and normal cerebrospinal fluid (CSF) composition.

A diagnosis of IIH was made. As there was no known exposure to exogenous substances associated with IIH and her visual acuity was preserved, her initial management consisted of a weight reduction diet, symptomatic headache treatment, and acetazolamide 500 mg twice daily.

The diagnosis of IIH includes the following criteria: (i) symptoms and signs of raised intracranial pressure (headaches, transient visual obscurations (TVOs), and horizontal diplopia due to unilateral or bilateral CN VI palsy), (ii) normal neuroimaging studies (MRI and MRV preferably; MRI may show small ventricles and occasionally an empty sella), and (iii) increased opening CSF pressure (greater than 250 mm H_2O) with normal composition (may show a low CSF protein). Patients may also complain of pulsatile tinnitus. Occasionally patients may present with oculomotor or trochlear nerve palsies or skew deviation.

Most common in obese young women, IIH is divided into two categories: primary (no identifiable pathogenesis) and secondary (cause of CSF pressure elevation identified). IIH has been associated with a variety of exogenous substances including tetracyclines, nalidixic acid, amiodarone, corticosteroids, danazol, lithium, hypervitaminosis A, isotretinoin, cyclosporine, indomethacin, and growth hormone. IIH has also been reported in association with pregnancy, menarche, systemic lupus erythematosus, Addison disease, corticosteroid withdrawal, hypoparathyroidism, thyroid replacement, uremia, severe anemia, high-flow arteriovenous malformations, radical neck dissection, and other disorders of cerebral venous drainage. Differential diagnosis of patients presenting with bilateral swollen optic discs should always encompass papilledema due to an intracranial mass lesion, papillitis, anterior ischemic optic neuropathy (AION), pseudopapilledema, optic nerve head drusen, bilateral optic nerve tumors, and malignant hypertension. MRI and MRV are obtained to exclude an intracranial mass lesion or cerebral venous thrombosis. CSF studies are needed to exclude inflammatory/infectious disorders or leptomeningeal malignancy.

Uncontrolled papilledema may result in progressive peripheral visual field constriction or nerve fiber bundle defects. The goal of treatment is visual preservation and consists of weight reduction for those patients who are overweight and diuretics such as acetazolamide or furosemide. For those patients who have deterioration of their visual function related to optic nerve dysfunction, proposed surgical procedures consist of optic nerve sheath fenestration or lumboperitoneal or ventriculoperitoneal shunting.

SELECTED REFERENCES

Brazis PW, Lee AG. Elevated intracranial pressure and pseudotumor cerebri. *Curr Opin Ophthalmol* 1998;9(6):27–32.

Corbett JJ, Savino PJ, Thompson HS, et al. Visual loss in pseudotumor cerebri. Follow-up of 57 patients from five to 41 years and a profile of 14 patients with permanent severe visual loss. *Arch Neurol* 1982;39:461–474.

Digre KB, Corbett JJ. *Practical viewing of the optic disc.* Boston: Butterworth-Heinemann, 2003.

Headache Classification Subcommittee of the International Headache Society. The international classification of headache disorders: 2nd edition. *Cephalalgia* 2004;24(Suppl 1):9–160.

SEE QUESTIONS: 145, 146, 160, 161, 162

CASE 102

TRIGEMINAL NEURALGIA

OBJECTIVES

- To present a typical patient with idiopathic trigeminal neuralgia (tic douloureux).
- To review relevant applied anatomy of the trigeminal nerve (CN V).
- To review management guidelines for patients with trigeminal neuralgia.

VIGNETTE

A 48-year-old man complained of episodic bursts of sharp, shooting left-sided facial pain.

CASE SUMMARY

Our patient had multiple episodes of severe, brief (few seconds), stabbing, unilateral (left-sided only) facial pain, affecting predominantly the dermatomal zones innervated by the maxillary (V2) and mandibular (V3) branches of the trigeminal nerve (CN V), and to a lesser extent the dermatomal zone innervated by the ophthalmic (V1) branch. The episodes of pain were frequently triggered by painless sensory stimuli such as a draft of cold wind, chewing, or even a kiss. The episodes were repetitive, usually three to four in a given day. Between attacks, he had no symptoms. Neurologic examination was normal.

Our patient provided an accurate description of a paroxysmal unilateral painful condition, with periods of remission, affecting the trigeminal nerve and typical of trigeminal neuralgia. The nucleus of the trigeminal nerve stretches from the midbrain (mesencephalic nucleus) through the pons (principal sensory and motor nucleus of V) to the upper cervical spinal cord region (nucleus of the spinal tract of the trigeminal nerve), where it becomes continuous with Lissauer tract. The nucleus of the spinal tract of the trigeminal nerve is divided into a pars oralis, a pars interpolaris, and a pars caudalis.

The trigeminal nerve (CN V), the largest of the cranial nerves, exits laterally at the level of the mid-pons, and its three divisions—ophthalmic (V1), maxillary (V2), and mandibular (V3)—proceed toward the gasserian ganglion located in Meckel cave of the petrous bone in the middle cranial fossa. From there, the ophthalmic division (V1) exits the cranium via the superior orbital fissure, the maxillary division (V2) exits through the foramen rotundum, and the mandibular division (V3) exits via the foramen ovale. The trigeminal nerve provides sensory innervation of the face and supplies the muscles of mastication.

Trigeminal neuralgia (tic douloureux or Fothergill disease) is the most frequent type of facial neuralgia. More common with advanced age, trigeminal neuralgia affects women more commonly than men. The most commonly affected dermatomal zones are innervated by V2 and V3 together. This pattern is more common than involvement of V2 or V3 alone. The V1 dermatome is the least affected. The right side tends to be affected more commonly than the left. Trigeminal neuralgia in a young patient should raise the suspicion of multiple sclerosis.

The pathogenesis of idiopathic trigeminal neuralgia is uncertain. Many cases of idiopathic trigeminal neuralgia have been attributed to pulsations of an aberrant vascular (venous or arterial) loop causing areas of focal demyelination of the trigeminal nerve root entry zone (REZ) into the pons leading to ephaptic transmission of impulses. Secondary forms of trigeminal neuralgia may be due to mass lesions, (e.g., acoustic neuroma and clivus chordomas) or meningeal inflammation. Pontine demyelinating lesions at the REZ of the trigeminal nerve have been demonstrated in multiple sclerosis patients with trigeminal neuralgia.

Diagnosis of trigeminal neuralgia is purely clinical, and is usually made by history alone. As in our patient, the neurologic examination findings are normal in patients with idiopathic trigeminal neuralgia. MRI of the brain is useful to exclude an intracranial lesion or other causes of symptomatic trigeminal neuralgia. The sensitivity of MRA in localizing a vascular compression remains low. Blood count, liver functions tests, and serum sodium are routinely obtained.

Medical management of patients with trigeminal neuralgia should be attempted first. Carbamazepine is the most effective medication; most patients respond to 200 to 800 mg daily in two or three divided doses, although higher doses, up to 2,400 mg daily, may be needed. Other alternatives include oxcarbazepine, phenytoin, valproic acid, baclofen, gabapentin, lamotrigine, or clonazepam. If medical therapy is not successful, surgical therapy should be entertained. One of the most effective procedures is the microvascular decompression (MVD or Jannetta procedure) of vascular elements from the trigeminal nerve. Percutaneous procedures include radiofrequency trigeminal gangliolysis (PRTG), retrogasserian glycerol rhizotomy (PRGR), and balloon microcompression (PBM). An increasingly popular noninvasive outpatient procedure is stereotactic gamma knife radiosurgery (GKS).

SELECTED REFERENCES

Barker FG, Janetta PJ, Bissonette DJ. The long-term outcome of microvascular decompression for trigeminal neuralgia. *N Engl J Med* 1996;334:1077–1083.

Biller J, ed. *Practical neurology*, 4th ed. Philadelphia: Lippincott Williams & Wilkins, Wolters Kluwer Health, 2012.

Burchile KV, Slavin KV. On the natural history of trigeminal neuralgia. *Neurosurgery* 2000;46:152–154.

Krafft RM. Trigeminal neuralgia. *Am Fam Physician* 2008;77(9):1291–1296.

Tenser RB. Trigeminal neuralgia: mechanisms of treatment. *Neurology* 1998;51(1):17–19.

SEE QUESTIONS: 62, 63, 133, 134, 146, 177

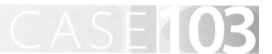

ATYPICAL FACIAL PAIN

OBJECTIVES

- To analyze the clinical features of atypical facial pain.
- To review the differential diagnosis of atypical facial pain.
- To summarize management guidelines for patients with atypical facial pain.

A 47-year-old woman complained of refractory constant left-sided facial pain of 8-year duration. Neurologic examination was normal.

CASE SUMMARY

Our patient had an 8-year history of a predominantly unilateral, dull, and unrelenting left-sided facial pain that did not follow the anatomical boundaries of the trigeminal nerve. The pain was described as a deep aching and burning on the left side of her face, ear, and lateral aspect of her neck. Occasionally, it was described as sharp and/or shooting. The pain was not aggravated by chewing, swallowing, talking, touching the face at a specific point (trigger point), or lateral movements of the jaw. There was no history of odontalgia. The pain was not related to biting or hot and cold foods. She had no ipsilateral conjunctival injection, nasal congestion, or other autonomic symptoms. She did not have nausea, photophobia, or sonophobia. There was no history of zoster or associated facial sensory loss. Due to the almost continuous nature of her deep and intense facial pain, she became very irritable and experienced recurrent depression. Her sleep was not affected.

She saw a variety of medical specialists. Initially she was thought to have a sinus infection. Then, she was diagnosed with trigeminal neuralgia. Treatment with appropriate doses of carbamazepine was unsuccessful. The diagnosis of trigeminal neuralgia was subsequently rejected by a neurosurgeon whom she consulted for a peripheral block by means of alcohol injections. Eventually, she had all her teeth removed without any benefit. Besides carbamazepine, numerous medications including tricyclic antidepressants, indomethacin, nonopioid analgesics, and finally opioid analgesics were tried but without satisfactory results. Neurologic and physical examination were normal. She had no trigger points. The temporomandibular joints were normal. There was no tenderness on palpation of the supraorbital and infraorbital foramina.

Based on her history of unrelenting facial pain with ill-defined anatomical boundaries, and after extensive investigations that excluded other possible structural causes of protracted facial pain, our patient was diagnosed with atypical facial pain. Despite its wide clinical acceptance as a separate entity, there are no well-accepted diagnostic criteria of atypical facial pain. The general characteristics of atypical facial pain resemble those described by our patient. Although mostly unilateral, a bilateral occurrence is not rare. The cause of atypical facial pain remains unknown. Atypical facial pain must be distinguished from trigeminal neuralgia (tic douloureux), temporomandibular joint syndrome, migraines, cluster headaches, paroxysmal hemicrania, short-lasting unilateral neuralgiform headache attacks with conjunctival injections and tearing (SUNCT) syndrome, temporal arteritis, postherpetic neuralgia, glossopharyngeal neuralgia, trigeminal neuropathy, dental pain, otitis media, neoplastic processes of the maxillary sinus or nasopharynx, and pain of psychological origin.

Diagnosis and management with atypical facial pain are challenging. Pharmacologic interventions include tricyclic antidepressants, gabapentin, lamotrigine, clonazepam, transcutaneous nerve stimulation, sphenopalatine ganglion block, psychotherapy, and behavioral approaches. After many strategies of pharmacologic combinations were attempted without major success, a combination of gabapentin and the synthetic prostaglandin E1 analog misoprostol (Cytotec) has decreased our patient's pain to tolerable levels, improving her quality of life.

SELECTED REFERENCES

Biller J, ed. *Practical neurology*, 4th ed. Philadelphia: Lippincott Williams & Wilkins, Wolters Kluwer Health, 2012.

Koopman JS, Dieleman JP, Huygen FJ, et al. Incidence of facial pain in the general population. *Pain* 2009;147(1–3):122–127.

Qual G. Atypical facial pain—a diagnostic challenge. *Aust Fam Physician* 2005;34(8):641–645.

Reder AT, Arnason BG. Trigeminal neuralgia in multiple sclerosis relieved by a prostaglandin E analogue. *Neurology* 1995;45:1097–1100.

Reik L. Atypical facial pain: a reappraisal. *Headache* 1985;25:30–32.

Turp J, Gobetti JP. Trigeminal neuralgia versus atypical facial pain: a review of the literature and case report. *Oral Surg Oral Med Oral Path Oral Radiol Endod* 1996;81:424–432.

SEE QUESTIONS: 63, 133, 134, 159, 177

SECTION 13

EPILEPSY AND SPELLS

CASE 104

PARTIAL COMPLEX SEIZURES

OBJECTIVES

- To review the classification of epilepsies and epileptic syndromes.
- To describe localizing signs of partial seizures.
- To describe common treatment options of complex partial seizures.

VIGNETTE

An 18-year-old man was evaluated because of recurrent "spells" since the age of 11.

CASE SUMMARY

 Our patient was an 18-year-old man with a history of complex partial and secondarily generalized seizures. He had had seizures since age 11. His seizures had been refractory to topiramate, oxcarbazepine, and levetiracetam. While being monitored with a video electroencephalography (EEG), he had a complex partial seizure. During the ictal phase, he had sudden onset of a motionless stare and became unresponsive. Next, a tonic abducting posture of both hands was noted. Initially, his right hand was held in a dystonic posture. Some mild lip smacking was noted. He then became restless and exhibited some purposeless hand movements. No sustained gaze deviation was noted. During the postictal phase, he had difficulty speaking and finding words, suggesting postictal dysphasia. A complex automatism was noted in his attempt to use the remote control.

An epileptic seizure is a transient and reversible alteration of movements, sensation, awareness, or behavior caused by a paroxysmal, abnormal, and excessive neuronal discharge. One isolated seizure is not defined as epilepsy. Among patients with a single seizure, only approximately 25% will experience an *unprovoked* recurrence within 2 years, that is, in the absence of triggers or risk factors. Epilepsy is typically defined as two or more recurring seizures not provoked by any triggers, including intracranial infections, drug withdrawal, acute metabolic changes, or fever.

The International League Against Epilepsy (ILAE) classification system for seizures divided seizures into two broad categories: partial (focal) seizures and generalized seizures. Partial seizures start in specific locations in the cerebral cortex and are associated with focal ictal and interictal changes during an EEG. Generalized seizures are characterized by generalized involvement of both the cerebral hemispheres from the beginning of the seizure and have no consistent focal areas of ictal onset.

Partial seizures can become secondarily generalized tonic–clonic seizures. Partial seizures are further subdivided into simple partial and complex partial seizures. Consciousness remains intact during a simple partial seizure, whereas consciousness is impaired during a complex partial seizure.

For etiology, the terms idiopathic (unknown cause), symptomatic (identifiable cause), and cryptogenic (hidden or occult cause) have been used, but newer concepts in classifications of the epilepsies are being proposed. Complex partial seizures are the most common seizure type in adults, and the temporal lobe, particularly the medial temporal lobe, is the most common site of epileptogenic focus. There appears to be a strong relationship between complicated febrile seizures during early childhood or infancy and the later development of medial temporal lobe epilepsy. Lateralizing signs can often predict the side of abnormality or epileptogenic region in patients with partial epilepsy.

Forced and sustained head deviation and asymmetric tonic limb posturing of the upper extremity (sometimes creating a "figure 4 sign") often indicate a contralateral epileptogenic region. Unilateral upper extremity automatisms may predict an ipsilateral seizure focus. Postictal dysphasia usually indicates a dominant-hemisphere seizure. A variety of additional ictal clinical signs have lateralizing or even localizing value (Table 104.1). This patient's ictal and postictal behavior would suggest a left temporal lobe focus.

TABLE 104.1   LATERALIZATION VALUE OF ICTAL OR POSTICTAL CLINICAL SIGNS

Ictal Clinical Signs	Lateralizing Value
Ictal tonic–clonic movements	Contralateral
Ictal head rotation	Contralateral
Ictal arm extension ("figure 4 sign")[a]	Contralateral to extended arm
Ictal visual aura or unilateral somatosensory sensation	Contralateral
Ictal nystagmus, fast phase	Contralateral
Last clonus of a secondarily generalized tonic–clonic seizure	Ipsilateral (85%)
Ictal spitting, nausea, vomiting, urinary urge	Nondominant temporal lobe
Ictal or postictal aphasia	Dominant hemisphere
Ictal or postictal speech or repetitive vocalizations	Nondominant hemisphere
Postictal oral automatisms	Nonlocalizing
Postictal unilateral manual automatism	Nonlocalizing
Ictal pallor and cold shivers	Dominant temporal lobe
Postictal unilateral nose wiping	Ipsilateral to the wiping hand
Automatism with preserved consciousness	Nondominant temporal lobe
Peri-ictal unilateral headache	Ipsilateral

[a]The "figure 4 sign" consists of asymmetric tonic limb posturing whereby one elbow is extended while the other is flexed during the tonic phase of the seizure. The seizure focus is contralateral to the extended elbow.

The temporal lobe is the most common site of origin for partial seizures. Mesial temporal sclerosis is the most common abnormality seen on magnetic resonance imaging (MRI) images of the brain in patients with temporal lobe epilepsy. Our patient's MRI showed evidence of bilateral mesial temporal sclerosis and cortical dysplasia of the right anterior temporal region. EEG showed frequent independent epileptiform discharges over both anterior midtemporal regions. Ictal single photon emission computed tomography (SPECT) scan during video EEG demonstrated hyperperfusion over the right temporal region. Subsequent positron emission tomography (PET) scan showed no focal deficits.

The first-line treatment of complex partial seizures is medical therapy with any number of antiepileptic drugs (AEDs). Although monotherapy is attempted first, combination of AEDs may be needed. For patients with medically refractory complex partial seizures, surgical treatment should be considered. Several surgical procedures are available. If, after extensive evaluation, a single epileptogenic focus is found that does not involve eloquent section of the cortex, resective surgery may be an option. Resection of the medial temporal lobe is the most common surgical procedure for treatment of medically refractory complex partial seizures. Due to discordance between electrographic and neuroimaging data, our patient did not have surgery.

SELECTED REFERENCES

Berg AT. Risk of recurrence after a first unprovoked seizure. *Epilepsia* 2008;49(Suppl 1):13–18.

Berg AT, Scheffer IE. New concepts in classifications of the epilepsia: Entering the 21st century. Critical Care Review and Invited Commentary. *Epilepsia* 2011;52(6):1058–1062.

Commission on Classification and Terminology of the International League Against Epilepsy. Proposal for revised clinical and electrographic classification of epileptic seizures. *Epilepsia* 1981;22:489–501.

Commission on Classification and Terminology of the International League against Epilepsy. Proposal for revised classification of epilepsies and epileptic syndromes. *Epilepsia* 1989;30:388–399.

French JA, Williamson PD, Thadnai VM, et al. Characteristics of medial temporal lobe epilepsy. I. results of history and physical examination. *Ann Neurol* 1993;34:774–780.

Kotagal P, Bleasel A, Geller E. et al. Lateralizing value of asymmetric tonic limb posturing observed in secondarily generalized tonic-clonic seizures. *Epilepsia* 2000;41(4):457–462.

Siebe S. Blume WT, Girvin JP, Eliasziw M. A randomized, controlled trial of surgery for temporal-lobe epilepsy. *N Engl J Med* 2001;345:311–318.

SEE QUESTIONS: 6, 7, 8, 9, 21, 22, 23, 24, 25, 98, 99, 100, 101, 198, 222, 224, 236, 237

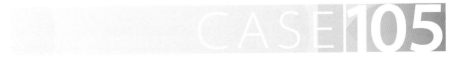

PARTIAL SEIZURES WITH ELEMENTARY SYMPTOMATOLOGY

OBJECTIVES

- To define simple partial seizures.
- To discuss the use of folic acid in women taking antiepileptic drugs.
- To discuss the management of epilepsy in pregnancy.

VIGNETTE

A 33-year-old woman had two episodes of right arm and forearm jerking movements lasting 2 to 5 minutes about 3 years prior to this evaluation. Three months later, she had an 18-hour episode of continuous jerking involving her lower abdomen and right arm. Two years later, she had a 10-minute episode of jerking movements involving her right foot followed by loss of consciousness and postictal confusion. A month later, she had another 10-minute episode characterized by right foot jerking movements. Since the last event, she had noted impaired dexterity of her right foot and tripping episodes while walking upstairs. She had no history of perinatal problems, meningitis, or encephalitis.

CASE SUMMARY

 Our patient had simple partial seizures manifested by elementary motor (clonic) symptomatology. Initially, only her right arm was affected, but with her second spell, both her right arm and lower abdomen were involved. She discontinued antiepileptic drug (AEDs) use for an attempted pregnancy. Her next spell consisted of a partial seizure (right foot) followed by secondary generalization. AEDs were restarted. After her last spell, she reported residual decreased dexterity of right foot movements.

Examination showed a decreased rate of right foot tapping associated with brisk muscle stretch reflexes on the right leg. MRI of the brain showed two areas of increased signal in intensity involving the left hemisphere near the central sulcus. The exact nature of these lesions had not been defined and did not progress on subsequent imaging studies. She planned to become pregnant again.

For women who require AEDs during their reproductive years, several concepts should be kept in mind. Seizure frequency increases in approximately 17% to 33% of pregnancies, metabolism of AEDs changes during pregnancy, and risk of fetal malformation for women with epilepsy taking AEDs is about twice that of the general population. Whichever AED is deemed appropriate for the type of seizures, efforts should be aimed at controlling seizures with monotherapy. Several AEDs, especially the enzyme-inducing ones, decrease the effectiveness of hormonal contraception. This should be thoroughly discussed in order to avoid unwanted pregnancies. All women of childbearing age on AEDs should be taking daily folic acid supplementation, at a dose of 4 mg/day, to lessen the chance of birth defects, especially neural tube defects. If a woman taking an AED desires to become pregnant and wishes to discontinue AEDs (and this may be clinically appropriate if seizure control has been adequate), conversion to monotherapy to the lowest effective dose should be considered.

A change to an alternative AED should not be undertaken during pregnancy for the sole purpose of reducing teratogenic risk. For women who are pregnant and taking an AED, prenatal testing with AFP levels at 14 to 16 weeks and fetal ultrasound at 16 to 20 weeks should be offered. If appropriate, amniocentesis for amniotic α-fetoprotein (AFP) levels can be done. This may be especially useful in patients taking carbamazepine, divalproex sodium, or valproic acid given the increased risk of neural tube defects noted with these medications. Close monitoring of AED levels during pregnancy and at least through the eighth week postpartum is necessary.

Changes in drug levels may be noted, and adjustments to drug doses may be appropriate as weight changes and drug pharmacokinetic alterations occur during pregnancy. Although the need for prenatal vitamin K in women with epilepsy during pregnancy is somewhat controversial, vitamin K is often given during the last month of pregnancy if the patient is taking enzyme-inducing AEDs, in order to prevent hemorrhagic disease in newborn, as these AEDs can decrease vitamin K–dependent clotting factors. If no oral vitamin K is given during pregnancy, parenteral vitamin K is often given to the mother as soon as possible after onset of labor. All neonates of women with epilepsy receive vitamin K at the time of birth. Breast-feeding is not contraindicated, but one must be aware of possible neonatal sedation if the mother is taking sedating AEDs.

Our patient followed previous recommendations with fetal ultrasounds during pregnancy and frequent monitoring of AED levels. She also received vitamin K, had an uneventful pregnancy, and delivered a healthy child.

SELECTED REFERENCES

Delgado-Esweta AV, Janz D. Consensus guidelines; preconception counseling, management, and care of the pregnant woman with epilepsy. *Neurology* 1992;42:149–160.

Harden CL, Pennell PB, Koppel BS, et al. American Academy of Neurology; American Epilepsy Society. Practical Parameter Update: management issues for women with epilepsy. Focus on pregnancy (an evidence-based review). Vitamin K, folic acid, blood levels, and breastfeeding. Report of the quality standards subcommittee of the American Academy of Neurology and American Epilepsy Society. *Neurology* 2009;73(2):142–149.

Koch S, Loesche G, Jafer-Roman E, et al. Major birth malformations and antiepileptic drugs. *Neurology* 1992;42(Suppl 5):132–140.

Practice parameter: management issues for women with epilepsy (summary statement from the Quality Standards Subcommittee of the American Academy of Neurology). *Neurology* 1998;51:944–948.

Prevention of neural tube defects, results of the Medical Research Council Vitamin Study. MRC Vitamin Study Research Group. *Lancet* 1991;338:131–137.

SEE QUESTIONS: 6, 7, 8, 9, 20, 21, 22, 23, 24, 25, 98, 99, 100, 101, 105, 198, 222, 226, 227, 236, 237, 238

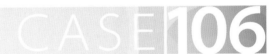

TUBEROUS SCLEROSIS COMPLEX

OBJECTIVES

- To review the main clinical manifestations of tuberous sclerosis complex (TSC).
- To discuss the genetic basis of TSC.
- To discuss the ancillary evaluation of patients with TSC.
- To summarize treatment guidelines for patients with TSC.

VIGNETTE

A 40-year-old man has had epileptic seizures since the age of 3 years.

CASE SUMMARY

 Our patient had a history of intellectual disability, epileptic seizures, and facial angiofibromas in a butterfly distribution over the nose, cheeks, and chin, characteristic of the TSC (Fig. 106.1). TSC is inherited as an autosomal dominant trait, although the rate of spontaneous mutation is high. TSC has been identified in all races and in all parts of the world. Two genes, *TSC1* on chromosome 9q34, encoding for protein product hamartin, and *TSC2* on chromosome 16p13, encoding for the protein product tuberin, have been identified. TSC affects almost every organ system, most commonly the brain, skin, eyes, kidneys, heart, and lungs. More than 80% of individuals with TSC will have epileptic seizures at some point in their life. Seizures are the initial manifestation of TSC in 90% of individuals. Most common neurologic manifestations are partial or generalized seizures including infantile spasms during the first years of life, usually before the age of 3. Other neurologic manifestations include intellectual disability, hydrocephalus, autism, and pervasive developmental and other behavioral disorders.

The most commonly found central nervous system (CNS) lesions are cortical tubers, subependymal nodules, and subependymal giant cell astrocytomas (SEGAs) adjacent to the foramen of Monro. Common skin manifestations include ash-leaf spots or hypomelanotic macules (better appreciated with a Wood lamp), facial angiofibromas (cutaneous hamartoma), shagreen patches (leathery plaque), and nontraumatic ungual or periungual fibromas (Koenen tumors). Ocular manifestations include retinal hamartomas or

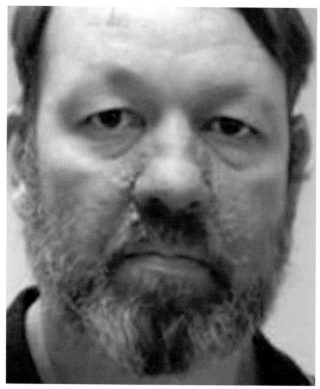

Figure 106.1 Patient with tuberous sclerosis complex showing characteristic facial angiofibromas in a butterfly distribution over the nose, cheeks, and chin.

astrocytomas, retinal achromatic patches, and colobomas of the iris, lens, and choroid. Renal manifestations consist of angiomyolipomas and autosomal dominant polycystic kidney disease, isolated renal cysts; hematuria, arterial hypertension, and renal failure may develop in severe cases. Cardiac rhabdomyomas may be focal or diffuse and may be asymptomatic or cause outflow obstruction, abnormal valve function, decreased contractility, or cardiac arrhythmias. The two most common lung lesions are single or multiple pulmonary cysts and lymphangioleiomyomatosis; spontaneous pneumothorax is a rare complication.

Minor features of TSC include pitting of the dental enamel, gingival fibromas, "confetti" skin lesions, hamartomatous rectal polyps, and bone cysts. Intracranial aneurysms have been reported in a small number of patients.

Magnetic resonance imaging (MRI) of the brain is recommended for the evaluation and follow-up of cortical tubers, subependymal nodules, and SEGAs. Electroencephalography (EEG) may demonstrate hypsarrhythmia in an infant with infantile spasms. Funduscopy may show retinal hamartomas or astrocytomas. Echocardiography is indicated for the detection of cardiac rhabdomyomas. Renal angiomyolipomas and polycystic changes can be demonstrated by renal ultrasound, computed tomography (CT), or MRI. Chest roentgenography or chest CT is indicated for the evaluation of lung cysts and lymphangioleiomyomatosis. Testing to determine genetic mutations with DNA probes is now available. Epileptic seizures are treated with standard antiepileptic drugs (AEDs), although the rate of medically refractory seizures is quite high among these patients. A ketogenic diet may be considered. Neurosurgery consultation may be required in cases of raised intractable seizures.

SELECTED REFERENCES

Beltramello A, Puppins G, Bricolo A, et al. Does the tuberous sclerosis complex include intracranial aneurysm? A case report with a review of the literature. *Pediatr Radiol* 1999;29(3):206–211.

Biller J, ed. *Practical neurology*, 4th ed. Philadelphia: Lippincott Williams & Wilkins, Wolter Kluwer Health, 2012.,

Jansen FE, vnan Huffelen AC, Algra A, et al. Epilepsy surgery in tuberous sclerosis: A systematic review. *Epilepsia* 2007;48:1477–1484.

Roach ES, Gomez MR, Northrup H. Tuberous sclerosis complex consensus conference: revised clinical diagnostic criteria. *J Child Neurol* 1998;13:624–628.

SEE QUESTIONS: 6, 7, 8, 9, 21, 22, 23, 24, 25, 98, 99, 100, 101, 105, 142, 176, 198, 222, 224

CASE**107**

EPILEPSIA PARTIALIS CONTINUA

OBJECTIVES

- To illustrate a typical case of progressive myoclonic encephalopathy (PME).
- To list the most common etiologies of PME.
- To highlight the treatment strategies for PME.

VIGNETTE

This 49-year-old man, previously healthy, was the victim of a collision by a drunk driver while he was bicycling 5 months prior to this assessment. His traumatic brain injury was severe and included a subarachnoid hemorrhage and hemorrhagic contusions of the brain. He demonstrated incremental improvements in speech and ability to interact with others as part of his rehabilitation program when, 4 months after his injury, he sustained a fall, which was followed by the appearance of rhythmic facial movements on the right side of his face and palate associated with deterioration in swallowing, speech, and memory. He could no longer swallow liquids and acted confused. He became unable to cooperate with further rehabilitation efforts and was sent to a nursing home. An electroencephalography (EEG) showed diffuse slowing but no epileptiform activity.

CASE SUMMARY

Our patient demonstrated rhythmic facial and palatal movements, affecting speech and swallowing. Despite a negative EEG, this is the classic phenomenology of epilepsia partialis continua (EPC). Indeed, an EEG-fMRI study was required to confirm the epileptic focus in the homuncular facial region on the left hemisphere. Although patients retain consciousness, and could carry on normal activities otherwise, the disorder can greatly affect function in those with traumatic brain injury, affecting speech and swallowing, and jeopardizing critical rehabilitation.

EPC is considered a simple partial motor form of status epilepticus, whereby focal clonic activity, often rhythmic or semirhythmic, remains localized to a body region. The abnormal movements should last for at least 60 minutes to qualify as status, but, in the case of EPC, it can last days, weeks, or even months before adequate recognition and treatment. Diagnosis can be delayed in part because a diagnostic EEG can be negative if the epileptic focus is small enough to fall beyond the resolution of a 20-electrode routine EEG. Positron emission tomography (PET) and single photon emission computed tomography (SPECT) scanning may be helpful, when available, to ascertain the cortical/subcortical area of hypometabolism or decreased blood flow, when the brain MRI is normal. A high index of suspicion is required in order to recognize the disorder as epileptic despite a mute or nondiagnostic EEG.

Some cases of EPC have been recognized in patients with subacute measles encephalitis, mostly in immunosuppressed patients, and in Rasmussen syndrome, an autoimmune chronic encephalitis associated with antibodies to glutamate receptor subtype 3, which tends to affect children between the ages of 3 and 15 years and often requires hemispherectomy due to its intractability to antiepileptic drugs and corticosteroids. Most adult-onset EPC develop in the context of static injuries (cortical dysplasia and arteriovenous malformation, traumatic brain injury, and stroke), neoplasms, encephalitides, metabolic disorders, mitochondrial disorders, intoxications, and multiple sclerosis.

The first-line treatment of EPC is based on antiepileptic drugs. Phenytoin and phenobarbital have been reported as more effective than carbamazepine or valproate. Oral corticosteroid therapy and immunosuppression may be of some benefit in cases refractory to antiepileptic drugs.

SELECTED REFERENCES

Bien CG, Elger CE. Epilepsia partialis continua: semiology and differential diagnoses. *Epileptic Disord* 2008;10(1):3–7.

Zupanc ML, Handler EG, Levine RL, et al. Rasmussen encephalitis: epilepsia partialis continua secondary to chronic encephalitis. *Pediatr Neurol* 1990;6(6):397–401.

SEE QUESTION: 340

CASE 108

FRONTAL LOBE EPILEPSY

OBJECTIVES

- To illustrate a case of frontal lobe epilepsy (FLE).
- To review the diagnostic pitfalls associated with this disorder.

(Case courtesy of Dr. David Ficker, University of Cincinnati)

VIGNETTE

This 46-year-old man had unusual spells for approximately 20 years. These consisted of episodes of fear, cold feeling, and well-formed speech ("Oh my God"). He was able to ambulate during these spells. The initial frequency was of 15 to 20 per day. The episodes occurred during the day and at night, while awake. His evaluation during an admission to the Epilepsy Monitoring Unit, as shown in the video, showed one such event in the absence of epileptiform activity.

CASE SUMMARY

Our patient demonstrated unusual events consisting of purportedly voluntary movements and intelligible vocalization of religious connotation, which were interpreted as psychogenic. This impression could have persisted given his ability to respond, even if inappropriately, to verbal commands during these spells; his resumption of normal behavior, including reading, immediately thereafter; and his seemingly counterintuitive postspell amnesia. Furthermore, his brain magnetic resonance imaging (MRI) and prior ictal electroencephalographs (EEGs) were normal. It was the brief appearance of right frontal beta discharges at the outset of his last video-EEG-documented spell, which prompted the diagnosis of right frontal lobe epilepsy, fitting with the localizing value of a well-formed ictal speech (see Table 104.1). Treatment with carbamazepine brought marked reduction in the frequency of the spells, a response that was further optimized with the later addition of phenytoin.

FLE is characterized by seizures with complex, often bizarre or violent rocking axial and pelvic movements, bipedal and bimanual activity, more typically occurring during sleep and often accompanied by normal EEG waveforms (the epileptic typically occupies the mesial surface of the frontal lobes) and neuroradiological findings. These features make FLE difficult to distinguish from other nonepileptic nocturnal paroxysmal events, such as parasomnias (Table 108.1) and psychogenic seizures. FLE could present in a variety of phenotypes, including as absencelike seizures, complex partial-type seizures, postural tonic spasms and a number of "parasomnic" behaviors, such as repetitive rocking or rolling, ambulation ("agitated somnambulism," "hypermotor" and/or pseudoperiodic movements). Hence, FLE needs to be distinguished from non-rapid eye movement parasomnias such as sleep–wake transition disorders (rhythmic movement disorder, sleeptalking, and nocturnal leg cramps) and arousal disorders (sleepwalking, sleep terrors, and confusional arousals), as well as from rapid eye movement (REM) sleep behavior disorder.

TABLE 108.1   **DIFFERENCES BETWEEN NOCTURNAL FRONTAL LOBE EPILEPSY VERSUS PARASOMNIAS**

Clinical Features	NFLE	Parasomnias
Age at onset	>11 y (throughout adulthood)	Usually <10 y (some adult cases)
Events/month	Around 30	<4
Clinical course	Increasing or stable	Decreasing: most disappear in adolescence
Movement semiology	Stereotypic	Polymorphic
	Two or three repetitive types of attacks	No motor pattern
Event onset	Any time during the night	First third of the night
	Stage 2, NREM (65%)	Stage 3 and 4 NREM
Event duration	<1 min (prolonged episodes possible)	Several minutes

NFLE, nocturnal frontal lobe epilepsy; NREM, non-rapid eye movement.
Adapted from Zucconi M, Ferini-Strambi L. NREM parasomnias: arousal disorders and differentiation from nocturnal frontal lobe epilepsy. *Clin Neurophysiol* 2000;111(Suppl 2):S129–S135.

The common prevalence of symptoms during sleep, as the second video case illustrates, prompted early inaccurate reports of FLE patients as *paroxysmal hypnogenic dystonia*, supported on a phenomenological description of "brief, occasionally painful *dystonic spasms* during non-REM sleep." The familial variant of this *hypnogenic dystonia* was later reclassified as a form of familial frontal lobe epilepsy, labeled as autosomal dominant nocturnal frontal lobe epilepsy (ADNFLE), and attributed to a mutation in the $\alpha4$ subunit of the neuronal nicotinic receptor gene *CHRNA4* (20q), with subsequent mutations found in genes coding for the $\alpha2$ and $\beta2$ subunits of the acetylcholine receptor (*CHRNA2* and *CHRNB2*). Novel loci have been reported on 15q, 3p, and 8q.

 Case 108, Video 2: This 61-year-old man was referred to the Epilepsy Monitoring Unit for unknown spells for about 2 years. He had no warning, and would vocalize, repetitively shout (often saying "help me!"), and engage in violent movements such as thrashing, with falls if he stood. These episodes occur both during daytime and at night, several times per week, and lasted about 2 minutes each. He would quickly return to normal. He was amnestic for these events. Zonisamide did not provide symptomatic control.

 **Case 108, Video 3:** The same patient in a different event, demonstrating similar symptoms, almost stereotypically similar to the prior one. This time the event occurred during stage 2 of sleep, helping reach the final diagnosis of nocturnal FLE. (*Case courtesy of Dr. David Ficker, University of Cincinnati*).

SELECTED REFERENCES

Bisulli F, Vignatelli L, Provini F. Parasomnias and nocturnal frontal lobe epilepsy (NFLE): lights and shadows–controversial points in the differential diagnosis. *Sleep Med* 2011;12(Suppl 2):S27–S32.

Zucconi M, Ferini-Strambi L. NREM parasomnias: arousal disorders and differentiation from nocturnal frontal lobe epilepsy. *Clin Neurophysiol* 2000;111(Suppl 2):S129–S135.

SEE QUESTIONS: 341, 342

CASE 109

COUGH SYNCOPE

OBJECTIVES

- To illustrate an unusual cause of neurally mediated syncope.
- To discuss the presumed pathophysiology of cough syncope.
- To highlight potential risks associated with cough syncope.

VIGNETTE

A 51-year-old man had recurrent episodes of syncope associated with coughing.

CASE SUMMARY

Our patient had recurrent episodes of syncope after prolonged episodes of coughing. He had a history of non-Hodgkin lymphoma diagnosed 6 years previously, treated with chemotherapy and autologous stem cell transplant. He was diagnosed with mantle cell lymphoma. He did not have a history of reactive airway disease and had not been treated with angiotensin-converting enzyme (ACE) inhibitors. A pacemaker had been previously deployed after an episode of syncope that occurred while coughing while driving his car, but he was never found to have any cardiac rhythm abnormality or cardiac conduction defect. On neurologic examination, he had evidence of a sensorimotor polyneuropathy with generalized areflexia, and impaired position and vibration sense in both legs.

He had a normal awake and sleep electroencephalography (EEG). Video EEG was unremarkable. Echocardiography showed no evidence of intracardiac infarct or vegetations. There was normal left ventricular ejection fraction. Computed tomography (CT) of the neck showed subtle-appearing focus of decreased density with a rim of increased density involving the right sternocleidomastoid, probably related to prior biopsy in this region. CT angiogram of the neck demonstrated no evidence of arterial stenosis or occlusion. Chest x-ray was unremarkable. EMG/nerve conduction velocities (NCVs) showed a moderate–severe sensory motor polyneuropathy in the lower limbs with mixed axonal and demyelinating features. Cultures of nasopharyngeal aspirate were positive for *Bordetella pertussis* by DNA polymerase chain reaction (PCR) and negative for *Bordetella parapertussis* and also negative for *Bordetella holmesii*.

Our patient was diagnosed with cough-induced syncope associated with *Bordetella pertussis* and received a 5-day course of azithromycin.

Syncope is defined by a rapid onset and temporary loss of consciousness and postural tone, usually accompanied by falling, followed by spontaneous and complete recovery. In the United States, 3% to 5% of all emergency room visits are due to syncope. Syncope has been broadly classified into the following categories: *neurally mediated syncope* (neurocardiogenic syncope), *orthostatic hypotension, cardiac arrhythmias, structural heart disease, vascular disease, metabolic/miscellaneous, psychogenic*, and *unknown.*

Cough syncope is unusual. First described by Charcot in 1876, using the term laryngeal spasm, it belongs to the heterogeneous group of neurally mediated syncope. Variants of neurally mediated syncope include *vasovagal syncope, carotid sinus hypersensitivity*, and *situational syncope* (cough, swallow, sneeze, micturition/postmicturition, defecation, postprandial, etc.). Cough syncope follows a series of coughs or even a single cough. The syncope is generally brief, lasting only seconds, and recovery is rapid. Brief rhythmic or clonic activity–like movements during the episodes have been observed, but no epileptiform activity has been reported.

The exact mechanism of cough-induced syncope is not known. It has been attributed to stimulation of vagal afferents in the upper airways in addition to a withdrawal of peripheral sympathetic tone leading to a decreased venous return, resulting in bradycardia, vasodilation, and ultimately in presyncope or syncope. During vigorous coughing, there is increase in the intrathoracic and intra-abdominal pressures. These pressure changes are transmitted via the great veins to the intracranial compartment causing a temporary rise in intracranial pressure (ICP) enough to decrease the cerebral perfusion pressure (CPP). As a consequence, there is critical impairment of cerebral blood flow (CBF) causing syncope. Cough can also cause brady- and tachyarrhythmias, and rarely, cough-induced syncope may be mediated by a complete heart block effected through extreme vagal responses. Cough is commonly encountered in patients receiving ACE inhibitors; cough syncope has been reported in a patient on ACE inhibitors with essential hypertension. Moreover, cough syncope has been reported in association with *Bordetella pertussis* infection, a condition that has recent significance among adults throughout the United States, although not often considered in the differential diagnosis of chronic cough in adults.

Cough syncope can have tragic consequences and be responsible for automobile accidents. Patients must be properly counseled.

▶ **Case 109, Video 2:**

SELECTED REFERENCES

Bock JM, Burtis CC, Poetker DM, et al. Serum immunoglobulin G analysis to establish a delayed diagnosis of chronic cough due to *Bordetella pertussis. Otolaryngol Head Neck Surg* 2012;146(1):63–67.

De Maria AA Jr, Westmoreland BF, Sharbrough FW. EEG in cough syncope. *Neurology* 1984;34(3):371–373.

Hart G, Oldershaw PJ, Cull P, et al. Syncope caused by cough-induced complete atrioventricular block. *Pacing Clin Electrophysiol* 1982;5(4):564–566.

Jayarajan A, Prakash O. Cough syncope induced by enalapril. *Chest* 1993;103:327–328.

Mattle HP, Nirkko AC, Baumgartner RW, et al. Transient circulatory arrest coincides with fainting in coughing syncope. *Neurology* 1995;45(3):498–501.

McCorry DJP, Chadwick DW. Cough syncope in heavy good vehicle drivers. *QJM* 2004;97(9):631–632.

Seiji Y, Takuro N. Cough syncope syndrome caused by pertussis. *J Japan Soc Int Med* 2003;92(7):131–134.

SEE QUESTIONS: 343, 344

SECTION 14

SLEEP MEDICINE

CASE 110

OBSTRUCTIVE SLEEP APNEA

OBJECTIVES

- To review common causes of excessive daytime sleepiness.
- To outline treatment strategies for obstructive sleep apnea.
- To recognize common features of narcolepsy.

VIGNETTE

A 71-year-old man with history of chronic obstructive pulmonary disease (COPD), atrial fibrillation, internal carotid artery stenosis, transient ischemic attacks (TIAs), secondary polycythemia, and essential tremor was evaluated because of excessive snoring. The interview was conducted after the patient had received treatment for the underlying condition.

CASE SUMMARY

Our patient presented with excessive daytime sleepiness. Other than hypothyroidism, overmedication, metabolic encephalopathy, and depression, the patient should be evaluated for a sleep disorder.

Sleep disorders are prevalent and underrecognized, have costly implications, and can be very serious. Fortunately, sleep disorders are very treatable. For example, obstructive sleep apnea (OSA) is estimated to be more prevalent than asthma. In 1990 in the United States, there were 200,000 motor vehicle accidents as a result of falling asleep at the wheel. Approximately 31% of all drivers have fallen asleep at the wheel at least once in their lifetime. Nearly one-third of all heavy trucking accidents in which the driver is injured are due to the driver falling asleep at the wheel. A number of major industrial catastrophes, including the Exxon *Valdez*, Three Mile Island, and Chernobyl, have been associated with sleepiness-related errors in judgment or performance in the workplace.

The United States National Highway Traffic Safety Administration cites drowsiness as a cause of 108,000 police-reported crashes annually involving 76,000 injuries and 1,500 deaths. Thirty million Americans are estimated to suffer from chronic sleep disorders, of which 95% are considered to be underdiagnosed and untreated. In addition, another 20 or 30 million Americans are estimated to experience sleep-associated problems. A survey in 1990 suggested the direct cost of sleepiness and sleep disorders to the American public was $16 billion with indirect costs of $160 billion.

OSA is a common syndrome classically presenting as excessive daytime sleepiness and fatigue. OSA is an independent risk factor for cardiovascular disease. Patients are at risk for cardiovascular manifestations of chronic intermittent hypoxia (hypertension, pulmonary hypertension, arrhythmia, and cor pulmonale). OSA has also been associated with atrial fibrillation and insulin resistance. Moreover, OSA increases the risk of stroke or death from any cause, independent of other risk factors, including arterial hypertension. Patients are classically obese, often with underlying chronic pulmonary disease. Another group of patients with OSA has anatomic problems with the upper airway leading to obstruction (large adenoids; palate and pharyngeal problems; short, stocky, muscular necks; small chins). Patients with OSA snore heavily. They are usually unaware of problems with nighttime sleep, but in fact have poor quality of sleep.

Presumably, the obstruction produces hypoxia, which interferes with achieving deep stages of sleep (hypoxia causes arousal). Patients wake up frequently for brief periods and never achieve adequate length of deep (stages III and IV) sleep. Occasionally they present with early-morning headaches due to hypercapnia and occasionally memory impairment or personality change due to hypoxia. Simple observation of sleep will make the diagnosis, but a nighttime sleep study will quantify the severity of obstruction and hypoxia. Therapy depends on the severity. Weight loss is an effective and simple therapeutic measure. Following diagnosis, most patients are treated with positive airway pressure to eliminate obstruction (biPAP).

Central sleep apnea is a less common and less well-understood disorder usually related to disorders affecting the brainstem respiratory centers. A polysomnogram is required to make this diagnosis. Failure of automatic control of ventilation (Ondine curse) is perhaps the most severe form.

Narcolepsy is a chronic sleep disorder characterized by a tetrad of symptoms as follows:

1. Sleep attacks—sudden-onset sleep that patients are unable to resist
2. Cataplexy—sudden loss of muscle tone without loss of consciousness provoked by a strong emotional stimulus. Laughing is the strongest emotional trigger of cataplexy.
3. Hypnagogic hallucinations—stereotyped vivid dreams while falling asleep or awakening (hypnopompic)
4. Sleep paralysis—common in the general population. Episodes of inability to move while falling asleep or waking, often frightening to the patient

Narcolepsy has a hereditary basis. About 90% of narcoleptic patients have human leukocyte antigen (HLA) DR2/DQ1, present in less than 30% of the general population. Current insights into the pathophysiology of narcolepsy indicate that hypocretin is markedly deficient in narcoleptics. Onset of narcolepsy is variable, but it often begins in adolescence, and the evaluation requires a multiple sleep latency test (MSLT). This study is done in the electroencephalography (EEG) or sleep lab and consists of monitoring EEG and eye movements as the patient lies down in a dark room for five trials or naps in 1 day. The length of time required for the onset of EEG-confirmed sleep is averaged (the average sleep latency). This will document and quantify the degree of excessive daytime sleepiness. Most narcoleptics enter rapid eye movement (REM) sleep within minutes of falling asleep. This finding usually establishes the diagnosis. These patients are managed with scheduled naps and usually prescribed CNS stimulants such as caffeine, amphetamine, and modafinil.

SELECTED REFERENCES

Barthlen GM. Sleep-disordered breathing. In: *Sleep disorders:* Continuum, Philadelphia 2002;8:147–155.

Ip MSM, Lam B, Ng MMT, et al. Obstructive sleep apnea is independently associated with insulin resistance. *Am J Respir Crit Care Med* 2002;165(5):670–676.

Krahn LE, Black JL, Silber MH. Narcolepsy: new understanding of irresistible sleep. *Mayo Clinic Proc* 2001;76:185–194.

Nishimo S, Okuro M. Emerging treatment s for narcolepsy and its related disorders. *Expert Opin Emerg Drugs* 2010;15(1):139–158.

Yaggi HK, Concato J, Kernan WN, et al. Obstructive sleep apnea as a risk factor for stroke and death. *N Engl J Med* 2005;353:2034–2041.

SEE QUESTIONS: 124, 125, 126, 130, 131, 132, 206

CASE **111**

LOWER-BODY PARKINSONISM (GAIT APRAXIA)

(OBJECTIVES)

■ To present a patient with a diagnostically challenging gait disorder.
■ To briefly review disorders commonly associated with lower-body–predominant parkinsonism (vascular parkinsonism, normal pressure hydrocephalus, and progressive supranuclear palsy).

(VIGNETTE)

A 76-year-old woman with a prior subcortical infarct was evaluated due to progressive decline in her ability to walk.

(CASE SUMMARY)

 Our patient had a prior subcortical infarct and consulted us due to her severe gait difficulty and frequent falls. She did not complain of headaches, nausea, vomiting, or visual difficulties. She had no history of subarachnoid hemorrhage (SAH), meningitis, cranial radiation, cranial surgery, or head trauma. Despite her severe gait disorder, our patient could move her legs fairly well, particularly when lying on her back. She did not have ataxia or overt muscle weakness.

Although she was able to stand, she had marked difficulty in lifting her feet and walked as if her feet were glued to the floor. Arm swing during walking was relatively preserved, and she did not have resting tremor, bradykinesia, or rigidity. Turning was difficult, and it took several steps. Her gait difficulties and falling episodes persisted despite a trial of levodopa/carbidopa. Magnetic resonance imaging (MRI) showed no widening of cerebrospinal fluid (CSF) spaces at the high convexity, ventricular enlargement, or leukoaraiosis.

On T2-weighted images, there was no evidence of increased signal in the periventricular areas. There was no thinning or upward bowing of the corpus callosum. There was no prominent flow void noticed in the aqueduct and third ventricle. Isotope cisternography was reported as showing a "mixed pattern."

Our patient had considerable difficulties in using her legs to walk out of proportion to that of other movements of her lower limbs when seated or lying, suggestive of apraxia of gait, a higher-level gait disorder diffusely localized to the medial frontal cortex or, in selected cases, higher brainstem structures (involving the pedunculopontine nucleus), and caused by a variety of frontal-predominant disorders, such as microangiopathic brain disease (vascular parkinsonism), hydrocephalus (e.g., normal pressure hydrocephalus and obstructive hydrocephalus), or neurodegenerative disorders highly selective to the frontal lobes and mesencephalic regions (frontotemporal dementia with parkinsonism and progressive supranuclear palsy).

Vascular parkinsonism applies to a *lower-half* parkinsonian disorder distinguished by hesitant, shuffling gait, with a wide base and variable stride length, with postural instability but no festination (progressive increase in cadence at the expense of shortening stride length). These patients have little to no arm rigidity, tremor, or bradykinesia, and exhibit no impairment in speech, facial gestures, or arm swing during gait. The response to levodopa is usually poor. Progression tends to be in a stepwise fashion. Pyramidal tract signs and pseudobulbar affect are common findings. A subcortical dementia almost invariably emerges. Vascular risk factors (such as hypertension, hypercholesterolemia, hyperhomocysteinemia, diabetes mellitus, sedentarism, or coagulopathies) are typically identified. There classically are T2-weighted confluent punctate hyperintensities on brain MRI in the periventricular and deep white matter, sometimes with associated enlargement of the perivascular spaces (Virchow-Robin spaces), particularly in the basal ganglia.

Hydrocephalus may be due to disorders of CSF production, circulation, or absorption. Some forms of hydrocephalus cannot be properly classified according to that scheme, as is the case of normal pressure hydrocephalus (NPH). NPH is a clinical entity seen in older subjects and characterized by ventriculomegaly and normal CSF pressure (with higher nocturnal pressures reported). The risk for NPH increases after SAH, meningitis, intracranial surgery, or head trauma, but in a large number of patients, the cause is unknown. NPH is characterized by progressive gait disturbance (shuffling, small steps, and broad based), urinary incontinence due to bladder detrusor overactivity, memory loss, and large ventricles, and it is confirmed with a favorable response to CSF diversion procedures. Gait impairment should be the most prominent and often the earliest manifestation of true NPH, and postural reflexes must be preserved. Distinguishing the gait disorder encountered among patients with NPH from other disorders of gait, particularly vascular parkinsonism, encountered in older adults may be challenging, but several features are helpful (Table 111.1). Improvement of gait and cognitive function following large-volume (40 to

TABLE 111.1 CLINICAL FEATURES DISTINGUISHING PARKINSON DISEASE FROM NPH AND VASCULAR PARKINSONISM

	Parkinson Disease	NPH and Vascular Parkinsonism
Base of ambulation	Narrow base	Wide base
Arm swing	Absent in affected side	Preserved
Sensory cues	Improve gait	Do not improve or worsen gait
Festination	Often present	Typically absent
Response to levodopa	Characteristic	Absent

50 mL) lumbar puncture (almost 100% specificity although only 30% sensitivity) or a 3-day continuous external lumbar drainage (about 80% specificity but higher sensitivity, at 50%) help predict eventual response to ventriculoperitoneal shunt placement, the definitive treatment. Flow void of the third ventricle, Evans' ratio, cisternography, and white matter abnormalities are generally unreliable in forecasting outcome to shunting.

Our case is most suggestive of primary progressive freezing of gait (PPFG), a severe form of isolated gait apraxia or "higher-level gait disorder" that results in freezing of gait and later in postural instability, when other motor or general parkinsonian features are generally absent. This is a heterogeneous disorder but the most common neuropathological correlate is progressive supranuclear palsy (PSP). The disorder falls within the spectrum of the so-called pure akinesia gait freezing (PAGF), which has been defined as the gradual onset of freezing of gait, absent limb rigidity and tremor, no sustained response to levodopa, and no dementia or ophthalmoplegia within 5 years from symptom onset. Most of these individuals end up developing features of PSP and are confirmed to have the disease at autopsy.

SELECTED REFERENCES

Adams RD, Fisher CM, Hakim S, et al. Symptomatic occult hydrocephalus with "normal" cerebrospinal fluid pressure. A treatable syndrome. *N Engl J Med* 1965;273:117–126.

Gupta D, Kuruvilla A. Vascular parkinsonism: what makes it different? *Postgrad Med J* 2011;87(1034): 829–836.

Shprechen D, Schwalb J, Kurlen R. Normal pressure by hydrocephalus. Diagnosis and treatment. *Curr Neurol Neurosci Rep* 2008;8(5):271–376.

Williams DR, Holton JL, Strand K, et al. Pure akinesia with gait freezing: a third clinical phenotype of progressive supranuclear palsy. *Mov Disord* 2007;22(15):2235–2241.

SEE QUESTIONS: 160, 161, 345, 346

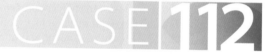

CASE **112**

VASCULAR PARKINSONISM AND NORMAL PRESSURE HYDROCEPHALUS

OBJECTIVES

- To illustrate a classical presentation of vascular parkinsonism (VaP) and a suspected presentation of VaP, whose response to fluid diversion and eventual neuropathology demonstrated normal pressure hydrocephalus (NPH).
- To recognize the imaging features suggestive of vascular parkinsonism and normal pressure hydrocephalus, recognizing the large overlap between these disorders.

VIGNETTES

▶ **Case 112, Video 1:** This 75-year-old woman had a 3-year stepwise progression of gait, balance, and cognitive impairment, with falls and requirement of a walker after 2 years from symptom onset. She had arterial hypertension, hypercholesterolemia, diabetes, and was a smoker.

▶ **Case 112, Video 2:** This 80-year-old man had a 2.5-year staggering progression of gait and balance impairment, sudden-onset freezing of gait hospitalizations, falls, and urinary incontinence. He had hypertension, hypercholesterolemia, Ménière disease; he accumulated a 60 pack/year history of smoking.

CASE SUMMARY

Both of these patients have a similar history of stepwise deterioration of gait over several years and shared several vascular risk factors. The initial working diagnosis was that of a lower-body parkinsonian syndrome, which was most suggestive of VaP. Both patients showed signal abnormalities in the periventricular and deep white matter, which further supported that assertion (Figs. 112.1 and 112.2).

However, in Patient 2 the degree of "small vessel disease" noted on magnetic resonance imaging (MRI) was of lesser magnitude than in Patient 1, and the extent of associated ventriculomegaly somewhat greater. These considerations were overshadowed by a heavy vasculopathic history and a stepwise deterioration suggesting strokelike events. Nevertheless and acquiescing to requests by his family physician, Patient 2 underwent a 3-day external lumbar drainage procedure, which in fact demonstrated a 40% gain in gait velocity and optimization of all of his gait parameters, as well as improvements in most of his cognitive endpoints, which had collectively crossed into the realm of moderate dementia prior to the procedure

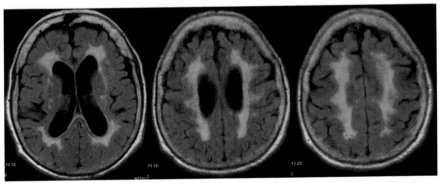

Figure 112.1   FLAIR axial brain MRI of Patient 1, showing severe confluent periventricular and deep white matter hyperintensity, with associated enlargement of the lateral ventricles and mild to moderate cortical atrophy.

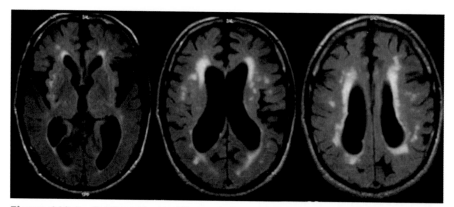

Figure 112.2 FLAIR axial brain of Patient 2, showing moderate confluent periventricular and cotton-shaped deep white matter hyperintensities, with associated enlargement of the lateral ventricles and moderate-to-severe cortical atrophy.

(see third video). As a result, this patient underwent a ventriculoperitoneal shunt placement. Unfortunately, bowel perforation at the abdominal end of the shunt emerged as an immediate postoperative complication and the patient succumbed to septic peritonitis. Brain autopsy demonstrated typical findings previously reported in NPH, namely, dilatation of the lateral and third ventricles associated with fibrous thickening of the leptomeninges, gaps in the ependymal lining, and periventricular gliosis. Despite our clinical prediction, there was no direct evidence of the "small vessel" ischemic disease suggested by imaging (which would have included gliosis, perivascular pallor, hyaline thickening, and widening perivascular spaces).

A closer reevaluation of the brain MRI of Patient 2 in the previously neglected apical cuts (Fig. 112.3) showed no extension of the same sulcal widening appreciated in lower cuts, thus suggesting a pattern of pseudoatrophy with enlarged sulcation due to entrapped spinal fluid rather than true parenchymal atrophy. In fact, the brain weight of this patient was a healthy 1,400 mg and the post hoc volumetric analysis on his brain MRI also supported the absence of atrophy despite such appearance on first glance.

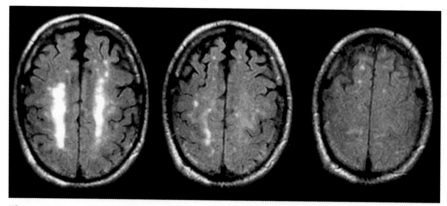

Figure 112.3 Upper axial cuts of the same brain MRI on Patient 2 (compare with Figure 112.2). Note the lack of sulcal widening that in the apical cortical regions, which suggested brain atrophy (and corresponding ex vacuo hydrocephalus) in the lower cuts.

TABLE 112.1   CLINICAL FEATURES OF GAIT IN VaP AND NPH

Common to NPH and VaP	Presumed Unique to NPH	Presumed Unique to VaP
• Reduced gait velocity • Reduced stride length • Diminished step height • Increased step width • Freezing of gait • Gait apraxia ("frontal ataxia" or "magnetic foot") • Preserved arm swing • Poor response to external cues • Poor response to levodopa	• Broad-based gait with outwardly rotated feet	• Upright posture with "wooden appearance," reduced hip extension, reduced knee flexion • Lack of festination (i.e., hastening steps with progressively shortened stride)

Adapted from Espay AJ, Narayan RK, Duker AP, et al. Lower-body parkinsonism: reconsidering the threshold for external lumbar drainage. *Nat Clin Pract Neurol* 2008;4(1):50–55.

Thus, several lessons emerged from these two cases. The gait pattern of lower-body parkinsonian disorders may be clinically indistinguishable, even if subtle differences have been reported (Table 112.1). Vascular pathology cannot be readily surmised from neuroimaging, unless the burden of evidence is overwhelming (Patient 1). Even in these cases, caution should be exercised as the clinicopathological correlations are scant for the reliable distinction between VaP and NPH. Finally, a dose of humility is always helpful in cases of lower-body parkinsonism where the burden of historical evidence may lead the clinician down the garden path (Patient 2). Hypertension and vascular disease are often associated features within an NPH–VaP continuum.

▶ **Case 112, Video 3:** The gait of Patient 2 before and after a 3-day external lumbar drainage (ELD) procedure, whereby CSF was drained at a rate of 10 mL/hour. There was a 17% improvement in cadence, a 40% improvement in gait velocity, and a 29% improvement in stride length.

SELECTED REFERENCES

Dunn L. "Normal pressure hydrocephalus": what's in a name? *J Neurol Neurosurg Psychiatry* 2002;73:8.
Espay AJ, Narayan RK, Duker AP, et al. Lower-body parkinsonism: reconsidering the threshold for external lumbar drainage. *Nat Clin Pract Neurol* 2008;4(1):50–55.
Marmarou A, Bergsneider M, Black P, et al. Guidelines for the diagnosis and management of idiopathic normal pressure hydrocephalus. *Neurosurgery* 2005;57(suppl):S2-1–S2-S2.

SEE QUESTIONS: 347, 348

CASE 113

HEMIPLEGIC GAIT/SPASTICITY

OBJECTIVES

- To illustrate common disabilities associated with spasticity.
- To analyze characteristic features of a spastic gait.
- To briefly summarize available management strategies for spasticity.

VIGNETTE

At the age of 39, this 46-year-old man with history of arterial hypertension, diabetes, dyslipidemia, and obesity had an infarct in the right posterior limb of the internal capsule. Further evaluation demonstrated a patent foramen ovale (PFO) and an atrial septal aneurysm (ASA).

CASE SUMMARY

Due to a right posterior limb of the internal capsule infarct with subsequent disruption of the corticospinal tract, our patient was left with a disabling spastic left hemiparesis. As a result of his spasticity, he had numerous complaints including inadequate use of his affected hand and leg, impaired walking, curling of his left toes, scraping of the floor with the outer edge of his left foot, excessive callous formation of his left foot, pain, and occasional flexor spasms. In addition to his left hemiparesis, he also had signs of spasticity characterized by increased muscle tone, clasp-knife phenomenon, hyperreflexia, clonus, and a Babinski sign. He had a characteristic spastic hemiparetic gait. There was spastic adduction and internal rotation of the left shoulder, flexion at the elbow, and a clenched left fist. The left leg was externally rotated at the hip. The left knee was extended and stiff. The left foot was plantar flexed and inverted (equinovarus). He had a tendency to circumduct and scuff the left foot.

Damage to the upper motor neurons results in muscles that are initially weak and flaccid, but eventually become hypertonic, particularly manifested as spasticity and hyperactivity of the muscle stretch reflexes. *Spasticity* is defined as an increase in muscle tone due to hyperexcitability of the stretch reflex and is characterized by a velocity-dependent increase in tonic stretch reflexes. Spasticity results from upper motor neuron impairment and can be cerebral or spinal in origin. Common causes of cerebral spasticity include cerebrovascular disease, demyelinating disease, and cerebral palsy. Common causes of spasticity of spinal cord origin include cervical spondylotic myelopathy, traumatic spinal cord injury, demyelinating disease, tumoral myelopathies, spinal cord vascular malformations, nutritional myelopathies, and tropical and hereditary spastic paraparesis.

Spasticity predominates on the antigravitational muscles. Weakness of the muscles of the upper extremity is most marked in deltoid, triceps, wrist extension, and finger extension. This predilection for involvement of the extensors and supinators explains the pronation and flexion tendencies of the upper extremity. The spastic wrist is flexed, and often it may have a radial deviation. Weakness of the muscles of the lower extremities is most marked in hip flexion, knee flexion, foot dorsiflexion, and eversion. Equinovarus is the most common pathologic posture of the foot.

Spasticity may be present even in cases of only minimal weakness. Certain pathologic reflexes and signs appear. One of the most common is the extensor plantar reflex or Babinski sign characterized by extension of the great toe and fanning of the other toes. Clonus can often be elicited at the ankle or wrist. The superficial reflexes (abdominal reflexes and cremasteric reflex in men) are absent or suppressed on the affected side. If the lesion occurs above the level of the pyramidal decussation, these signs will be detected on the opposite side of the body; if it occurs below the pyramidal decussation, the signs will be detected on the same side. A commonly used scale to assess the degree of spasticity is the modified Ashworth Scale, which grades resistance to passive movement.

A variety of strategies are available for the management of spasticity. Physical therapy is of paramount importance in these patients. Medications that are useful for the management of spasticity are the GABAergic drugs baclofen, tizanidine, and benzodiazepines. Other oral agents used to treat spasticity are dantrolene and gabapentin. Selected patients can benefit from injections of botulinum toxin, which inhibits the release of acetylcholine at the neuromuscular junction, into specific muscles. In paraplegic patients with severe and disabling spasticity, intrathecal baclofen administration may be useful in ameliorating severe spasticity and urinary urgency. Lumbar intrathecal phenol administration has been proposed in managing spasticity in patients with advanced multiple sclerosis. One of the most effective neurosurgical treatments for spasticity is selective dorsal rhizotomy.

SELECTED REFERENCES

Ashworth B. Preliminary trial of carisoprodal in multiple sclerosis. *Practitioner* 1964;192:540–542.

Biller J, ed. *Practical neurology*, 4th ed. Philadelphia: Lippincott Williams & Wilkins, Wolters Kluwer Health, 2012.

Brazis PW, Masdeu JC, Biller J. *Localization in clinical neurology*, 4th ed. Philadelphia: Lippincott Williams & Wilkins, Wolters Kluwer Health, 2001.

Simpson DM, Alexander DN, O'Brien CF, et al. Botulinum toxin A in the treatment of upper extremity spasticity: a randomized, double blind placebo controlled trial. *Neurology* 1996;46:1306–1310.

Thompson AJ, Jarrett L, Lockley L, et al. Clinical management of spasticity. *J Neurol Neurosurg Psychiatry* 2005;76:459–463.

SEE QUESTIONS: 30, 55, 87

CASE 114

HEMIPARKINSONIAN GAIT

OBJECTIVES

- To recognize a typical case of hemiparkinsonism and distinguish it from the hemiparetic case reviewed in the prior case.
- To highlight the importance of reaching the correct diagnosis for prompt initiation of appropriate therapy.

VIGNETTE

This 56-year-old woman complained of left arm pain and left shoulder pain for 11 years prior to this evaluation. Her left foot started to "stick up" about 5 years ago. For the last 2 years, she noted greater difficulty with walking and slowness, which forced her to walk "on the ball of her feet." She had experienced no falls but felt as though her "weight shift" to the right made her stumble more often. She had also been more anxious and depressed, for which fluoxetine was prescribed to no avail. Recently, she noted a bit of tremor on the left hand when holding her arms outstretched. She admitted to mild hyposmia, occasional urinary frequency, and hot flashes, which she attributed to menopause.

CASE SUMMARY

Our patient showed a left hemiparkinsonian gait, which has many of the attributes of the hemiparetic gait but a notable exception: the affected arm is extended, rather than flexed at the elbow, and there was no wrist flexion or thumb adduction. This patient was incorrectly suspected of having had a stroke. Instead, she had an asymmetric bradykinesia and rigidity (her right hemibody was not normal, despite her subjective perception), which had very slowly progressed over 10 years, with normal cognitive function and no atypical motor features aside from hyperreflexia. She also demonstrated the presence of a striatal toe, a spontaneous dorsiflexion of the first toe, which may be confused with the reflexive dorsiflexion of Babinski. These findings were most consistent with the diagnosis of Parkinson disease (PD), surprisingly benign given the lack of appropriate treatment over a decade. A genetic cause of her PD, likely parkin, was suspected given her relatively early age at onset (46 years), her hyperreflexia, and the report of PD in her father.

This case was instructive because it demonstrated that a benign form of PD may continue to appear as hemiparkinsonism and mimic a hemiparetic gait if it remains undiagnosed after many years. Upon levodopa initiation, the patient showed excellent response with normalization of her gait (see second video). Of great interest was her prompt development of motor complications. Within 5 months from treatment initiation, and 1 month after reaching the dose of 800 mg/day of levodopa divided in four doses, she reported wearing off after only 2 hours of "on" time after each dose and had to add a fifth dose, still with insufficient coverage during the day. She noted that the effect of levodopa, once clinically effective after about

50 minutes from each dose, thoroughly relaxed her. She had developed mild peak-dose levodopa-induced dyskinesias, predominantly affecting the left limbs and cervical region, intermixed with wearing off-related left-hand dystonia, tightening of her thighs, and reemergence of gait impairment (see third video). Hence, over the next few months, she required higher individual doses of levodopa, a reduction in the interdose interval, and the addition of extended-release ropinirole. Entacapone paradoxically aggravated her symptoms and was promptly discontinued. Increases beyond 300 mg of levodopa per dose created intolerable dyskinesias and was therefore not relied upon as a strategy to minimize the "off" periods before amantadine, introduced as an antidyskinetic strategy, became part of her treatment regimen.

One misconception in the treatment of PD is that the initiation of levodopa should be delayed because "the clock" for the development of motor complications "begins to tick" once levodopa is initiated. The theory goes that by relying on the lower-potency dopamine agonists (ropinirole, pramipexole, and rotigotine) or MAO-B inhibitors (selegiline and rasagiline), wearing off and dyskinesias are delayed. This case illustrates that such "clock" is timed on disease onset. The development of motor fluctuations and dyskinesias are a greater function of disease duration than of cumulative dosage of levodopa exposure. Also, in cases of diagnostic doubt such as in this case, when diagnosis remained elusive for over a decade, response to levodopa should be ascertained promptly in order to support the diagnostic impression of PD, particularly when other parkinsonian disorders may also be considered in the differential diagnosis.

Intriguingly, a recent case–control study has shown that left-sided onset of parkinsonism, such as that shown by this patient, is an independent predictor of a "benign" phenotype of PD, defined as a duration of disease greater than 20 years while retaining independent ambulation and remaining free of dementia. The biological reason for a differential effect of disease lateralization remains unclear but is of scientific interest.

A final note, marked and sustained hemiparkinsonism should also make one suspicious for the corticobasal syndrome (more rapid progression, associated apraxia, cortical sensory loss in the affected hand, and poor response to levodopa), a lesion in the contralateral basal ganglia (also more rapid progression and poor response to levodopa), or hemiparkinsonism–hemiatrophy syndrome (hemispheric and body hemiatrophy).

▶ **Case 114, Video 2:** Normalization of gait is demonstrated after treatment initiation with Levodopa. Patient is shown 4 months after earlier video, once the dose had been titrated up to 200 mg four times a day for optimization of function.

▶ **Case 114, Video 3:** Sustained benefit documented 6 months after the last video (10 months after initiation of levodopa treatment). Mild, as of yet, non-troublesome peak-dose dyskinesias can be appreciated, though the video is taken 2.5 hours after the last dose of levodopa, when wearing off is expected to bring on dystonia in the left hand, thigh soreness, and reemergence of gait impairment.

SELECTED REFERENCES

Hametner E, Seppi K, Poewe W. The clinical spectrum of levodopa-induced motor complications. *J Neurol* 2010;257(Suppl 2):S268–S275.

Munhoz RP, Espay AJ, Morgante F, et al. Long-duration Parkinson's disease: role of lateralization of motor features. *Park Related Disord* 2013;19(1):77–80.

Tessitore A, Russo A, Cirillo M, et al. Hemiparkinsonism and hemiatrophy syndrome: a rare observation. *Clin Neurol Neurosurg* 2010;112(6):524–526.

SEE QUESTIONS: 349, 350

CASE 115

ADULT-ONSET DYSTONIC GAIT

OBJECTIVES

- To recognize a typical case of adult-onset foot dystonia, which is typically secondary to lesions contralateral brain hemispheric lesions.
- To recognize the clinical features suggestive of a dystonic gait.

VIGNETTE

This 50-year-old woman noted some "pressure" in the bottom of her right foot about 4 months prior to her evaluation. In relatively short sequence thereafter, she started limping and feeling tightness in her right thigh, relieved with exercise, and clumsiness in the right leg. She reported a recent motor vehicle collision whereby she rear-ended another car as she could not move the right foot away from the accelerator promptly enough. Over the past few weeks, she has noted episodes when the right arm is drawn up with the hand clenched.

CASE SUMMARY

Our patient shows right foot plantar flexion and inversion activated during walking, which are relieved when the motor program changes (e.g., during marching, or when walking backward), and disappears at rest. This task-specific, action-induced phenomenon is referred to as dystonia. Most adult-onset focal dystonias occur in the upper body (cervical, cranial, or brachial regions). Onset of dystonia in the foot at the age of 50 years suggested a secondary cause and deserves further evaluations.

Additional examination findings demonstrated generalized hyperreflexia with right leg spasticity, right ankle clonus, and right weakness of proximal and distal muscles of the leg to a greater extent than the arm (see second video). These findings were consistent with an upper motor neuron syndrome. Furthermore, the presence of a jaw jerk and mild to moderate cortical sensory loss (mild right agraphesthesia and astereognosis) pointed in the direction of a left hemispheric lesion, affecting the parietal cortex and disrupting

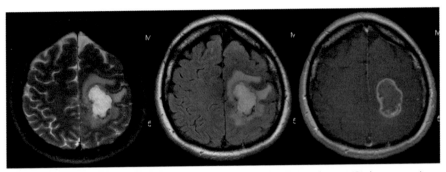

Figure 115.1   Axial T2-weighted, FLAIR, and T1-postgadolinium brain MRI demonstrating a confluent left posterior frontal lesion with ring enhancement and perilesional edema, suggestive of a primary malignancy or metastatic lesion.

the corticospinal system. Although a form of motor neuron disease could not initially be ruled out, a brain magnetic resonance imaging (MRI) demonstrated a large ring-enhancing lesion in the left frontoparietal region, near her motor strip (Fig. 115.1). A functional MRI showed her corticospinal track to be located along the anterior border of this lesion, which, upon stereotactic biopsy, was revealed to be a glioblastoma multiforme, World Health Organization (WHO) grade IV. Radiation and chemotherapy were initiated. Given the eloquent location of the tumor, resection of the tumor was not deemed feasible.

Stereotyped and repetitive action-induced abnormal posturing or "twisting," which may abate at rest and with sensory tricks, defines dystonia. Dystonic disorders are classified into primary and secondary forms. Adult-onset primary dystonia is typically focal and involves upper-body segments in the form of cranial dystonia (blepharospasm, oromandibular and lingual dystonia, and spasmodic dysphonia), cervical dystonia (previously referred to as spasmodic torticollis), and task-specific hand dystonia (also referred to as writer's cramp). These are the disorders highly responsive to chemodenervation with botulinum toxin injections.

Lower limb dystonia in adults is rarely a primary disorder. Isolated foot dystonia is a common presenting feature among younger-onset or genetic forms of Parkinson disease. Foot dystonia associated with pyramidal or other abnormalities, such as illustrated by our case, should raise suspicion for a space-occupying lesion (Table 115.1). Compared to primary

TABLE 115.1   FEATURES SUGGESTIVE OF SECONDARY LIMB DYSTONIA

History of Prior Insult	Perinatal Hypoxia, Drug Exposure, Head Trauma, Encephalitis
Clinical features of dystonia	Hemidystonia
	Dystonia at rest from onset[a]
	Atypical site for age at onset (cranial onset in children, leg onset in adults)
Associated clinical findings	Parkinsonism
	Upper motor neuron features
	Sensory deficits
	Ataxia
	False weakness or sensory loss, inconsistent or incongruent movements[a]
Other signs or symptoms	Dysarthria, deafness, cognitive impairment, neuropathy, dysautonomia

[a]These features are suggestive of a psychogenic etiology.

dystonia, adult-onset secondary dystonia more frequently generalizes or remains hemidystonic. In these cases, brain (and, in selected cases, spinal cord) neuroimaging is mandatory.

▌ **Case 115, Video 2:** The rest of examination is shown.

SELECTED REFERENCES

Bressman SB. Dystonia genotypes, phenotypes, and classification. *Adv Neurol* 2004;94:101–107.
Evatt ML, Freeman A, Factor S. Adult-onset dystonia. *Handbook Clin Neurol* 2011;100:481–511.
Pont-Sunyer C, Martí MJ, et al. Focal limb dystonia. *Eur J Neurol* 2010;17(Suppl 1):22–27.

SEE QUESTIONS: 351, 352

CASE 116

PSYCHOGENIC GAIT

◖ **OBJECTIVES** ◗

- To recognize the most common presentation of psychogenic gait in order to avoid unnecessary investigations and coordinate appropriate management.
- To list the various recognized phenotypes of psychogenic gait.
- To describe features of psychogenic disorders.

◖ **VIGNETTE** ◗

This 70-year-old man suddenly developed bilateral leg tremors about a year prior to this evaluation. The tremors were present mostly when sitting throughout the day. Two months later, as he was tried on levetiracetam, the tremors were suddenly "transferred to the upper body" and mostly disappeared in the legs. He also developed intermittent jerking of the left arm, but may also have similar jerking of the right. About 4 months later, he started to experience stumbling with walking although he had no falls. This problem kept him from playing golf. He had been treated for depression and anxiety for about 2 years but reported that trials with paroxetine, escitalopram, and venlafaxine were of no benefit to him. He continued to work at his own health insurance company but admitted to a growing list of unfinished responsibilities and problems with personnel.

CASE SUMMARY

 Our patient showed classic features of both psychogenic tremor and ataxia. The tremor was of variable frequency, amplitude, and distribution, and was readily suppressed in either limb when a complex task was performed in a different limb. Indeed, his tremor disappeared in the right hand when the left one was performing finger tapping, but reappeared when the task ceased. Similarly, his left foot tremor was suppressable and when tapping was performed accurately, both hands were tremorless.

He demonstrated the classic psychogenic pattern of buckling, the most common pattern of isolated psychogenic gait, followed by astasia–abasia. Abnormal gait can be an isolated psychogenic manifestation or associated with other psychogenic movement disorders (PMD), most commonly psychogenic tremor and psychogenic dystonia. In a series of 118 patients with psychogenic gait disorders, excessive slowing of gait was the most common pattern (18.6%), followed by dystonic gait (17.8%), bizarre gait (11.9%), astasia–abasia (11.9%), and buckling of the knee (7.6%). Among those with pure psychogenic gait, buckling of the knee was the most common pattern (31.3%), followed by astasia–abasia (18.8%). The proportion of pure psychogenic gait was 5.7% of PMD but increased to 42.3% when including other psychogenic features.

Psychogenic tremor, the most common PMD, can be positively diagnosed (i.e., not by exclusion of other diseases but by application of clinical criteria) by demonstrating variability in the frequency, distribution, and amplitude of the tremor, rapid onset (and offset, when paroxysmal), incongruent topographical change (e.g., stopping in the leg but appearing in the head), suppressibility by performance of complex tasks in other body parts, and, most convincingly when suppressibility is not achieved, entrainability of the tremor to a clinician-provided rate. A previous history of minor injury, including motor vehicle accidents or surgical procedures is often elicited as trigger. Our patient had sufficient features to qualify as clinically definite psychogenic tremor, associated with psychogenic knee-buckling–type gait impairment. Supportive features were multiple additional symptoms, symptom fluctuation, and previous documented psychiatric disturbances. He underwent extensive counseling and cognitive behavioral therapy sessions with a clinical psychologist.

SELECTED REFERENCES

Baik JS, Lang AE. Gait abnormalities in psychogenic movement disorders. *Mov Disord* 2007;22(3): 395–399.

Bressman SB. Dystonia genotypes, phenotypes, and classification. *Adv Neurol* 2004;94:101–107.

Espay AJ. Psychogenic movement disorders. In: Gálvez-Jiménez N, Tuite PJ, eds. *Unusual causes of movement disorders*. Cambridge, UK: Cambridge University Press, 2010.

Espay AJ. Psychogenic movement disorders: patterns of practice. In: Hallett M, ed. *Psychogenic movement disorders and other conversion disorders*. Cambridge, UK: Cambridge University Press, 2012.

SEE QUESTIONS: 353, 354

SECTION 16

NEURO-ONCOLOGY

CASE 117

LEPTOMENINGEAL MALIGNANCY (LYMPHOMA)

OBJECTIVES

- To recognize the presentation and manifestations of leptomeningeal malignancy.
- To outline the appropriate differential diagnosis and diagnostic workup for a chronic progressive polyradiculopathy and mononeuritis multiplex.
- To illustrate classic cerebrospinal fluid (CSF) findings in leptomeningeal malignancy.
- To emphasize the importance of a thorough diagnostic workup for patients with progressive polyradiculopathy and mononeuritis multiplex.

VIGNETTE

A 38-year-old man had a subacute progressive afebrile illness characterized by right thigh numbness and itching followed by right lower back pain, left foot numbness and itching, left lower extremity burning pain, left hand numbness, and deep left elbow and upper back pain. Subsequently, he had tingling of his right toes and severe stabbing pain in his left hand. This was followed by left arm and right thigh weakness, left face weakness, and then right face weakness. He then complained of bilateral circumoral numbness. During the course of his illness, he lost 25 pounds. Two months prior to onset of this illness, he had high fever, chills, and night sweats lasting 2 days.

CASE SUMMARY

Our patient presented with 6 months of multifocal sensory neuro-pathic/radiculopathic features, and pain followed by multiple cranial neuropathies. Sensory symptoms and signs followed a peripheral or cranial nerve distribution, and his weakness was of a lower motor neuron type. Neurophysiologic studies showed evidence of a patchy sensory motor peripheral neuropathy consistent with mononeuritis multiplex.

Differential diagnosis of multifocal radiculopathies and peripheral and cranial neuropathies should raise suspicion for a variety of chronic inflammatory or infiltrating conditions including infectious diseases such as Lyme disease, syphilis, cryptococcal meningitis, tuberculous meningitis, and leprosy. In addition, autoimmune inflammatory conditions known to cause mononeuritis multiplex include neurosarcoidosis, polyarteritis nodosa, other connective tissue diseases, and vasculitides. The spectrum of malignancy with carcinomatous meningitis can be one of the more difficult diagnoses to establish with certainty. CSF analysis has notoriously limited sensitivity and requires, in many patients, multiple samplings with high-volume spinal fluid.

Patients with immune-mediated chronic inflammatory polyradiculoneuropathy tend not to have such a patchy multifocal stuttering course. They rather have a clinical picture of a more symmetric and steadily progressive sensory and motor dysfunction. Patients with classical aggressive carcinomatous meningitis typically have low CSF glucose content (although other conditions listed previously could also be associated with low CSF glucose), and the CSF cytology can establish the diagnosis in many patients. Differential diagnosis of a polyradiculoneuropathy includes diabetes, vasculitic neuropathies, neurosarcoidosis, multiple myeloma, or a variety of immune-mediated disorders.

Neuroimaging studies in our patient showed little in the way of meningeal enhancement. Initial CSF studies showed an elevated CSF protein content, a mild lymphocytic pleocytosis, and a normal or marginally low glucose value. Initial CSF cytology was normal. Because of the patient's progressive clinical course, he had a more extensive diagnostic evaluation including a total body computed tomography (CT) scan, which demonstrated widespread lymphadenopathy. Lymph node biopsy showed B-cell lymphoma. Clinically, lymphomas are divided into Hodgkin lymphoma and non-Hodgkin lymphomas. Central nervous system (CNS) involvement with lymphomas is rare. Flow cytometry has improved the sensitivity of conventional cytology for the identification of leptomeningeal disease in aggressive B-cell non-Hodgkin lymphomas.

Management included systemic chemotherapy with cyclophosphamide, Adriamycin, and prednisone. The use of vincristine was problematic due to the presence of underlying peripheral neuropathy/radiculopathy and concerns of possible superimposed neurotoxicity.

As the blood–brain barrier serves to limit access to systemic drugs for treatment of malignancy, it is not uncommon for CNS metastases to be more resistant to systemic therapy. For this reason, radiation therapy and intrathecal chemotherapy are often necessary for the management of meningeal metastatic disease. Our patient responded favorably to systemic chemotherapy for several months. Systemic recurrence has led to an alternative therapy, stem cell transplantation.

SELECTED REFERENCES

Biller J, ed. *Practical neurology*, 4th ed. Philadelphia: Lippincott Williams & Wilkins, Wolters Kluwer Health, 2012.

Posner JB. *Neurologic complications of cancer*. Philadelphia: FA Davis Co., 1995.

Quijano S, Lopez A, Manuel SJ, et al. Identification of Leptomeningeal disease in aggressive B-cell non-Hodgkin's lymphoma: improved sensitivity of flow cytometry. *J Clin Oncol* 2009;27(9):1462–1469.

Roos KL. Carcinomatous meningitis. In: *Meningitis (100 maxims in neurology)*. New York: Oxford University Press, 1996:182–198.

SEE QUESTIONS: 137, 151, 154, 155, 194, 215

CASE 118

PARANEOPLASTIC CHOREA

OBJECTIVES

- To recognize the presentation of paraneoplastic chorea.
- To outline the appropriate differential diagnosis and diagnostic workup for a rapidly progressive movement disorder.
- To illustrate the management strategies for paraneoplastic disorders.

(Case courtesy of Dr. David Houghton, University of Louisville.)

VIGNETTE

This 75-year-old woman reported gait instability and involuntary movements for about 18 months preceding her evaluation. She also felt "wobbled" when walking, had difficulty negotiating stairs and curbs, and started to fall in any direction within 6 months, prompting the need for a walker. Her family noted "wiggling of her fingers" and "wrinkling" of her forehead as early as 3 months after the onset of gait problems. Although she was initially unaware, the abnormal movements progressed dramatically over 6 months to involve her face, trunk, and limbs. She was also noted to have word-finding difficulties, poor concentration, and decreased attention, interspersed with angry outbursts and generalized apathy. Of note, she had accumulated a 50-pack per year smoking history. She had no family history of similar neurological problems.

CASE SUMMARY

Our patient presented with progressive ataxia; axial-predominant chorea (face > head > trunk and limbs); cognitive impairment (Montreal Cognitive Assessment, 22/30); stocking-glove hypesthesia to temperature, vibration, and position; and patellar hyperreflexia and jaw jerk. The differential diagnosis for a subacute, progressive, late-onset chorea and ataxia with neuropsychiatric features includes metabolic, hereditary, autoimmune, and paraneoplastic disorders (Table 118.1).

A brain MRI demonstrated no cerebellar atrophy but abnormal T2-weighted and FLAIR hyperintensity in the putamen and periventricular region (Fig. 118.1). Additional investigations showed normal blood count, creatine kinase, liver profile, serum and urine copper, ceruloplasmin, antinuclear antibody (ANA), double-stranded DNA (dsDNA), rheumatoid factor (RF), thyroid-stimulating hormone (TSH)/T3/T4, and antiphospholipid antibody panel, except for an "inconclusive" immunoglobulin G (IgG) anticardiolipin (17, normal less than 15). There were no acanthocytes on blood smear, and her lipoprotein electrophoresis was normal. Genetic testing was negative for Huntington disease (HD) and dentatorubral-pallidoluysian atrophy (DRPLA). Symptomatic treatment with amantadine yielded minimal improvement, but tetrabenazine, titrated to a dose of 25 mg three times a day, led to marked improvement of her chorea, although with mild parkinsonian features as a drug-related complication.

TABLE 118.1   SELECTED CAUSES OF LATE-ONSET SUBACUTE, PROGRESSIVE, GENERALIZED CHOREA

Hereditary	Immune-Mediated	Metabolic
Huntington disease (HD)	Antiphospholipid antibody syndrome	Hypocalcemia
Neuroacanthocytosis	Sjögren	Hyperparathyroidism
Dentatorubral-pallidoluysian atrophy (DRPLA)	Polyarteritis nodosa	Hyperglycemia
HD-like phenocopies	Behcet disease	Fahr disease
	Paraneoplastic	

Anti-CRMP-5 antibody in serum was markedly elevated, at 1:61,440 (abnormal titers range reported, 120 to 61,440), leading to the diagnosis of paraneoplastic chorea. Further evaluation revealed the presence of a small-cell lung carcinoma.

Paraneoplastic chorea is most often associated with small-cell lung carcinoma and anti-CRMP-5. Conversely, 11% of patients with anti-CRMP-5 antibodies have chorea, 47% sensory neuropathy, 26% ataxia, and 25% subacute dementia, in isolation or combined with other features. CRMP-5-associated chorea tends to affect the face and limbs almost universally. Neuropathy, ataxia, and limbic features (behavioral disturbances) are less prevalent. The disorder improves with the removal of the underlying tumor and after chemotherapy and steroids, but tends to be unresponsive to plasmapheresis. Other paraneoplastic movement disorders are more commonly associated with specific antibodies (Table 118.2).

Of note, isolated bilateral putaminal T2/FLAIR hyperintensity, as noted in our patient, is a typical neuroimaging feature of paraneoplastic limbic encephalitis caused by CRMP-5 neuronal antibodies. Other causes of bilateral isolated putaminal hyperintensity include glutaric aciduria type I and Leigh syndrome.

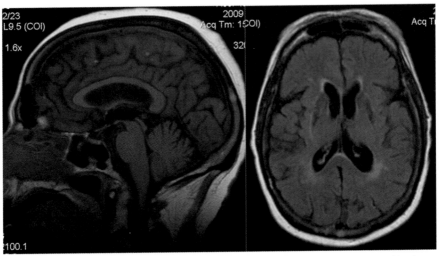

Figure 118.1   Midsagittal T1-weighted and axial FLAIR brain MRI showing normal brain and cerebellar volume but high intensity around the putamen and periventricular regions, bilaterally. Putaminal volume appears reduced.

TABLE 118.2 **PARANEOPLASTIC PHENOTYPE AND ASSOCIATED ANTIBODIES**

Paraneoplastic Phenotype	Most Common Antibodies	Most Common Malignancies
Chorea	Anti-CRMP-5	Small-cell lung cancer
Parkinsonism	Anti-Ma2	Testicular cancer
Cerebellar ataxia	Anti-Ri, Anti-Yo	Breast cancer
Cerebellar tremor	Anti-Yo	Breast cancer, ovarian cancer
Ataxia and pseudoathetosis	Anti-Hu	Small-cell lung cancer

SELECTED REFERENCES

Biller J, ed. *Practical neurology*, 4th ed. Philadelphia: Lippincott Williams & Wilkins, Wolters Kluwer Health, 2012.

Espay AJ, Biller J. *Concise neurology*. Philadelphia: Lippincott Williams & Wilkins, Wolters Kluwer Health, 2011.

Panzer J, Dalmau J. Movement disorders in paraneoplastic and autoimmune disease. *Curr Opin Neurol* 2011;24(4):346–353.

Vernino S, Tuite P, Adler CH, et al. Paraneoplastic chorea associated with CRMP-5 neuronal antibody and lung carcinoma. *Ann Neurol* 2002;51:625–630.

Yu Z, Kryzer TJ, Griesmann LE, et al. CRMP-5 neuronal autoantibody: marker of lung cancer and thymoma-related autoimmunity. *Ann Neurol* 2001;49:146–154.

SEE QUESTIONS: 311, 355, 356, 357

SECTION 17

NEUROLOGIC EMERGENCIES/URGENCIES

CASE 119

ACUTE CEREBELLAR INFARCTION (PICA) WITH EARLY HYDROCEPHALUS

OBJECTIVES

- To highlight pitfalls in the diagnosis of acute cerebellar infarction.
- To review the clinical presentation of acute cerebellar infarction in the posterior inferior cerebellar artery (PICA) territory.
- To review the potential serious consequences of large edematous cerebellar infarctions.
- To discuss management guidelines for these patients.

VIGNETTE

A 41-year-old woman with untreated hyperlipidemia and a history of cigarette smoking was evaluated at the emergency room 3 days previously because of new-onset nausea, vomiting, and disequilibrium. Diagnosed with flu and depression, she was sent home in a wheelchair, to be readmitted a day later because of occipital headaches and increasing gait unsteadiness.

CASE SUMMARY

Our patient had an acute cerebellar infarction involving the territory of the PICA. Fortunately, despite the initial misdiagnosis, she had a good clinical outcome.

The brainstem, cerebellum, and labyrinths are supplied by the vertebrobasilar arterial system. The areas of the cerebellum supplied by the PICA are extremely variable. There are several different patterns of PICA territory cerebellar infarctions. If the medial branch is affected, involving the vermis and vestibulocerebellum, the clinical findings include prominent vertigo, ataxia, and nystagmus. If the lateral cerebellar hemisphere is involved, patients can have vertigo, gait ataxia, limb dysmetria and ataxia, nausea, vomiting, conjugate or dysconjugate gaze palsies, miosis, and dysarthria.

Cerebellar infarction accounts for 2% to 3% of the 600,000 ischemic stroke cases seen annually in the United States. Cerebellar infarctions are more common than cerebellar hemorrhages, accounting for 85% of all cerebellar strokes. If the cerebellar infarction is large with associated mass effect and compression of the brainstem and fourth ventricle, altered consciousness and hydrocephalus or herniation may occur. There is also a syndrome of dorsolateral medullary and cerebellar infarction that may be caused by a vertebral artery occlusion or a medial PICA occlusion. Although a PICA occlusion can be the cause of Wallenberg (lateral medullary) syndrome, Wallenberg syndrome is more often caused by an intracranial vertebral artery occlusion.

Emergency room physicians should have a low threshold for obtaining consultation with a neurologist or neurosurgeon in patients who present with isolated vertigo or with vertigo, imbalance, and nausea and who also have cerebrovascular risk factors. Failure to assess gait on examination is frequently found on cases of misdiagnosis. Because not all signs of stroke are recorded as deficits on the National Institute of Health Stroke Scale (NIHSS), physicians should be reminded that a zero on the NIHSS does not rule out a stroke. Cerebellar strokes may be misdiagnosed as peripheral vestibulopathies migraines, toxic encephalopathies, gastroenteritis, or the "flu." As many as 25% of patients with cerebrovascular risk factors presenting to an emergency room with isolated vertigo, nystagmus, and postural instability have an infarction involving the inferior cerebellum.

Magnetic resonance imaging (MRI) and magnetic resonance angiography (MRA) are the preferred neuroimaging modalities for evaluating these patients. If MRI is unavailable or contraindicated, computed tomography (CT) with fine cuts through the posterior fossa is required. Careful attention to the status of the brainstem cisterns and fourth ventricle is required.

Patients with cerebellar infarction should be admitted to an intensive care unit or a dedicated stroke unit. In cases of space-occupying edematous cerebellar infarction with mass effect where fourth ventricular compression and hydrocephalus are the primary concerns, some neurosurgeons prefer to perform an external ventricular drainage. However, this procedure may be associated with a risk of upward cerebellar herniation through the free edge of the tentorial incisura. For this reason, others favor posterior fossa decompressive surgery by means of an occipital craniectomy.

SELECTED REFERENCES

Edlow JA, Newman-Token DE, Savitz SI. Diagnosis and initial management of cerebellar infarction. *Lancet Neurol* 2008;7(10):951–964.

Martin-Schild S, Albright KC, Tanksley J, et al. Zero on the NIHSS does not equal the absence of stroke. *Ann Emerg Med* 2011;57:42–45.

Norrving B, Magnusson M, Holtas S. Isolated acute vertigo in the elderly: vestibular or vascular disease? *Acta Neurol Scand* 1995;91:43–48.

Pfefferkorn T, Eppinger U, Linn J, et al. Long-term outcome after suboccipital decompressive craniectomy for malignant cerebellar infarction. *Stroke* 2009;40:3045–3050.

Savitz SI, Caplan LR, Edlow JA. Pitfalls in the diagnosis of cerebellar infarction. *Acad Emerg Med* 2007;14:63–68.

SEE QUESTIONS: 19, 55, 68, 92, 95, 143, 183

CASE 120

IATROGENIC EMERGENCIES

OBJECTIVES

■ To highlight common pitfalls in the management of Parkinson disease (PD), restless legs syndrome (RLS), dementia with Lewy bodies, and frontotemporal dementia, which can lead to acute symptomatic worsening of these disorders.
■ To review the mechanisms behind such complications and list strategies to prevent their occurrence.

VIGNETTE

This 65-year-old woman with a 4-year history of PD and early dementia developed severe nausea and vomiting after a dose increase in levodopa to minimize episodes of off-related freezing of gait. At the emergency room, she was given promethazine (Phenergan), which had sufficient antiemetic effect to allow her discharge to home. While at home, she developed episodes of full-body flailing, which were captured by her husband on her cell phone and transmitted to us (the clip shown). The patient had to return to the emergency room, where administration of diphenhydramine (Benadryl) abated the complication.

CASE SUMMARY

This PD patient developed promethazine-induced acute dystonic reaction expressed as dramatic worsening of preexistent levodopa-induced dyskinesias. This patient was already functionally brittle given the presence of diphasic dyskinesias and freezing of gait in the "off" state alternating with tolerable peak-dose levodopa-induced dyskinesias in the "on" state, developing in the background of early dementia. Dyskinetic manifestations are exacerbated by promethazine and other phenothiazines. Prompt administration of drugs with anticholinergic properties is necessary to abort this iatrogenic complication.

Prochlorperazine and metoclopramide are two commonly used antiemetics and, compared to antipsychotics, have remained under the radar as causes of acute dystonic reaction and symptomatic worsening in PD patients. These agents have dopamine receptor–blocking properties for which, together with antipsychotics, they are termed *neuroleptics*. Drugs in the neuroleptic category include the phenothiazines fluphenazine and prochlorperazine as well as the substituted benzamides: metoclopramide, sulpiride, tiapride, and clebopride. The blockade of striatal D2 receptors is believed to be responsible for the development of acute dystonic reactions and drug-induced parkinsonism. Metoclopramide administered as antiemetic strategy, particularly in patients with acute renal failure, is a common cause of acute dystonic reactions in the ICU setting (see second video). Appropriate antiemetic control in PD can be safely achieved with domperidone, a peripheral dopamine antagonist, or ondansetron, a selective serotonin 5-HT$_3$ receptor antagonist.

While diphenhydramine can be beneficial in PD patients with dyskinetic complications, this drug can be detrimental in patients with RLS. A dramatic increase in symptoms similar to those documented after promethazine in our patient with PD can be seen after the use of diphenhydramine in patients with RLS who, when poorly controlled, may be given this "sedative" in the emergency setting. Diphenhydramine is notorious for greatly increasing the severity of RLS and often forces the admission of these acutely worsened RLS patients into psychiatry units. It is probable that patients with presumed "allergy" to diphenhydramine may in fact have subclinical RLS, unmasked by the exposure to this antihistaminic agent.

Two additional examples of dramatic, if paradoxical, worsening of function are psychotic exacerbation following antipsychotic administration (typically, but not always, with drugs other than quetiapine and clozapine) in patients with early, often unrecognized dementia with Lewy bodies and the acute behavioral and cognitive worsening after the administration of cholinesterase inhibitors in patients with frontotemporal dementia. Frontotemporal dementia (FTD) patients have no cholinergic loss compared to Alzheimer disease, PD dementia, and dementia with Lewy bodies; thus, the increased cholinergic tone produced by cholinesterase inhibitors disrupts a precarious neurotransmitter balance and leads to behavioral decompensation. Antipsychotic-induced worsening of psychosis ("neuroleptic sensitivity") and cholinergic-induced deterioration of cognition, when encountered serendipitously in emergency settings, can be held as diagnostic clues in favor of dementia with Lewy bodies and FTD, respectively.

▶ **Case 120, Video 2:** This 38-year-old man with end-stage renal disease was given metoclopramide 10 mg three times a day, scheduled over 2 weeks, before severe tongue protrusion dystonia, a hallmark of acute dystonic reaction, developed. This prompted measures to prevent tongue laceration or biting. The complication resolved after discontinuation of metoclopramide and administration of diphenhydramine.

SELECTED REFERENCES

Espay AJ. Toxic movement disorders: the approach to the patient with a movement disorder of toxic origin. In: Dobbs M, ed. *Clinical neurotoxicology.* Amsterdam, The Netherlands: Saunders, Elsevier, 2009:Chapter 10, 115–130.

Espay AJ, Lang AE. *Common movement disorders pitfalls: case-based teaching.* New York: Cambridge University Press, 2012.

SEE QUESTIONS: 358, 359, 360, 361

SECTION 18

BORDERLAND BETWEEN NEUROLOGY AND PSYCHIATRY

CASE 121

CONVERSION DISORDER (PSYCHOGENIC GAIT)

OBJECTIVES

- To present a typical psychogenic gait phenotype.
- To list the various recognized phenotypes of psychogenic gait.

VIGNETTE

A 22-year-old woman was admitted after sudden onset of leg buckling when she attempted to stand and walk. She was 2 months postpartum. Review of systems was normal. The patient admitted to feeling overwrought with the stressors of a new baby and her engagement to the baby's father.

CASE SUMMARY

Is her gait dysfunction organic in nature? Despite full strength, normal muscle tone, unremarkable muscle stretch reflexes, and normal sensory and cerebellar examination, our patient had a bizarre and rather spectacular gait disorder characterized by exaggerated effort, variability with distraction, excessive slowness or hesitation in walking, and sudden buckling of her knees without falling. Her gait pattern did not resemble a hemiparetic, ataxic, shuffling, steppage, or scissor type of gait abnormality. The sudden-onset, markedly incongruent features, and inconsistent phenotype were consistent with a clinically definite psychogenic ataxia.

The proportion of isolated psychogenic gait is about 6% of psychogenic movement disorders, but increases to 42% when considering it as part of a complex psychogenic presentation. Somatoform disorders represent a psychiatric condition because the physical

247

symptoms present in this disorder cannot be fully accounted for by a medical disorder, substance use, or another mental disorder. Specific somatoform disorders include (a) somatization disorder, (b) conversion disorder, (c) factitious disorder, (d) malingering, (e) hypochondriasis, (f) somatoform pain disorder, and (g) body dysmorphic disorder. As stated in the *Diagnostic and Statistical Manual of Mental Disorders,* fourth edition *(DSM-IV)*, conversion disorder involves symptoms or deficits affecting voluntary motor or sensory function that suggest a neurological or other general medical condition.

Gait disorders are very common in the very old and in the very young. Knee buckling and astasia–abasia are the most common patterns of isolated psychogenic gait. The phenotype of psychogenic gait when mixed with other psychogenic manifestations include, in decreasing order of frequency, excessive slowing of gait, dystonic gait, bizarre gait, astasia–abasia, and buckling of the knees. The chair test has been proposed as a potentially useful diagnostic test in patients suspected of psychogenic gait disorders. In this test, patients are asked to sit in a swivel chair with wheels and to propel the chair forward and backward. While patients with psychogenic ataxia show a preserved ability to propel a chair forward when seated, patients with organic gait impairment cannot (i.e., these patients perform equally when walking or propelling a swivel chair).

SELECTED REFERENCES

Baik JS, Lang AE. Gait abnormalities in psychogenic movement disorders. *Mov Disord* 2007;22(3):395–399.

Biller J, ed. *Practical neurology*, 4th ed. Philadelphia: Lippincott Williams & Wilkins, Wolters Kluwer Health, 2012.

Lemperet T, Brandt T, Dieterich M, et al. How to identify psychogenic disorders of stance and gait. *J Neurol* 1991;238:140–146.

Okun MS, Rodriguez RL, Foote KD, Fernandez HH. The "chair test" to aid in the diagnosis of psychogenic gait disorders. *Neurologist* 2007;13(2):87–91.

Sudarsky L. Psychogenic gait disorders. *Semin Neurol* 2006;26(3):351–356.

SEE QUESTIONS: 252, 362, 363, 364

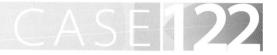

CASE 122

SOMATIZATION DISORDER (PSYCHOGENIC STUTTERING)

OBJECTIVES

- To review the somatoform disorders.
- To demonstrate a presentation of conversion disorder.
- To distinguish somatization from factitious disorder and malingering.

VIGNETTE

One month after clipping of an unruptured basilar tip aneurysm, this 43-year-old woman, recently divorced, experienced difficulty producing speech. She also had recent hospitalizations because of unexplained abdominal pain, chest pains, and syncope.

CASE SUMMARY

Six weeks following clipping of an asymptomatic, unruptured, basilar tip aneurysm, our patient had changes with her speech. At first, she was unable to speak at all. She improved, although fluency remained impaired, with frequent stuttering. She also had difficulty remembering "sequential things," by which she meant she had to read instructions a number of times, such as those for getting to our clinic. She also could not remember recipes. She denied any sense of sadness or dysphoria and did not seem particularly disturbed or upset by the idea that her speech problem might become chronic and prevent her from returning to work. Postoperative magnetic resonance imaging (MRI) of the brain and catheter cerebral angiogram showed the basilar tip aneurysm clip, but they were otherwise unremarkable. Ears, nose, and throat (ENT) evaluation showed inconsistent glottal closure with laryngeal tremors.

There were some marked social stressors in our patient's recent past. Her husband reportedly left her abruptly after 24 years for another woman whom she did not know. She denied other prior stressors including financial pressures or health problems in her family or children. She had no previous problems at work with her colleagues. She reportedly liked her work, and denied any symptoms of obsessive–compulsive disorder, panic disorder, generalized anxiety disorder, schizophrenic disorder, bipolar disorder, or post-traumatic stress disorder.

Examination showed an awake, alert, and well-oriented woman who provided her own history. She was casually dressed, neatly groomed, and appeared her stated age. Speech was marked by stuttering on the initial clause of a sentence and on consonants. Upon beginning a phrase, her eyes rolled closed and her neck torqued (sometimes to the right and sometimes to the left). She squinted as well and occasionally experienced a whole-body jerk. Her mood appeared to be quite euthymic, and she smiled or laughed frequently, including during descriptions of traumatic events such as her husband leaving her. Assessment of effort with forced-choice recognition memory was unremarkable. Her thoughts in conversation were logical, sequential, and goal oriented. Her fund of general knowledge was high average and estimated intellectual endowment was average to high average based on word pronunciation.

Despite the speech abnormality, letter fluency was normal, as was confrontation naming. She could write well to dictation, but her writing was not particularly fluent and she wrote with great pressure on the pencil. Constructional praxis in assembling blocks to match a template was average to normal on the nondominant left. Specifically, her grip strength was 20 kg/in^2 on the right hand, which was somewhat inconsistent with the pressure she was applying with her pencil and to hand squeeze. Limb praxis appeared to be essentially normal.

The Minnesota Multiphasic Personality Inventory, MMPI-2, was administered, but the profile was invalid from overly positive self-presentation. That said, there were no obvious indications of depression. The clinical scales themselves were a 1 to 3 profile, which was associated with individuals who commonly convert psychological distress into somatic complaints. The remainder of the neurological examination was unremarkable.

In summary, our patient had a rather unusual and inconsistent speech pattern associated with incongruent paroxysmal axial movements with inconsistent blepharospasm and psychogenic oromandibular dystonic spasms, temporally associated with relevant psychological stressors despite a suggestion of *la belle indifférence*. These features were consistent with a psychogenic disorder, most likely due to somatization disorder.

Somatoform disorders represent a psychiatric condition because the physical symptoms present in this disorder cannot be fully accounted for by a medical disorder, substance use, or another mental disorder. Specific somatoform disorders include

(a) somatization disorder, (b) conversion disorder, (c) factitious disorder, (d) malingering, (e) hypochondriasis, (f) somatoform pain disorder, and (g) body dysmorphic disorder. Somatization disorder describes patients with excessive and persistent concern about multiple somatic complaints (in our patient, at least abdominal pain, chest pains, and fainting) for whom there is neither secondary gain nor intentional production of symptoms but deep conviction of illness. The multiple symptoms, which lack recognizable etiology, may include pain and gastrointestinal and sexual symptoms, in addition to at least one pseudoneurological symptom. These are out of proportion to the physical findings and may lead to multiple procedures and hospitalizations.

Speech manifestations of psychogenic disorders include dysphonia, aphonia, spasmodic dysphonia, and stuttering-like behavior. Less commonly, some individuals exhibit a pseudo-foreign dialect, infantile speech, prosodic disorders, or psychogenic mutism.

The patient was reassured that her symptoms were very real although not due to an underlying organic neurological or other organic disorder. She was subsequently referred to psychiatry and to a clinical psychologist for cognitive behavioral therapy.

SELECTED REFERENCES

American Psychiatric Association. Somatoform disorders. In: *Diagnostic and statistical manual of mental disorders*, 4th ed. Washington, DC: APA Press, 1994:452–457.

Baumgartner J, Duffy JR. Psychogenic stuttering in adults with and without neurologic disease. *J Med Speech Lang Pathol* 1997;5:75–95.

Boffeli TJ, Guze SB. The simulation of neurologic disease. *Psychiatric Clin North Am* 1992;15(Jun):301–310.

Espay AJ. Psychogenic movement disorders. In: Gálvez-Jiménez N, Tuite PJ eds. *Unusual causes of movement disorders*. Cambridge, England: Cambridge University Press, 2010.

Fink P, Sorensen L, Engberg M. Somatization in primary care. Prevalence, health care utilization, and general practitioner recognition. *Psychosomatics* 1999;40(Jul–Aug):330–338.

SEE QUESTIONS: 252, 362, 363, 364

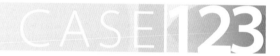

CASE 123

PSYCHOGENIC TREMOR

OBJECTIVES

- To demonstrate a typical presentation of psychogenic tremor.
- To briefly discuss distinguishing elements between organic and psychogenic tremor.

VIGNETTE

This 43-year-old woman dated the onset of her problems to 8 months previously, immediately following a complete hysterectomy, when she had two episodes of full-body convulsions, the second of which was without loss of consciousness. Since then, she has had unremitting tremor in the head, hands, and trunk with intermittent eyelid fluttering. She has also had stuttering. The tremor and stuttering have remained unchanged and kept her from working. She had enhanced anxiety prior to the hysterectomy, mostly related to stresses at her workplace and fear from retaliation by her supervisor. She was on a long list of medications (aripiprazole, propranolol, zolpidem, hydrocodone, and alprazolam) without perceived benefits in her tremor and underlying anxiety. She admitted to headaches but denied chest or abdominal discomfort. She had noted some unusual walking and unsteadiness but had not had falls. She was highly concerned about her problem and the lack of a clear diagnosis.

CASE SUMMARY

 Our patient had right-sided predominant tremor with variable amplitude, frequency, and severity; easily suppressible with complex tasks; and exhibiting a positive co-contraction sign on examination (co-contraction of antagonistic muscles in her forearm was needed for the reemergence of her tremor). These findings, along with a bizarre gait and the absence of any objective neurological deficits, formed the basis for a diagnosis of clinically definite psychogenic tremor. The etiology was most likely conversion disorder.

As the most common psychogenic movement disorders (PMD) phenotype, psychogenic tremor can be diagnosed with a clinically definite degree of certainty when the oscillating and rhythmic activity of a patient's limb can be shown to be variable in amplitude and distribution, distractible (suppressed by performance of complex tasks), entrainable when not distractible (its frequency changes to match the induced tapping rate of an unaffected limb), and capable of being modulated (altered in amplitude with nonphysiologic interventions, such as a vibrating tuning fork on the forehead).

We thoroughly discussed the psychogenic nature of her problem, the importance of accepting the diagnosis, and the need to establish a long-term relationship with a clinical psychologist with experience in stress-related and psychogenic movement disorders for application of cognitive behavioral therapy. Slow, cautious, and sequential withdrawal was recommended for each of her medications, with the exception of alprazolam if clinically significant anxiety disorder can be formally diagnosed. We welcome the opportunity of reviewing matters again in 6 months provided that (1) she had remained in regular psychological counseling with a psychologist with whom we regularly communicate, (2) she accepted the diagnosis fully and without reservations, and (3) she could demonstrate some gains in function at her next evaluation. She accepted these reevaluation criteria and was scheduled for reevaluation in 6 months. After 8 months of regular psychotherapy, she markedly improved, with rare relapses. She gained employment at a different company and felt strengthened and less vulnerable to the effects of her new responsibilities.

Effective communication, providing personal follow-up, and connecting patients to a mental health specialist are important elements in the management of patients with psychogenic disorders, also contributing to avoiding "doctor shopping" and minimizing iatrogenic harm. Neurologists are best poised to embrace PMD as a complex neurobehavioral disorder for which they have a primary role in establishing the diagnosis and coordinating management. Clinicians who engage in the discussion of patients' psychosocial problems are less likely to request investigations, refer patients elsewhere, or offer inappropriate drug treatments.

SELECTED REFERENCES

Espay AJ, Goldenhar LM, Voon V, et al. Opinions and clinical practices related to diagnosing and managing patients with psychogenic movement disorders: an International Survey of Movement Disorder Society Members. *Mov Disord* 2009;24(9):1366–1374.

Espay AJ. Psychogenic movement disorders. In: Gálvez-Jiménez N, Tuite PJ eds. *Unusual causes of movement disorders*. Cambridge, England: Cambridge University Press, 2010.

Lang AE, Voon V. Psychogenic movement disorders: past developments, current status, and future directions. *Mov Disord* 2011;26(6):1175–1186.

SEE QUESTIONS: 365, 366

BORDERLAND BETWEEN NEUROLOGY AND MEDICINE

CASE 124

POST–CARDIAC ARREST SYNDROME

OBJECTIVES

■ To present a survivor with postanoxic encephalopathy after out-of-hospital cardiac arrest due to ventricular fibrillation.
■ To describe the neurological aftermath of postanoxic encephalopathy at greater than 6 months' follow-up.
■ To describe the functional status and long-term neurological outcome post–cardiac arrest.

VIGNETTE

A 45-year-old-man with hypertension, dyslipidemia, and diabetes mellitus, complicated by diabetic retinopathy and prior left foot fourth and fifth digit amputation, had ventricular fibrillation cardiac arrest while working out at a fitness center. Advanced cardiac life support (ACLS) was initiated within 1 to 2 minutes. An automatic external defibrillator (AED) was applied, and the patient was shocked. Cardiopulmonary resuscitation (CPR) continued. An ambulance was present at the scene within 10 minutes. He remained unresponsive and was taken to a local hospital, where he had endotracheal intubation in the emergency department and taken to the cardiac catheterization laboratory where he was revascularized with a coronary artery stent to a 99% stenosed left anterior descending (LAD) artery. He remained intubated and was admitted to the intensive care unit (ICU). A therapeutic hypothermia protocol was promptly initiated. He received a beta-blocker and angiotensin-converting enzyme (ACE) inhibitor. He was extubated 3 days after admission. A recommendation for an internal cardiac defibrillator (ICD) depending on resolution of neurologic status was made.

The patient continued to have altered mental status attributed to anoxic brain injury with resulting post–cardiac arrest encephalopathy. Electroencephalogram (EEG) showed diffuse background slowing. Head computed tomography (CT) without contrast was unremarkable. There was normal gray–white matter differentiation throughout. Magnetic resonance imaging (MRI) of the brain demonstrated some scattered foci of increased signal on T2 and FLAIR images in the periventricular and subcortical white matter bilaterally.

During his hospitalization, his level of alertness began to improve with some purposeful movements and "nonsensical" speech according to family members. He was started on nasogastric feeds. He became febrile due to aspiration pneumonia. He also had renal insufficiency, likely due to contrast administration as well as sudden cardiac arrest with resulting kidney hypoperfusion.

At his family's request, he was transferred to our institution, where he had four additional coronary artery stents. Following cardiac stabilization, he was transferred for inpatient rehabilitation. Ongoing behavioral issues, cognitive impairment, apathy, and bladder and bowel incontinence delayed his evaluation by a few months after his cardiac arrest. A repeat EEG showed mild to moderate slowing of the background. There were no epileptiform discharges, EEG seizures, or focal abnormalities at any point during the recording.

CASE SUMMARY

 Our patient suffered an anoxic encephalopathy secondary to cardiac arrest with little improvement after 2 years. He is able to walk unassisted but does not engage in much spontaneous behavior or conversation, and his sister notes that, left to his own devices, he would probably simply lie in bed all day long. He is incontinent. He remains persistently disoriented, and his sister reports that he sometimes does not even respond to direct questioning. The patient could not tell where he is currently living and instead confabulated that he was living at home with his sister. He did not feel as though he had suffered any significant cognitive impairment.

Our patient was able to ambulate independently. He was rather avolitional and responded only to direct questioning. His affect seemed generally blunted. He was cooperative with all aspects of the interview and testing. Neuropsychological evaluation placed him into the range of mental retardation, 50 points below predicted premorbid levels of function. His cerebral performance category was considered to be a level 3 (Table 124.1). He appears to have a static postanoxic encephalopathy, with relative severe impairment of anterograde memory as the primary feature, but significant compromise of all other neurocognitive domains as well. The prognosis for any significant improvement in his neurobehavioral condition is poor.

TABLE 124.1 **CEREBRAL PERFORMANCE CATEGORIES (CPCs) SCALE**

CPC 1	Good cerebral performance: conscious, alert, able to work
CPC 2	Moderate cerebral disability: conscious, can carry out independent activities
CPC 3	Severe neurological disability: conscious, dependent on others for daily support
CPC 4	Coma or vegetative state
CPC 5	Death

From Cronberg T, Lilja G, Rundgren M, et al. Long-term neurological outcome after cardiac arrest and therapeutic hypothermia. *Resuscitation* 2009;80:1119–1123.

Hypoxic–ischemic brain injury, also known as hypoxic–ischemic encephalopathy, anoxic brain injury, or postresuscitation encephalopathy, refers to the neurologic aftermath of global reduction in oxygen delivery to the brain. Post–cardiac arrest brain injury is a common cause of mortality and morbidity.

A simple bedside prediction tool known as the Cardiac Arrest Survival Postresuscitation In-Hospital (CASPRI) score recently demonstrated the ability to identify patients with probably favorable neurological survival after in-hospital cardiac arrest. Eleven variables were identified with the greatest ability to predict a favorable neurological survival. These characteristics included younger age, initial cardiac arrest rhythm of ventricular fibrillation or pulseless ventricular tachycardia with a defibrillation time less than 2 minutes, baseline neurological status without disability, cardiac arrest location in a monitor unit, shorter duration of resuscitation, and absence of mechanical ventilation, renal/hepatic insufficiency, sepsis, malignant disease, and hypotension prior to cardiac arrest.

Susceptible areas of neuronal damage include the pyramidal neurons in the CA1 region of the hippocampi, cerebellar Purkinje cells, medium spiny striatal neurons, and pyramidal neurons in layers 3, 5, and 6 of the neocortex. The spectrum of clinical manifestations of post–cardiac arrest brain injury include coma, seizures, myoclonus, cognitive dysfunction, persistent vegetative state, secondary parkinsonism, cortical strokes, spinal cord strokes, and brain death.

The most common cause of hypoxic–ischemic encephalopathy is cardiac arrest. Our patient suffered an anoxic encephalopathy secondary to cardiac arrest secondary to ventricular fibrillation. He received therapeutic hypothermia. The efficacy of therapeutic hypothermia following cardiac arrest has been demonstrated in two randomized clinical trials. Both trials used external cooling to achieve targeted hypothermia, and in both trials, the initial rhythm was ventricular fibrillation.

SELECTED REFERENCES

Bernard SA, Gray TW, Buist MD, et al. Treatment of comatose survivors of out-of-hospital cardiac arrest with induced hypothermia. *New Engl J Med* 2002;346:557–563.

Chan PS, Spertus JA, Krumholz HM, et al. A validated prediction tool for initial survivors in in-hospital cardiac arrest. *Arch Intern Med*. Published online May 28, 2012.

Cronberg T, Lilja G, Rundgren M, et al. Long-term neurological outcome after cardiac arrest and therapeutic hypothermia. *Resuscitation* 2009;80:1119–1123.

Ewy GA, Kern KB, Sanders AB, et al. Cardiocerebral resuscitation for cardiac arrest. *Am J Med* 2006;119: 6–9.

The Hypothermia after Cardiac Arrest Study Group. Mild therapeutic hypothermia to improve the neurologic outcome after cardiac arrest. *N Engl J Med* 2002;346:549–556.

Nichol G, Thomas E, Callaway CW, et al. Regional variation in out-of-hospital cardiac arrest and outcome. *JAMA* 2008;300:1423–1431.

Nolan JP, Neumar RW, Adrie C, et al. Post-cardiac arrest syndrome: epidemiology, pathophysiology, treatment, and prognostication. A Scientific Statement from the International Liaison Committee on Resuscitation; the American Heart Association Emergency Cardiovascular Care Committee; the Council on Cardiovascular Surgery and Anesthesia; the Council on Cardiopulmonary Perioperative, and Critical Care; the Council on Clinical Cardiology; the Council on Stroke. *J Resuscitation* 2008;79(3):350–379.

SEE QUESTION: 367

CASE125

TETANY IN ELECTROLYTIC DERANGEMENT

. . . .

OBJECTIVES

■ To present a case of carpal spasm or tetany confused with paroxysmal dystonia.
■ To recognize the metabolic disturbances capable of generating tetany.
■ To list disorders that can be listed in the differential diagnosis.

VIGNETTE

This 66-year-old woman was evaluated for episodes of finger posturing. About 6 months ago, while sewing a button (she is a seamstress), she noted sudden onset of left thumb adduction and index finger extension, which was painful and lasted about 5 minutes. She had since several episodes, and the frequency increased over time, no longer requiring any manual work on her part. These were happening at anytime, almost every day, and were always painful but short lasting. Intriguingly, she had an episode of upward toe curling during each of her two pregnancies, 37 and 40 years ago, which did not recur until last a week prior to this evaluation. She was known to have hypertension, diabetes mellitus type II (with neuropathy), hypothyroidism, anxiety, chronic obstructive pulmonary disease, and sleep apnea. Her neurological exam was unremarkable, except for mild decreased sensation to temperature and vibration in the distal legs.

CASE SUMMARY

Our 66-year-old diabetic seamstress had intermittent painful hand posturing, with rapid-onset painful thumb adduction, slight metacarpophalangeal flexion, and interphalangeal finger extension. These painful episodes lasted less than 5 minutes and disappeared abruptly, as represented by the patient's account. The episodic nature, short duration, and accompanying pain were consistent with a peripheral nerve hyperexcitability syndrome and were reminiscent of muscle cramps rather than paroxysmal dystonia, which was the initial diagnosis. The combination of painful contractions of finger muscles resulting in thumb adduction, metacarpophalangeal flexion, and interphalangeal finger extension should be recognized as tetany or carpopedal spasm (sans *pedal* [foot]; isolated *carpal* spasm in this case), which is a peripheral neuromuscular disorder not to be confused with dystonia.

In different topographical distributions, other conditions worth considering are the tonic spasm of multiple sclerosis, neuromyotonia, and Lambert-Brody syndrome (exercise-induced pain, stiffness, and cramping in arm and leg muscles associated with impairment of relaxation).

Tetany applies to painful finger contractions resulting in thumb adduction, metacarpophalangeal flexion, and interphalangeal finger extension. It is associated with hypocalcemia as well as hypomagnesemia, hypokalemic alkalosis, and respiratory alkalosis. Tetany is classically triggered by hypocalcemia, but hypomagnesemia as well as metabolic and respiratory alkalosis can also induce it. Alkalotic states are capable of inducing tetany by binding calcium to proteins, thus lowering ionized calcium. In a paradoxical twist, metabolic alkalosis can also induce hypokalemia, which protects against tetany in the setting of hypocalcemia. Correction of hypokalemia alone can precipitate hypocalcemic tetany.

Our patient's ionized calcium was normal, but parathyroid hormone (PTH) and phosphorus were high while magnesium was low. Further investigations demonstrated that these changes were due to previously unrecognized renal insufficiency, likely a complication of her diabetes mellitus. Correction of the laboratory abnormalities and tighter management of her diabetes and renal insufficiency led to complete resolution of the tetany episodes. Antidystonic drugs or botulinum toxins, which were considered when her condition was suspected to represent dystonia, did not become part of her treatment strategy.

SELECTED REFERENCES

Espay AJ. Neurologic complications of electrolyte disturbances and acid/base balance. In: Aminoff MJ, Boller F, Swaab DF, eds. *Handbook of clinical neurology—systemic diseases*, 3rd series. Vol. I: The Neurological Complications of Systemic Diseases (Biller J, Ferro JM, sub-editors). Amsterdam, The Netherlands: Elsevier, 2013, in press.

Espay AJ, Lang AE. *Common movement disorders pitfalls: case-based teaching.* New York: Cambridge University Press, 2012.

Matustik MC. Late-onset tetany with hypocalcemia and hyperphosphatemia. *Am J Dis Child* 1986;140(9):854–855.

Narayan SK, Sivaprasad P, Sahoo RN, et al. Teaching video NeuroImage: Chvostek sign with Fahr syndrome in a patient with hypoparathyroidism. *Neurology* 2008;71(24):e79.

SEE QUESTIONS: 368, 369

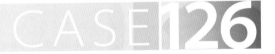

ACQUIRED NEUROMYOTONIA IN RHEUMATOLOGIC DISEASE

OBJECTIVES

- To present a case of acquired neuromyotonia confused with dystonia.
- To recognize that neuromyotonia may remain elusive until electromyographic features are ascertained.
- To highlight the importance of myokymia in steering evaluation for paraneoplastic, autoimmune, and genetic disorders.

VIGNETTE

This 23-year-old woman reported the onset of left thumb "twitches" at the age of 16 years. The movements were present at rest and during posture holding, most noticeable in the left hand. She also noted "twitching" of the thighs. These movements had progressed over the last 2 years, worsening toward the end of the day. Handwriting was associated with cramping of the right thumb. She was diagnosed with lupus at the age of 21 years. Besides the movements appreciated on the video, the rest of the neurological examination was normal.

CASE SUMMARY

 These movements were at different times considered to represent tremor, myoclonus, or dystonia. In reality, they were too slow for myoclonus, too fast for dystonia, and too dysrhythmic for tremor. The jerks were asynchronous, showed variable amplitude but barely moved the joints, were not influenced by positional changes, and had similar magnitude at rest and on posture. Hence, the movements did not fit the bill for any of the hyperkinetic movement phenotypes known to occur from central nervous system pathology (myoclonus, dystonia, and tics).

In this situation, a peripheral disorder should have been considered. Indeed, "cramps" and "twitches" belong to the umbrella of peripheral nerve hyperexcitability. In this patient, needle electromyogram (EMG) over forearm muscles revealed doublets and triplets, firing at a frequency of 40 Hz. These findings were diagnostic of myokymia or acquired neuromyotonia.

The patient developed recurrent episodes of knee pain and finger swelling followed by pain in the tarsal–metatarsal joints when she walked. Her antinuclear antibody (ANA) titer was 1:80, speckled pattern. A rheumatology consultation was requested, and after extensive investigations, she was diagnosed with mixed tissue connective disorder, an autoimmune disorder characterized by features of systemic lupus erythematosus, systemic sclerosis, and polymyositis. She was started on a short course of prednisone, which improved her arthritis and attenuated the movements (see second video). The appearance of comorbid facial myokymia further supported the underlying presence of peripheral nerve hyperexcitability as part of her autoimmune disorder.

Neuromyotonia or electric myokymia applies to the sustained muscle activity of peripheral nerve origin, which is defined electrophysiologically as spontaneous and EMG needle-induced irregular trains of doublets, triplets, and multiplets firing at a high intraburst frequency (150 to 300 Hz; neuromyotonic discharges) and at lower frequencies (less than 60 Hz; myokymic discharges). Away from joints they appear as visible rippling movements, slower than fasciculations, also referred to as "bag of worms." Acquired neuromyotonia can occur as an idiopathic autoimmune syndrome or as a paraneoplastic phenomenon (anti–voltage-gated potassium channel [VGKC] binding to CASPR2, also known as Isaac syndrome) and may be associated with other autoimmune disorders (thymoma, vitiligo, myasthenia gravis, Hashimoto thyroiditis, or penicillamine treatment), or appear within a genetic or other rheumatologic disorder. If disease-specific treatment does not yield adequate improvement of the neuromyotonia, one may consider a trial with carbamazepine or phenytoin, which can be effective through their interaction with voltage-gated sodium channels.

▶ **Video 2:** The patient is examined after an episode of pain and swelling in the knees and finger joints. The movements seem less prominent. The last segment demonstrates that her pain and swelling have been controlled with prednisone. Residual movements are also attenuated. Facial myokymia has newly appeared.

SELECTED REFERENCES

Maddison P. Neuromyotonia. *Clin Neurophysiol* 2006;117(10):2118–2127.

Rueff L, Graber JJ, Bernbaum M, et al. Voltage-gated potassium channel antibody-mediated syndromes: a spectrum of clinical manifestations. *Rev Neurol Dis* 2008;5(2):65–72.

Zhang YQ. Teaching video NeuroImages: regional myokymia. *Neurology* 2010;74(23):e103–e104.

SEE QUESTIONS: 370, 371

CLINICOPATHOLOGIC
CORRELATIONS

CASE 127

PRIMARY CNS ANGIITIS

OBJECTIVES

- To review the basic pathophysiology of the vasculitides.
- To review the clinical characteristics of primary central nervous system (CNS) angiitis.
- To discuss ancillary diagnostic tests in primary CNS angiitis.
- To review management principles in primary CNS angiitis.

VIGNETTE

A 30-year-old man had protracted severe headaches that he attributed to migraines. He also had binocular horizontal diplopia, worse when looking to the right, and numbness below the right eyelid that progressed to involve the right side of his skull.

He had numerous investigations including magnetic resonance imaging (MRIs), magnetic resonance angiography (MRAs), magnetic resonance venography (MRVs), and a catheter cerebral angiogram. MRI showed T2 signal hyperintensities involving the right cerebellar hemisphere. He was initially thought to have a brain tumor and was seen by a neurosurgeon who disagreed with the diagnosis.

Subsequent investigations suggested the possibility of a cerebellar venous thrombosis with compromised right cerebellar hemispheric venous drainage on a cerebral arteriogram done on June 2001. There was also a partial thrombosis of one of the right occipital veins draining into the right transverse sinus. Cerebrospinal fluid (CSF) analysis showed 18 white blood cells, a protein content of 46, and a glucose content of 62. There was some elevation of the immunoglobulin G (IgG) index and albumin index. The patient was treated with warfarin. Seemingly, attempts to discontinue warfarin were associated with reappearance of his headaches.

His symptoms waxed and waned and he had another hospitalization because of frequent vomiting and numbness on the right side of his forehead and right lower lid. He also had some dizziness and ringing in both ears. On November 2, 2001, he was hospitalized due to severe right occipital headaches. International Normalized Ratio (INR) on admission was 1.65. Neuroimaging studies obtained during that hospitalization are shown. One day after admission, he was taken to the operating room and had a left suboccipital craniotomy.

CASE SUMMARY

The vasculitides are characterized by blood vessel inflammation and necrosis. Four basic immunopathogenetic mechanisms have been proposed: (a) anaphylactic, (b) cytotoxic/cell activating, (c) immune complex, and (d) cell mediated. Injury can also occur by other pathways including cytokine-mediated, direct neutrophil involvement, genetically mediated, infectious, or environmental/chemical injury. More than one mechanism is likely to be involved in a particular vasculitis.

The diagnosis of vasculitis is often inferential, based on clinical presentation, presence of multisystem organ involvement, and abnormal serologic tests. Cerebral vasculitis should be considered when the stroke is recurrent, associated with encephalopathic changes, or accompanied by fever, weight loss, fatigue, arthralgias, myalgias, palpable purpura or other skin lesions, renal disease, multifocal neurological signs, anemia, hematuria, or elevated erythrocyte sedimentation rate (ESR).

Our patient was diagnosed with primary angiitis of the CNS. Primary angiitis of the CNS (aka: isolated CNS vasculitis, primary CNS vasculitis, or granulomatous angiitis of the nervous system) is a rare, noninfectious, granulomatous, necrotizing angiopathy of unknown cause. Primary angiitis of the CNS is characterized by predominant or exclusive involvement of the CNS. Men are more commonly affected than women (M:F = 7:3). Usual symptoms include headaches and altered mental status. Symptoms of predominant small and medium-sized cerebral blood vessel involvement may present as a mass lesion or as a multifocal encephalopathy. Small vessel strokes may occur over weeks to many months. Intracerebral hemorrhage and subarachnoid hemorrhage have been reported. The ESR is usually normal or minimally elevated. Other acute phase reactants are characteristically normal. CSF abnormalities include increased opening pressure, increased protein values, normal glucose level, and a discrete lymphocytic pleocytosis rarely exceeding 250 cells/mm³. In some cases, oligoclonal bands can be detected. Contrast-enhanced MRI studies are abnormal in over 90% of cases. Prominent leptomeningeal enhancement may be present. MRA lacks adequate resolution to show the medium-sized and small cerebral blood vessel involvement in this disorder. Catheter arteriography may show segmental arterial narrowing, vascular occlusions, peripheral aneurysms, vascular shifts, and avascular areas. Computed tomography (CT) may be entirely unremarkable. Brain/leptomeningeal biopsy is the gold standard of diagnosis. There is segmental inflammation and necrosis of leptomeningeal and parenchymal blood vessels. Leptomeningeal vessels are predominantly involved. Skip lesions are not uncommon. Thus, because of its focal nature, a negative biopsy result does not preclude the diagnosis of primary CNS angiitis. Early recognition and management is essential because of its progressive and often fatal course if untreated. Therapy consists of combined immunosuppressive therapy with long-term high-dose corticosteroids, with the addition of intermittent cyclophosphamide. Pulse cyclophosphamide has been successfully used in the treatment of primary CNS angiitis in children.

SELECTED REFERENCES

Biller J, Adams HP. Non-infectious granulomatous angiitis of the central nervous system. In: Toole JF, ed. *Handbook of clinical neurology.* Amsterdam: Elsevier Science, 1987:387–400.

Biller J, Grau RG. Cerebral vasculitis. In: Adams HP Jr, ed. *Handbook of cerebrovascular diseases.* 2nd ed. Revised and Expanded. New York: Marcel Dekker, 2005:Chapter 28, 653–680.

Biller J, Loftus CM, Moore SA, et al. Isolated central nervous system angiitis first presenting as spontaneous intracranial hemorrhage. *Neurosurgery* 1987;20:310–315.

Calabrese LH, Duna GF, Lie JT. Vasculitis in the central nervous system. *Arthritis Rheum* 1997;7: 1189–1201.

SEE QUESTIONS: 67, 68, 71, 104, 188, 216, 217

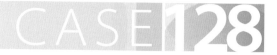

CASE 128

CEREBROTENDINOUS XANTHOMATOSIS

OBJECTIVES

- To review the main neurological features of cerebrotendinous xanthomatosis (CTX).
- To discuss the clinical course and progression of CTX.
- To review diagnostic criteria for CTX.
- To discuss management strategies for CTX.

VIGNETTE

A 64-year-old woman was evaluated 6 years previously due to progressive gait difficulties rendering her reliant on a cane for ambulation. More recently, she had been confined to a wheelchair. She had a history of chronic diarrhea, bilateral cataract surgery in her early thirties, and "lumps" involving both Achilles tendons.

CASE SUMMARY

Our patient had a history of progressive ataxia and short-term memory impairment, and surgery for early-onset adult cataracts. On neurologic examination, she had inappropriate jocularity, mild dysarthria, muscle stretch hyperreflexia, bilateral Babinski signs, mild intention tremor, dysdiadochokinesis, a wide-base unstable gait requiring the assistance of a cane, and inability to perform tandem walking. Neuropsychological testing showed widespread neurocognitive deficits with poor attention and concentration, dyscalculia, and impaired memory.

Serum cholestanol level was elevated at 1.60 mg/dL (normal 0.2 ± 0.2 mg/dL). Serum levels of methylmalonic acid, vitamin B$_{12}$, and vitamin E and genetic testing for commercially available spinocerebellar ataxias were all normal. Cultured fibroblasts were checked for 27-sterol hydroxylase deficiency. Treatment was initiated with chenodeoxycholic acid. She initially had some mild improvement, but this was followed by progressive neurologic deterioration with increasing ataxia, further sensory changes of her limbs, urinary incontinence, and a mild decline on repeat neuropsychological testing. Nerve conduction studies were consistent with a demyelinating neuropathy of the lower extremities.

MRI of the brain was remarkable for increased T2 and fluid-attenuated inversion recovery (FLAIR) signal abnormalities along the corticospinal tracts in the periventricular and subcortical white matter of both cerebral hemispheres, posterior limb of the internal capsules, cerebral peduncles, and pons. MRI of the spinal cord was normal. Magnetic resonance spectroscopy (MRS) showed decreased N-acetylaspartate peak and an increased amino acids versus lipids peak of 0.9 to 1.5 over the left basal ganglia. MRS of the right occipital region was normal.

She then became wheelchair bound and incontinent of urine and feces. Repeat neurologic examination showed decreased vibration and position sense in both feet. Atorvastatin was added to chenodeoxycholic acid in an attempt to prevent further neurologic deficits.

Cerebrotendinous xanthomatosis (CTX, van Bogaert disease) is a rare autosomal recessive disorder of bile acid synthesis caused by homozygous and compound heterozygous mutations in the sterol 27-hydroxylase gene (*CYP27*). The disorder is characterized by an accumulation of cholestanol and cholesterin in various tissues of the body. Onset of symptoms and signs usually occurs in childhood with a combination of chronic diarrhea and bilateral cataracts followed by the development of neurologic abnormalities. CTX is caused by a defect in the *CYP27A1* gene that codes for sterol 27-hydroxylate. Characteristic features of the disease in adults are progressive cerebellar ataxia in conjunction with tendinous xanthomas. Pyramidal, extrapyramidal, and cerebellar manifestations along with dementia are the predominant neurologic manifestations. Various other neurological manifestations have been described including seizures, psychosis, parkinsonism, chronic myelopathy, and peripheral neuropathy.

In addition to Achilles tendon xanthomas, tendon xanthomas may also be found on the patella, elbow, and hand or neck tendons. Tendon xanthomas seldom develop before age 20. Ophthalmologic findings other than cataracts include optic disc pallor, myelinated retinal nerve fibers, and signs of premature retinal aging. Elevated serum cholestanol and urine bile acid glucuronides help to confirm the diagnosis.

Early treatment of CTX is imperative. Primary treatment is with the oral administration of chenodeoxycholic acid. 3-hydroxy-3-methylglutaryl-CoA (HMG-CoA) reductase inhibitors may also be used as adjunctive therapy.

SELECTED REFERENCES

Barkhof F, Verrips A, Nesseling P, et al. Cerebrotendinous xanthomatosis: the spectrum of imaging findings and the correlation with neuropathological findings. *Radiology* 2000;219:869–876.

Chen W, Kubota S, Teramoto T, et al. Genetic analysis enables definite and rapid diagnosis of cerebrotendinous xanthomatosis. *Neurology* 1998;51:865–867.

Gallus G, Dotti MT, Federico A. Clinical and molecular diagnosis of cerebrotendinous xanthomatosis with a review of the mutations in the CYP27A1 gene. *Neurol Sci* 2006;27(2):143–149.

Kuriyama M, Tokimura Y, Fujiyama J, et al. Treatment of cerebrotendinous xanthomatosis: effects of chenodeoxycholic acid, pravastatin, and combined use. *J Neurol Sci* 1994;125(1):22–28.

Van Bogaert L, Scherer HJ, Epstein E. *Une forme cérébrale de la cholestérinose généralise.* Paris, France: Mason et Cie, 1937.

SEE QUESTIONS: 27, 251

CASE 129

POLYMYOSITIS/MYASTHENIA GRAVIS

OBJECTIVES

- To identify the principal causes of chronic progressive bulbar weakness.
- To demonstrate the value of clinical and laboratory data to distinguish myasthenia gravis (MG) from myositis.
- To outline acute and chronic treatment strategies for immune-mediated neuromuscular disorders.

VIGNETTE

Two years earlier, this 53-year-old woman had a left middle cerebral artery territory cardioembolic infarction due to atrial fibrillation/flutter. She was status post–catheter cardiac ablation a week prior to her stroke. She was treated with warfarin and had a good recovery. Subsequently she had a maze atrial procedure and warfarin was discontinued.

She then complained of progressive dysphagia and increased muscle weakness, involving mostly the proximal aspect of her extremities. She also had difficulty getting up from stairs, lifting objects above her shoulders, and brushing her hair. Furthermore, she had trouble climbing stairs and had muscle pain and tenderness when climbing stairs. There was no history of skin disease, lung disease, inflammatory arthritis, or Raynaud phenomenon.

CASE SUMMARY

Our patient presented with progressive and severe neuromuscular weakness including dysphagia and dyspnea. The first priority assessing a patient with speech, swallowing, or breathing difficulties is always to establish that their vital neuromuscular functions are secure. If overtly aspirating, choking frequently with meals, or losing weight precipitously, it is best to admit the patient on an urgent basis to formally assess swallowing function more thoroughly and adjust nutritional intake appropriately. Similarly, if any question arises about pulmonary status, it is best to deal with that on an urgent basis before pursuing further diagnostic tests.

At the bedside, a vigorous cough provides a rough estimate to the patient's pulmonary function. Taking a deep breath and then counting out loud is an excellent method of estimating the forced vital capacity (FVC). If the individual can count to 10 on one breath, the FVC is about 1 L. If the individual can count to 25 on one breath, then the estimated FVC is about 2 L. In general, patients with neuromuscular or respiratory failure who are acutely deteriorating should be considered as severe enough to warrant intubation and mechanical ventilation when the FVC drops below 15 mL/kg.

Our patient had evidence of proximal limb weakness as well as bulbar muscle weakness. Proximal and symmetric muscle weakness is characteristic of a myopathic process.

The oropharyngeal musculature can be affected in a variety of myopathies including inflammatory and immune-mediated conditions such as dermatomyositis, polymyositis, and inclusion body myositis. Both polymyositis and dermatomyositis can sometimes be associated with malignancies, including breast, lung, ovarian, and colon cancer, and lymphomas. The cancer risk is much greater with dermatomyositis.

At times, the degree of oropharyngeal weakness can be severe, and in some patients, it is the predominant feature. A thorough physical and laboratory work is strongly recommended in patients with suspected idiopathic inflammatory myositis. Elevation of serum creatine kinase and aldolase in our patient supported the diagnosis of a myopathic process. Electromyography (EMG) is usually abnormal in active polymyositis, with evidence of short-duration, low-amplitude, polyphasic potentials, fibrillations, and positive waves. Our patient had normal nerve conduction studies with no decremental response to 2-Hz repetitive stimulation. On EMG needle exam, there were fibrillations and small voluntary motor units, further supporting a myopathic process, whereas the presence of fibrillations indicated an active inflammatory myopathic process. This was corroborated with her muscle biopsy, which showed muscle fiber necrosis and inflammatory infiltrates consistent with polymyositis.

Because her bulbar weakness fluctuated, we also measured acetylcholine receptor antibodies, which were positive on serologic testing. Because false positives are exceedingly rare in a patient like ours with fluctuating bulbar muscle weakness, we also diagnosed her with myasthenia gravis (MG). Not surprisingly patients with one autoimmune neuromuscular disease have a greater chance of having other immune-mediated conditions including other neuromuscular disorders. MG and polymyositis may occur together, and in some instances, both may be precipitated by the administration of penicillamine. Our patient probably had both conditions, and inflammatory myopathy and MG. These patients should be carefully screened for thymoma or underlying or neoplasia.

Because she had severe bulbar weakness and a tendency for exacerbations over a period of a few days, we favored MG as the predominant mechanism accounting for her bulbar weakness. Therefore, cholinesterase inhibitors and immunosuppression were considered appropriate. Immunosuppressive drugs used in MG include high-dose long-term corticosteroids, azathioprine, mycophenolate, and cyclosporine. Short-term treatment for patients severely affected or acutely decompensated includes plasma and intravenous immunoglobulin (IVIG).

Treatment options for dermatomyositis and polymyositis consists of high-dose long-term prednisolone. Second-line treatments include azathioprine, methotrexate, cyclosporine, mycophenolate, and on rare occasions cyclophosphamide.

SELECTED REFERENCES

Behan Wm II, Behan PO, Dooyle D. Association of myasthenia gravis and polymyositis with neoplasma, infection, and autoimmune disorder. *Acta Neuropathologica* 1982;57(2–2):221–229.

Biller J, ed. *Practical neurology*, 4th ed. Philadelphia: Lippincott Williams & Wilkins, Wolters Kluwer Health, 2012.

Dalakas MC, Hohlfeld R. Polymyositis and dermatomyositis. *Lancet* 2003;362:(9388):971–982.

Kissell JT. Misunderstanding, misperceptions and mistakes in the management of the inflammatory myopathies. *Semin Neurol* 2002;22:41–51.

SEE QUESTIONS: 11, 17, 73, 74

CASE 130

MULTIPLE SYSTEM ATROPHY, CEREBELLAR TYPE

OBJECTIVES

- To review the main neurological features of multiple system atrophy, cerebellar type (MSA-C).
- To discuss the clinical course and progression of MSA-C.
- To review diagnostic pitfalls in a rapidly progressive cerebellar ataxia.

VIGNETTE

This 59-year-old woman had an 8-year history of progressive difficulty with walking, balance, and speech. The earliest reported difficulty was stiffness in her legs and staggering while walking. She tended to walk on the heels with support. She went on to have slurring of speech and difficulties with fine motor skills (eating and getting dressed) by 1 year from the initial gait difficulties. She then developed a left hand resting tremor and dystonia (she misattributed to "arthritis"), which was partially improved on levodopa, although her tremor and her ataxia continued to increase in severity. Given an intercurrent diagnosis of diabetes mellitus type 1, which required insulin, and her prior history of hypothyroidism, antibodies against glutamic acid decarboxylase (GAD) were requested. GAD-65 was 14.2 U/mL (normal range, 0.0 to 1.5). Anti-amphiphysin titers were 6.4 ($n < 0.8$). Repeat testing confirmed elevated anti-GAD antibodies but were negative for anti-amphiphysin. Brain magnetic resonance imaging (MRI) taken 3 years after symptom onset showed mild to moderate cerebellar atrophy (Fig. 130.1). Full body positron emission tomography (PET) scan was negative for malignancies, intravenous immunoglobulin (IVIG) treatment failed to deliver any benefits. Her condition was compounded by the development of severe orthostatic hypotension. She succumbed to her illness less than 8 years after symptom onset.

CASE SUMMARY

Our patient's relatively rapid progression of ataxia, parkinsonism, dystonia, and hyperreflexia, associated with elevated anti–glutamic acid antibodies, suggested an autoimmune disorder. Her type 1 diabetes and hypothyroidism suggested a pathogenic role for anti-GAD antibodies and the possibility that her deficits fell within the broad spectrum of the stiff person syndrome (SPS). However, further deterioration failed to declare into the typical ascending rigidity of SPS and instead deepened the ataxic phenotype and revealed a clearer olivopontocerebellar pattern of regional atrophy, as shown on a subsequent brain MRI, obtained 6 years after symptom onset (Fig. 130.2). This pattern of atrophy suggested the cerebellar form of multiple system atrophy (MSA-C) or a pseudosporadic variant of spinocerebellar ataxia, particularly Spinocerebellar ataxias (SCAs) 2, 3, 12, 17, or 21, whereby parkinsonism is known to emerge as part of the phenotype. Testing for these SCAs was negative.

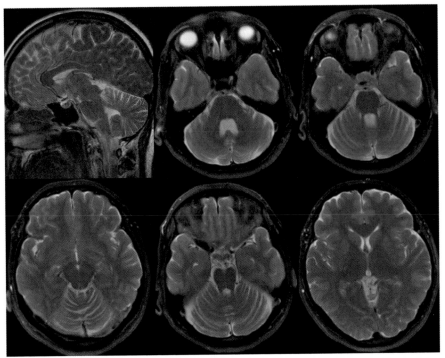

Figure 130.1 Brain MRI obtained 3 years after symptom onset showed cerebellar atrophy, with widening of the fourth ventricle and thinning of the superior cerebellar peduncle.

Postmortem neuropathologic studies demonstrated severe neuronal cell loss and gliosis predominantly in the pons, cerebellum, putamen, and inferior olivary nuclei with widespread alpha-synuclein–positive oligodendroglial cytoplasmic inclusions in these structures and globus pallidus, internal capsule, cerebellum, midbrain, pons, medulla, and spinal cord. These findings confirmed MSA-C as the etiology of our patient's ataxic and parkinsonian phenotype.

Multiple system atrophy is indeed a neurodegenerative oligodendrogliopathy associated with parkinsonian, cerebellar, autonomic, and pyramidal deficits, which typically manifests at an earlier age and progresses at a faster rate than the other two common atypical parkinsonisms (corticobasal degeneration and progressive supranuclear palsy). MSA is divided into two clinically identifiable "subgroups," the cerebellar type (MSA-C), previously known as sporadic olivopontocerebellar atrophy (sOPCA), and the parkinsonian type (MSA-P), previously termed striatonigral degeneration. Associated autonomic failure is predominantly central (preganglionic) and includes orthostatic hypotension (drop of 20 mm Hg systolic or 10 mm Hg diastolic), urinary incontinence, erectile dysfunction, anhidrosis, and respiratory dysfunction (sleep apnea, snoring, and inspiratory stridor). Dementia is not a feature of MSA but frontal lobe dysfunction usually develops.

This case also highlighted the potential pitfall of overreliance or misinterpretation of serologic testing. Although the antibodies against GAD were elevated, the levels were within the range expected for late-onset autoimmune diabetes mellitus type 1 (~100 U/mL) but far lower than those expected in SPS and also for the rare disorder of anti-GAD–associated cerebellar ataxia (often far greater than 5,000 U/mL). In the latter case, once high serum levels of anti-GAD antibodies, cerebrospinal fluid (CSF) should be evaluated for the presence

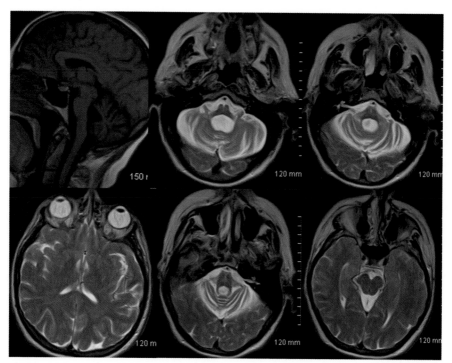

Figure 130.2   Brain MRI obtained 6 years after symptom onset showed a marked interval increase in regional atrophy confined to the pancerebellum, medulla, and pons (olivopontocerebellar). Note greater ex vacuo enlargement of the fourth ventricle compared to Figure 130.1.

of oligoclonal immunoglobulin G (IgG) bands and intrathecal synthesis of anti-GAD antibodies to further prove an autoimmune origin of the syndrome. The dramatic speed of atrophy documented by MRI over the span of 3 years supported a neurodegenerative rather than autoimmune pathology. Furthermore, the olivopontocerebellar pattern of atrophy, in a case of sporadic ataxia, is most often indicative of MSA than of any of the SCAs. Unfortunately no effective treatment for this form of ataxia is available and symptomatic treatment is only available for the associated comorbidity of orthostatic hypotension (liberalizing salt intake, use of thigh-high compressive leg stocking, head elevation at night, fludrocortisone, and midodrine).

SELECTED REFERENCES

Biller J, ed. *Practical neurology,* 4th ed. Philadelphia: Lippincott Williams & Wilkins, Wolters Kluwer Health, 2012.

Espay AJ, Biller J. *Concise neurology.* Philadelphia: Lippincott Williams & Wilkins, Wolters Kluwer Health, 2011.

Honnorat J, Saiz A, Giometto B, et al. Cerebellar ataxia with anti-glutamic acid decarboxylase antibodies: study of 14 patients. *Arch Neurol* 2001;58(2):225–230.

Vianello M, Tavolato B, Armani M, et al. Cerebellar ataxia associated with anti-glutamic acid decarboxylase autoantibodies. *Cerebellum* 2003;2(1):77–79.

SEE QUESTIONS: 27, 42, 373

NEOPLASTIC BRACHIAL PLEXOPATHY

OBJECTIVES

- To discuss the anatomy of the brachial plexus.
- To highlight the distinguishing features of radiation-induced versus neoplastic brachial plexopathy.

VIGNETTE

A 57-year-old woman with breast carcinoma developed right upper extremity weakness.

CASE SUMMARY

 This 57-year-old woman was evaluated for weakness of the right arm and hand. She had previously undergone a right mastectomy and chemotherapy for breast cancer. Because of recurrent tumor, she received additional chemotherapy and had radiation therapy to the right shoulder/axilla. She consulted us because of right arm and hand weakness and pain under her right scapula.

Examination showed no evidence of a Horner syndrome. There was atrophy of her right forearm and weakness of multiple muscles of the right upper extremity including the supraspinatus, deltoid, biceps, brachioradialis, triceps, wrist and finger extensors, finger flexors, and multiple intrinsic hand muscles. Triceps and wrist extensor weakness was especially severe. Muscle stretch reflexes in both arms were diffusely hypoactive. A trace triceps reflex was noted on the left, but none on the right. Pinprick sensation was diminished on the right thumb, middle finger, and medial forearm.

Electromyography (EMG)/nerve conduction studies were abnormal with acute denervation changes noted in muscles innervated by multiple nerves and mild abnormalities noted on median and ulnar motor and sensory nerve conductions. These findings were most indicative of an acute brachial plexopathy. No myokymia was noted. Magnetic resonance imaging (MRI) of the right axilla/brachial plexus demonstrated axillary lymphadenopathy. The patient was diagnosed with right brachial plexopathy due to metastatic lymphadenopathy.

The brachial plexus is divided into five major components: roots, trunks, divisions, cords, and branches (Fig. 131.1). The five roots arise from C5 through T1. The three trunks are named the upper, middle, and lower trunks. The three trunks separate into three anterior and three posterior divisions. The divisions unite to form three cords, named the posterior, lateral, and medial cords. The cords pass through the space of the first rib and clavicle and then give off the major terminal branches or peripheral nerves. Branches of the lateral cord consist of the musculocutaneous nerve and lateral head of the median nerve. Branches of the medial cord consist of the medial anterior thoracic nerve, medial cutaneous nerve of the arm, medial cutaneous nerve of the forearm, ulnar nerve, and median head of the median nerve. Branches of the posterior cord consist of the subscapular nerve, thoracodorsal nerve, axillary nerve, and radial nerve.

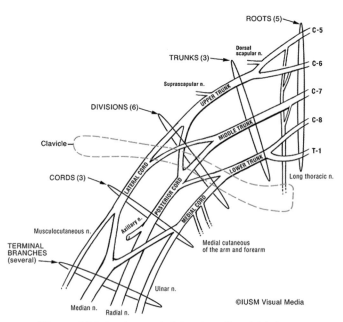

ROOTS (5)
C-5
Dorsal scapular n.
TRUNKS (3)
C-6
Suprascapular n.
C-7
DIVISIONS (6)
UPPER TRUNK
C-8
MIDDLE TRUNK
Clavicle
T-1
CORDS (3)
LOWER TRUNK
Long thoracic n.
LATERAL CORD
POSTERIOR CORD
Musculocutaneous n.
MEDIAL CORD
Axillary n.
Medial cutaneous of the arm and forearm
TERMINAL BRANCHES (several)
Ulnar n.
©IUSM Visual Media
Median n.
Radial n.

Figure 131.1   Anatomical drawing of brachial plexus.

Given the relatively complex anatomy of the brachial plexus, lesions can produce a multitude of different signs and symptoms, usually pain, weakness, and numbness of various parts of the affected shoulder, arm, and hand. A brachial plexopathy is a well-recognized complication of cancer, especially breast and lung cancer. Many of these patients have received radiation to the axilla or chest to treat their tumors. Distinguishing between a radiation-induced plexopathy and a neoplastic plexopathy is not straightforward. Early severe pain occurring in conjunction with signs and symptoms of brachial plexopathy would suggest a neoplastic process. Some have suggested that lower trunk lesions occur more frequently with tumors, whereas radiation injuries affect the upper plexus more frequently. A Horner syndrome is more common in neoplastic plexopathies, whereas lymphedema of the affected arm is more common in radiation injury of the brachial plexus. Patients with neoplastic brachial plexopathies tend to have more rapid progression of signs and symptoms compared to patients with radiation-induced plexopathies who often have a slowly progressive course and sensory symptoms such as weakness, paresthesias, and dysesthesias as the predominant presenting manifestations. There is little in the way of electrophysiologic studies to distinguish the two types of brachial plexopathy, except that myokymia on needle examination is more common in radiation-induced plexopathies. Radiologic imaging of the plexus with computed tomography (CT) or MRI may show discrete tumors or lymphadenopathy involving the plexus. In some instances, surgical exploration and biopsy of the brachial plexus are needed to distinguish between neoplastic-induced and radiation-induced brachial plexopathy.

SELECTED REFERENCES

Brazis PW, Masdeu JC, Biller J. *Localization in clinical neurology*, 6th ed. Philadelphia: Lippincott Williams & Wilkins, Wolters Kluwer Health, 2011.
Dropcho EJ. Neurotoxicity of radiation therapy. *Neurol Clin* 2010;2(1):217–234.

Harper CM, Thomas JE, Cascino TL, et al. Distinction between neoplastic and radiation-induced brachial plexopathy, with emphasis on the role of EMG. *Neurology* 1989;39:502–506.

Jaeckle KA. Neurologic manifestations of neoplastic and radiation-induced plexopathies. *Semin Neurol* 2010;30(3):254–262.

Kori SH, Foley KM, Posner JB. Brachial plexus lesions in patients with cancer: 100 cases. *Neurology* 1981;31:45–50.

SEE QUESTIONS: 4, 59, 79, 81, 229

REVIEW QUESTIONS
AND ANSWERS

1. A 50-year-old man complains of trouble chewing for the past year. He has a history of hypertension, cataract surgery, renal stones, and right bundle branch block (RBBB) on EKG (but no clinical cardiac symptoms). On examination, jaw closure is weak, with 4/5 neck flexion, deltoid, brachioradialis, and quadriceps strength (active movement against gravity and resistance—Medical Research Council 0 to 5/5 scale). No fatigability is found. His hands stiffen with repeated attempts at squeezing the examiner's fingers. Reflexes and sensation are preserved. Mild bilateral eyelid ptosis is noted with normal extraocular movements. What is the most likely clinical diagnosis?

A. Myasthenia gravis
B. Myotonic dystrophy
C. Polymyositis
D. Myotonia congenita
E. Amyotrophic lateral sclerosis

Answer: B

2. A 20-year-old woman has a 2-week history of bilateral eyelid ptosis and horizontal diplopia when driving home from work every day. She has no other complaints. Her office examination is normal, with no abnormal movements or fatigability of voice, neck, or limbs. However, after 1 minute of sustained upgaze, she develops 2 mm of bilateral asymmetric eyelid ptosis. Which of the following statements is most correct?

A. She has ocular myasthenia gravis.
B. She has progressive external ophthalmoplegia.
C. Her ocular symptoms may later progress into generalized myasthenia gravis.
D. She has thyroid ophthalmopathy.
E. She may have an internuclear ophthalmoplegia.

Answer: C

3. Select the most characteristic clinical feature or differential diagnosis in carpal tunnel syndrome (CTS).

A. Occurs with greater frequency in men and in the dominant hand
B. Sensory symptoms can be mimicked by the neurogenic thoracic outlet syndrome.
C. A Tinel sign has a high specificity as a clinical feature in CTS.
D. An early symptom of CTS is asymmetric nocturnal hand paresthesias.
E. A similar pattern of hand weakness can be seen in a C7 radiculopathy.

Answer: D

4. A clinical condition that could be confused with a retrohumeral radial neuropathy is

A. C8 radiculopathy
B. Anterior interosseus neuropathy
C. A lesion of the upper trunk of the brachial plexus
D. Posterior interosseus neuropathy
E. C6 radiculopathy

Answer: D

5. The differential diagnosis of a unilateral foot drop would include

A. S1 radiculopathy
B. Superficial peroneal mononeuropathy
C. Proximal sciatic mononeuropathy with involvement of the tibial nerve division
D. L4 radiculopathy
E. Deep peroneal mononeuropathy

Answer: E

6. Juvenile absence epilepsy is associated with
   A. Relatively high incidence of absence status
   B. Age of onset from 4 to 8 years
   C. Generalized tonic–clonic seizures in 40%
   D. Generalized 3-Hz spike wave pattern on EEG
   E. Numerous seizures (hundreds) per day

   Answer: A

7. In juvenile myoclonic epilepsy:
   A. Benzodiazepines are contraindicated due to the risk of seizure exacerbation.
   B. Seizure types include myoclonic jerks and generalized seizures; absence seizures do not occur.
   C. Treatment is lifelong, and seizures recur in virtually all patients after withdrawal of therapy.
   D. The syndrome is significantly more common in men than in women.
   E. Patients may be weaned off therapy after the age of 20, provided there has been a seizure-free period of at least 5 years.

   Answer: C

8. Common side effects associated with the use of topiramate in the treatment of epilepsy include all of the following *except*
   A. Weight loss
   B. Hepatotoxicity
   C. Elevated intraocular pressure
   D. Cognitive dysfunction
   E. Increased incidence of renal calculi

   Answer: B

9. Vagus nerve stimulation therapy for epilepsy is indicated in the following clinical situation
   A. First-line therapy for temporal lobe epilepsy due to mesial temporal sclerosis with documented hippocampal atrophy on MRI
   B. Adjunctive therapy for treatment-resistant idiopathic generalized epilepsy
   C. Alternative to temporal lobectomy in mesial temporal lobe epilepsy
   D. Adjunctive therapy for treatment-resistant focal epilepsy
   E. First-line therapy in extratemporal, nonlesional focal epilepsy with secondarily generalized tonic–clonic seizures

   Answer: D

10. A 30-year-old healthy man presents to the emergency room with a 3- to 4-day history of progressive tingling and numbness in both hands and feet. On examination, he has diffuse 4/5 strength (active movement against gravity and resistance—Medical Research Council 0 to 5/5 scale), distal more than proximal. Muscle stretch reflexes are absent. Sensory examination shows decreased pinprick in both hands and feet and normal position and vibration sense. Which of the following is the most likely diagnosis?
   A. Transverse myelitis
   B. Guillain-Barré syndrome
   C. Polymyositis
   D. Amyotrophic lateral sclerosis
   E. Myasthenia gravis

   Answer: B

11. A 30-year-old woman with a history of systemic lupus erythematosus (SLE) has a 3- to 4-week history of progressively worsening muscle weakness and myalgias. On examination, she has diffuse 4/5 strength (active movement against gravity and resistance—Medical Research Council 0 to 5/5 scale) in both upper and lower extremities, proximal more than distal. Muscle stretch reflexes and sensory examination are normal. Which of the following is the most likely diagnosis?
   A. Transverse myelitis
   D. Amyotrophic lateral sclerosis

B. Guillain-Barré syndrome
C. Polymyositis
E. Myasthenia gravis

Answer: C

12. A 30-year-old woman is seen in the emergency room with a 2-day history of progressively worsening tingling and numbness in both lower extremities. She lost control of her bladder since this morning and also has difficulties moving her legs. On examination, she has diffuse 2/5 strength (active movement with gravity eliminated—Medical Research Council 0 to 5/5 scale). Muscle stretch reflexes are hyperactive, and she has bilateral Babinski signs. There is a sensory level to pinprick at T10. Which of the following is the most likely diagnosis?

A. Transverse myelitis
B. Guillain-Barré syndrome
C. Polymyositis
D. Amyotrophic lateral sclerosis
E. Myasthenia gravis

Answer: A

13. A 30-year-old woman is seen in the emergency room because of binocular horizontal diplopia worse on looking to the right. She has also noticed droopy eyelids in the late hours of the day and admits being "dead tired" by the end of the day. Neurologic examination is normal except for minimal bilateral asymmetric eyelid ptosis and complaints of double vision on right gaze. Which of the following is the most likely diagnosis?

A. Transverse myelitis
B. Guillain-Barré syndrome
C. Polymyositis
D. Amyotrophic lateral sclerosis
E. Myasthenia gravis

Answer: E

14. Following surgery for a ruptured abdominal aortic aneurysm, a 60-year-old man developed bilateral lower extremity weakness. On examination, he has flaccid paraparesis with absent muscle stretch reflexes and no response to plantar stimulation. Sensory examination shows decreased pinprick sensation with a T10 sensory level. Position and vibration sense are preserved. Which of the following is the most likely diagnosis?

A. Transverse myelitis
B. Guillain-Barré syndrome
C. Brown-Séquard syndrome
D. Amyotrophic lateral sclerosis
E. Spinal cord infarction

Answer: E

15. A 50-year-old man has stiffness and twitching in most of his muscle groups, progressively getting worse for the last 2 months. On examination, he has fasciculations on his right deltoid and right gastrocnemius muscles, with wasting and weakness of the right hand interossei muscles. Muscle stretch reflexes are bilaterally hyperactive, and he has bilateral Babinski signs. Which of the following is the most likely diagnosis?

A. Transverse myelitis
B. Guillain-Barré syndrome
C. Polymyositis
D. Amyotrophic lateral sclerosis
E. Myasthenia gravis

Answer: D

16. A 30-year-old healthy man recently involved in a motor vehicle accident presents with neck pain radiating to the right shoulder, lateral aspect of the forearm, right thumb, and index finger. Neurologic examination shows diminished right biceps and brachioradialis reflexes. Which of the following is the most likely diagnosis?

A. Right carpal tunnel syndrome
B. Right C6 radiculopathy
C. Guillain-Barré syndrome
D. Parsonage-Turner syndrome
E. Cervical myelopathy

Answer: B

17. A 30-year-old woman has a 3-month history of numbness in both hands, more so in her right hand. The numbness is mainly nocturnal and on doing manual activities. The numbness fades away on gentle shaking of her hands. She has no neck pain or weakness. She has gained 40 pounds in the last 4 months. On examination, she has decreased pinprick sensation on her right thumb and index finger and a positive Tinel sign at both wrists. Which of the following pair of tests might better explain her clinical problem?

A. Sedimentation rate/ANA titer
B. MRI of cervical spine/CSF analysis
C. MRI of cervical spine/somatosensory evoked potentials
D. Acetylcholine receptor antibodies/chest CT
E. TSH/EMG and NCVs

Answer: E

18. Which of the following neurologic disorders carries the worst prognosis for survival whether treated or untreated?

A. Transverse myelitis
B. Guillain-Barré syndrome
C. Polymyositis
D. Amyotrophic lateral sclerosis
E. Myasthenia gravis

Answer: D

19. The most common symptom of cerebellar infarction is

A. Vertigo/dizziness
B. Diplopia
C. Paralysis of all volitional movements
D. Convergence retraction nystagmus
E. Head tilt

Answer: A

20. Transtentorial herniation may result in infarction of which of the following brain areas?

A. Supramarginal gyrus
B. Superior temporal gyrus
C. Hypothalamus
D. Bilateral inferior frontal gyrus
E. Temporo-occipital

Answer: E

21. The structure most responsible for the generation of absence seizures is

A. Hippocampus
B. Hypothalamus
C. Thalamus
D. Temporal lobe
E. Corpus callosum

Answer: C

22. Automatisms can occur in which of the following seizure types?

A. Myoclonic
B. Tonic
C. Absence
D. Generalized tonic–clonic
E. Simple partial

Answer: C

23. The prevalence of epilepsy in the United States is approximately

A. 250,000
B. 2.5 million
C. 1 million
D. 10 million
E. 20 million

Answer: B

24. Ethosuximide (Zarontin) is used mainly in which of the following seizure types?

A. Generalized tonic–clonic
D. Myoclonic

    B. Partial   **E.** Gelastic
    C. Absence

Answer: C

25. Complex partial seizures by definition refer to seizures that
    A. Manifest with convulsions
    B. Are prolonged
    C. Begin in childhood
    D. Are associated with an alteration of consciousness
    E. Are resistant to medications

Answer: D

26. A 5-year-old boy with Down syndrome has had two previous episodes of right facial droop and limp right arm following bouts of crying. The first two episodes resolved within a few hours. His parents brought him in this time because it has lasted more than 4 hours. In the ER he is crying intermittently, has a flattened right nasolabial fold, and pushes you away with the left arm but not the right. What is the most likely diagnosis?
    A. Stereotypical behavior typical of Down syndrome
    B. Todd paresis
    C. Migraine
    D. Moyamoya
    E. Brachial plexopathy

Answer: D

27. A 9-year-old girl has had progressive difficulty with balance over the past 3 years. She has dysarthria, scoliosis, and mild hearing loss. She has no muscle stretch reflexes and has decreased vibration sense at the toes. An older brother who had similar initial symptoms ended up in a wheelchair and died of a "heart attack" at age 22. What is the most likely diagnosis?
    A. Glutaric aciduria   **D.** Sea-blue histiocytosis
    B. Friedreich ataxia   **E.** MELAS
    C. Ataxia–telangiectasia

Answer: B

28. Ipsilateral paralysis of adduction of the right eye on volitional gaze with monocular nystagmus of the abducting left eye indicates a lesion of which of the following anatomical structures?
    A. Right medial longitudinal fasciculus   **D.** Left central tegmental tract
    B. Left medial longitudinal fasciculus   **E.** Dentatorubral tract
    C. Right central tegmental tract

Answer: A

29. Which of the following is the most common cause of ischemic stroke in children?
    A. Moyamoya disease   **D.** Kawasaki disease
    B. Cardiac disease   **E.** Homocystinuria
    C. Progeria

Answer: B

30. Paradoxical embolization leading to transient ischemic attacks or stroke is a complication of which of the following disorders?
    A. Turner syndrome   **D.** Interrupted aortic arch
    B. Coarctation of the aorta   **E.** Williams syndrome
    C. Rendu-Osler-Weber syndrome

Answer: C

31. Which of the following organisms infecting the CNS is most common among cardiac transplant patients?

A. *Neisseria meningitidis*
B. *Streptococcus pneumoniae*
C. *Escherichia coli*
D. *Aspergillus fumigatus*
E. *Pseudomonas aeruginosa*

Answer: D

32. Which of the following is a significant risk factor for stroke associated with coronary artery bypass graft (CABG)?

A. Male gender
B. Hypercholesterolemia
C. Left ventricular hypertrophy
D. Aortic arch atherosclerosis
E. Hyperhomocysteinemia

Answer: D

33. Facio-pharyngo-laryngo-glosso-masticatory supranuclear palsy results from bilateral infarction of which of the following structures?

A. Brainstem tegmentum
B. Central tegmental tract
C. Opercula and insula
D. Medial temporo-occipital region
E. Parietooccipital region

Answer: C

34. Anosognosia for cortical blindness results from lesions of which of the following regions?

A. Bilateral parietooccipital
B. Bilateral medial temporo-occipital
C. Basal forebrain
D. Bioccipital (area 17)
E. Diagonal band of Broca

Answer: D

35. The pain and temperature component of the trigeminal lemniscus originates from which of the following anatomical structures?

A. Pars rostralis
B. Pars interpolaris
C. Pars caudalis
D. Aberrant fibers of Dejerine
E. Nucleus solitarius

Answer: C

36. Which of the following pathways decussate at the medullocervical junction?

A. Conjugate horizontal gaze system
B. Dorsal tegmental decussation of Meynert
C. Corticobulbar axons to nuclei of cranial nerves III and IV
D. Corticobulbar axons to nuclei of cranial nerves V, VI, and VII
E. Pyramidal tract

Answer: E

37. When the head of an infant is slowly turned to one side, the normal response is characterized by which of the following features?

A. Extension of the arm and leg on the side to which the head is turned
B. Flexion of the arm and leg on the side to which the head is turned
C. Flexion of both arms and legs
D. Extension and pronation of both arms
E. Extension of both legs

Answer: A

38. Ipsilateral loss of the corneal reflex in the Wallenberg lateral medullary syndrome results from involvement of which of the following anatomical structures?

A. Descending sympathetic tract
B. Spinal trigeminal nucleus
C. Lateral spinothalamic tract
D. Central tegmental tract
E. Reticular substance

Answer: B

39. Which of the following sensory modalities is mediated by both dorsal and ventral column pathways?

A. Pain
B. Temperature
C. Touch
D. Vibration
E. Position

Answer: C

40. A 63-year-old woman with Parkinson disease experiences troublesome peak-dose levodopa-induced dyskinesias after each dose of carbidopa/levodopa 25/100, 2 tablets po q.i.d., every 4 hours apart during the day. Her dyskinesias are followed by wearing off with freezing and tremor for about 45 minutes to 1 hour between each dose cycle. What would be the most appropriate management plan for this patient?

A. Decrease the frequency of levodopa to 100 mg po t.i.d.
B. Increase the interdose interval without decreasing the q.i.d. frequency.
C. Add amantadine and optimize levodopa.
D. Add a dopamine agonist and optimize levodopa.
E. Add selegiline and optimize levodopa.

Answer: C

41. A 78-year-old man with an 18-year history of Parkinson disease is brought to the emergency department with visual hallucinations and agitation. He takes a combination of several antiparkinsonian medications including amantadine, levodopa, selegiline, and pramipexole. He does not take other medications with potential to cause encephalopathy. Infectious and metabolic derangements were ruled out. What would be the most appropriate medication adjustment to control his hallucinations and agitation in this patient?

A. Add risperidone to control the hallucinations and agitation.
B. Stepwise discontinuation of antiparkinsonian medications as needed in the following order: (1) amantadine, (2) selegiline, (3) pramipexole, and (4) levodopa
C. Stepwise discontinuation of antiparkinsonian medications as needed in the following order: (1) selegiline, (2) pramipexole, (3) amantadine, and (4) levodopa
D. Add olanzapine and discontinue amantadine, selegiline, and pergolide.
E. Add an acetylcholinesterase inhibitor and olanzapine.

Answer: B

42. A 60-year-old woman with a 2-year history of speech difficulties, stiffness, and frequent falls comes to the clinic for evaluation. On examination, there was no tremor, but axial-predominant rigidity was present, with slow and hypophonic speech and decreased eye blinking rate. Neurophthalmic examination showed square-wave jerks but normal slow pursuit and saccadic eye movements. There was impaired vertical eye response to the optokinetic strip. She also showed echolalia and a tendency for motor perseveration. Which of the following is the most likely diagnosis?

A. Progressive supranuclear palsy
B. Parkinson disease
C. Corticobasal degeneration
D. Multiple system atrophy
E. Dementia with Lewy bodies

Answer: A

43. A 65-year-old hypertensive woman with a history of diabetes and hyperlipidemia develops abrupt, painless, monocular visual loss of her right eye. On examination, visual acuity is 20/50 OD and 20/20 OS. The superior aspect of her right optic nerve head is edematous. Visual fields show an inferior altitudinal defect. Which of the following is the most likely diagnosis?

A. Posterior ischemic optic neuropathy
B. Central retinal artery occlusion
C. Branch retinal artery occlusion
D. Anterior ischemic optic neuropathy
E. Central retinal vein occlusion

Answer: D

44. Which of the following neurological disorders has been associated with the use of sildenafil (Viagra)?

    A. Cluster headaches   **D.** Myopathy
    B. Tics   **E.** Anterior ischemic optic neuropathy
    C. Peripheral neuropathy

Answer: E

45. Which of the following is the accepted time for treating irreversible retinal ischemia?

    A. 180 minutes   **D.** 72 hours
    B. 24 hours   **E.** 96 hours
    C. 48 hours

Answer: A

46. Typically, most strokes in patients with Fabry disease (alpha-galactosidase-A deficiency) are characterized by which of the following?

    A. Hemorrhagic nature
    B. Predominant involvement of the carotid circulation
    C. Predominant involvement of the vertebrobasilar circulation
    D. Predominant involvement of the spinal cord
    E. Predominantly in women

Answer: C

47. Which of the following vessels supplies the midbrain, thalamus, and medial aspect of the temporal lobes and occipital lobes?

    A. Anterior cerebral artery   **D.** Posterior communicating artery
    B. Middle cerebral artery   **E.** Anterior choroidal artery
    C. Posterior cerebral artery

Answer: C

48. Which of the following vessels supplies anatomical structures on both sides of the midline?

    A. Anterior cerebral artery   **D.** Central artery of Percheron
    B. Middle cerebral artery   **E.** Recurrent artery of Heubner
    C. Posterior cerebral artery

Answer: D

49. A preserved level of consciousness in patients with the locked-in syndrome indicates sparing of which of the following anatomical structures?

    A. Pontine tegmentum
    B. Paramedian pontine reticular formation (PPRF)
    C. Medial longitudinal fasciculus (MLF)
    D. Central tegmental tract
    E. Midbrain tectum

Answer: A

50. Atherosclerotic occlusive disease of the vertebrobasilar circulation affects predominantly which of the following vessels?

    A. Distal third of the basilar artery
    B. Vertebral artery siphon (V3)
    C. Distal intracranial vertebral arteries and proximal and middle segment of basilar artery
    D. Distal subclavian arteries
    E. Posterior inferior cerebellar arteries

Answer: C

51. Ipsilateral conjugate gaze palsy and internuclear ophthalmoplegia result from a lesion simultaneously involving which of the following anatomical structures?

    A. Paramedian pontine reticular formation (PPRF) and medial longitudinal fasciculus (MLF)

B. Sixth nerve fascicle and medial longitudinal fasciculus (MLF)
C. Sixth nerve fascicle and rostral interstitial nucleus of the medial longitudinal fasciculus (riMLF)
D. Mollaret triangle and periaqueductal gray matter
E. Medial longitudinal fasciculus (MLF) and central tegmental tract

Answer: A

52. A congruous homonymous hemianopia with macular sparing is most often seen with occlusion of which of the following vessels?

A. Anterior choroidal artery   **D.** Posterior communicating artery
B. Posterior cerebral artery   **E.** Recurrent artery of Heubner
C. Posterior choroidal artery

Answer: B

53. Following coronary artery bypass graft (CABG), a patient presents with simultanagnosia, optic ataxia, and apraxia of gaze. Which of the following is the most likely diagnosis?

A. Bilateral parietooccipital infarcts   **D.** Bilateral orbitofrontal infarcts
B. Midbrain infarct   **E.** Left Mesial temporal lobe infarct
C. Paramedian thalamic infarcts

Answer: A

54. Which of the following is the most common cause of posterior cerebral artery (PCA) occlusion?

A. PCA dissection   **D.** Vertebrobasilar fibromuscular dysplasia
B. Transtentorial herniation   **E.** Antiphospholipid antibody syndrome
C. Cardioembolism

Answer: C

55. Which of the following manifestations may increase the risk that patients may mistake the time of stroke onset?

A. Left hemiparesis   **D.** Dissociated sensory loss
B. Ataxia   **E.** Left homonymous hemianopia
C. Internuclear ophthalmoplegia

Answer: E

56. Numbness, tingling, and painful hypersensitivity of the anterolateral thigh down to the upper patellar region are most characteristic of which of the following conditions?

A. L4 radiculopathy   **D.** Lateral femoral cutaneous neuropathy
B. L5 radiculopathy   **E.** Femoral neuropathy
C. Obturator neuropathy

Answer: D

57. Which of the following is the most common entrapment neuropathy?

A. Posterior interosseus syndrome   **D.** Deep ulnar nerve at the wrist
B. Suprascapular nerve entrapment   **E.** Radial nerve at the humerus
C. Carpal tunnel syndrome

Answer: C

58. A 60-year-old man has acute onset of severe low back pain, numbness of both legs, and inability to void. On neurological examination, there is flaccid paraparesis and loss of pain and temperature sensation below the nipple line with sparing of touch, vibration, and position sense. Which of the following is the most likely diagnosis?

A. Syringomyelia
B. Spinal cord infarction
C. Viral myelitis

D. Spinal cord meningioma
E. Subacute combined degeneration (B_{12} deficiency)

Answer: B

59. Heterochromia of the iris in a patient with a Horner syndrome is indicative of which of the following?

A. Preganglionic lesion
B. Lesion occurrence before 2 years of age
C. Postganglionic lesion
D. Raeder paratrigeminal syndrome
E. Pancoast tumor

Answer: B

60. Which of the following clinical features distinguishes fulminant hepatic failure from chronic portosystemic encephalopathy?

A. Tremor   **D.** Agitation
B. Asterixis   **E.** Confusion
C. Cerebral edema

Answer: C

61. A 30-year-old man with Guillain-Barré syndrome should be intubated when the forced vital capacity drops below how many milliliters per kilogram?

A. 5   **D.** 40
B. 15   **E.** 50
C. 30

Answer: B

62. Which of the following is the most likely diagnosis in a 30-year-old woman with new-onset bilateral asynchronus trigeminal neuralgia?

A. Syringobulbia
B. Basilar artery aneurysm
C. Brainstem glioma
D. Multiple sclerosis
E. Nasopharyngeal carcinoma

Answer: D

63. Which of the following clinical features *excludes* the diagnosis of idiopathic trigeminal neuralgia?

A. Mandibular trigeminal distribution
B. Normal facial sensation
C. Age group 60 to 70 years
D. Right-sided predominance
E. Loss of corneal reflex

Answer: E

64. The sudden onset of vertigo while trying to sit up suddenly, associated with rotatory nystagmus beating toward the downmost ear, with latency and limited duration is characteristic of which of the following disorders?

A. Otosclerosis   **D.** Benign paroxysmal positional vertigo
B. Ménière disease   **E.** Vertebrobasilar ischemia
C. Acoustic neuroma

Answer: D

65. Episodic vertigo, fluctuating hearing loss, tinnitus, and aural fullness are characteristic of which of the following disorders?

A. Otosclerosis   **D.** Benign paroxysmal positional vertigo

B. Ménière disease   **E.** Vertebrobasilar ischemia
C. Acoustic neuroma

Answer: B

66. Which of the following stroke syndromes is *not* at risk for intracranial hypertension?
  A. Main stem of middle cerebral artery occlusion
  B. Internal carotid artery occlusion
  C. Paramedian pontine infarction
  D. Aneurysmal subarachnoid hemorrhage
  E. Intracerebral hemorrhage

Answer: C

67. Which of the following parameters should be the primary goal of intracranial pressure (ICP) management in a monitored patient with an acute stroke?
  A. ICP < 20 mm H_2O; cerebral perfusion pressure > 70 mm Hg
  B. ICP < 50 mm H_2O; cerebral perfusion pressure > 100 mm Hg
  C. ICP < 80 mm H_2O; cerebral perfusion pressure > 100 mm Hg
  D. ICP < 70 mm H_2O; cerebral perfusion pressure > 20 mm Hg
  E. ICP < 100 mm H_2O; cerebral perfusion pressure > 30 mm Hg

Answer: A

68. Administration of mannitol for elevated intracranial pressure in a monitored patient should aim for which of the following serum osmolality values (mOsm)?
  A. <250   **D.** <320
  B. <280   **E.** <350
  C. <300

Answer: D

69. Which of the following medications should be started on arrival in patients with aneurysmal subarachnoid hemorrhage?
  A. Nifedipine   **D.** Nitroglycerin
  B. Nimodipine   **E.** Sodium nitroprusside
  C. Labetalol

Answer: B

70. Arterial hypotension during the first hours after thrombolysis for acute ischemic stroke should raise the concern for which of the following diagnoses?
  A. SIADH   **D.** Hemopericardium and cardiac tamponade
  B. Central salt-wasting syndrome   **E.** Pulmonary embolus
  C. Dehydration

Answer: D

71. Which of the following is the most common cause of spontaneous subarachnoid hemorrhage?
  A. Ruptured cerebral arteriovenous malformation   **D.** Vasculitides
  B. Ruptured cerebral aneurysm   **E.** Illicit drug use
  C. Coagulopathies

Answer: B

72. Which of the following is the most common location of saccular intracranial aneurysms?
  A. Ophthalmic artery   **D.** Basilar apex
  B. Pericallosal artery   **E.** Origin of posterior inferior cerebellar artery
  C. Anterior communicating artery

Answer: C

73. A 50-year-old man presents with complaints of fatigue and subjective weakness. Symptoms have been present for approximately 4 months. On examination, there is no atrophy or fasciculations and muscle strength testing is grossly normal. The patient has been a farmer for 30 years, drinks two beers a day, and has smoked one and a half packs of cigarettes per day for 35 years. Which of the following elements in his review of systems, if positive, would assist in focusing the diagnosis?

A. Low back pain
B. Intermittent right upper quadrant pain
C. Dry mouth
D. Remote exposure to pesticides
E. Tinnitus

Answer: C

74. The above patient agrees to undergo EMG/NCS for further evaluation. Which of the following, if any, might confirm the clinical suspicion?

A. Low amplitudes in motor nerve conduction studies
B. Absent median sensory action potential
C. Incremental response seen in CMAP with high-frequency (50 Hz) repetitive stimulation
D. A and C
E. None of the above

Answer: C

75. A 65-year-old man presents with a 4-year history of progressive wasting and weakness of both upper extremities. There is no history of neck trauma or injury. His symptoms began in his right arm and spread to involve the left arm about 1 year ago. There is no pain and no sensory complaints. He has no dysarthria or dysphagia. On examination, there is severe diffuse atrophy with weakness in muscles involving the median, ulnar, and radial nerves bilaterally. Laboratory data demonstrate normal ESR, TSH, Ca^{2+}, and elevated GM1 antibodies. The next step you would take with this patient is

A. Repeat laboratory values in 6 months
B. Schedule EMG/NCS, cervical spine MRI, and brain MRI
C. Counsel the patient that he probably has ALS and nothing can be done
D. Discuss the risks and benefits of immunotherapy and plan for a course of either IVIG or plasmapheresis
E. Recommend an intense course of physical therapy to build up arm strength

Answer: D

76. A 6-month-old infant presents in the pediatric neurology clinic with failure to thrive. The infant is in the 1% range for weight, 50% for height and head circumference. The patient's mother reports that her infant has a difficult time feeding and a weak high-pitched cry but is otherwise alert, responsive, and has a responsive smile. On examination, the patient cannot raise his head from a prone position and has decreased tone (floppy) in all extremities. An EMG performed earlier in the day showed denervation with fibrillations and positive waves, with large rapid-firing motor units in all muscles evaluated. You discuss with the parents

A. Brain MRI to evaluate for cerebral palsy
B. Fibroblasts for mucopolysaccharidoses
C. EEG for infantile spasms
D. Survival motor neuron gene testing for SMA
E. Muscle biopsy for nemaline rod myopathy

Answer: D

77. A 35-year-old woman with genetically proven myotonic dystrophy presents to your clinic. Her chief complaint is fatigue. She has not seen a physician in several years. She complains of bilateral foot drop and distal hand stiffness but has no other problems. She finished high school at 19 years of age and took one semester of college work. She is recently married. She reports that her father wears braces and uses CPAP at night. You recommend for the patient

A. No need to worry, that everything appears fine
B. Many myotonics are fatigued and she should "take it slow."
C. Baseline EKG, overnight polysomnography, and genetic counseling
D. MRI of the brain, EEG, and respiratory therapy
E. As a patient with myotonic dystrophy, she has decreased mental capacity and should appoint a power of attorney.

Answer: C

78. Which of the following angiopathies is caused by mutations in the notch 3 gene?

A. Fabry disease   D. Susac syndrome
B. CADASIL   E. Fibromuscular dysplasia
C. Moyamoya

Answer: B

79. A 45-year-old man is unable to flex the distal phalanx of the thumb and index finger. There is no sensory loss. Which of the following is the most likely diagnosis?

A. Carpal tunnel syndrome   D. Radial neuropathy at the spiral groove
B. Posterior cord brachial plexopathy E. C6 radiculopathy
C. Anterior interosseus syndrome

Answer: C

80. Which of the following is the most common location of ulnar nerve compression?

A. Axilla   D. Wrist
B. Arm   E. Palm
C. Elbow

Answer: C

81. Following a bout of alcoholic intoxication, a 25-year-old man developed weakness of right wrist and finger extension and right brachioradialis, with preservation of triceps and deltoid function. Which of the following is the most likely diagnosis?

A. Posterior interosseus syndrome   D. Radial sensory neuropathy
B. Radial neuropathy at the spiral groove E. C8 radiculopathy
C. Posterior cord brachial plexopathy

Answer: B

82. Following a weekend of archery competition, a 35-year-old woman complains of difficulty combing her hair. Examination shows winging of the medial border of the scapula. Which of the following nerves is most likely affected?

A. Axillary   D. Long thoracic
B. Suprascapular   E. Musculocutaneous
C. Spinal accessory

Answer: D

83. Which of the following is *not* a feature of a common peroneal neuropathy?

A. Foot drop   D. Weakness of ankle eversion
B. Weakness of ankle dorsiflexion E. Weakness of plantar flexion
C. Weakness of toe dorsiflexion

Answer: E

84. The spinal accessory nerve exits the cranium through which of the following anatomical structures?

A. Hypoglossal canal   D. Foramen lacerum

B. Jugular foramen
C. Stylomastoid foramen
E. Foramen rotundum

Answer: B

85. An 18-month-old child presented with macrocrania. CT scan demonstrated cystic dilatation of the fourth ventricle, cerebellar vermian dysgenesis, and hydrocephalus. Which of the following is the most likely diagnosis?

   A. Chiari I malformation
   B. Aqueductal stenosis
   C. Joubert syndrome
   D. Alexander disease
   E. Dandy-Walker malformation

Answer: E

86. Which of the following dementias have parietotemporal hypometabolism with sparing of the occipital cortex on FDG-PET scans?

   A. Dementia with Lewy bodies
   B. Alzheimer disease
   C. Dementia associated with Parkinson disease
   D. Huntington disease
   E. Corticobasal degeneration

Answer: B

87. Which of the following is the treatment of choice in patients with disabling upper limb poststroke spasticity?

   A. Clonidine
   B. Benzodiazepines
   C. Botulinum toxin A
   D. Phenytoin
   E. Phenobarbital

Answer: C

88. Which risk factor is most prevalent in patients with ischemic stroke?

   A. Cigarette smoking
   B. Diabetes mellitus
   C. Hyperlipidemia
   D. Hypertension
   E. Prior transient ischemic attacks

Answer: D

89. Which of the following symptomatic patients with hemispheric ischemia would benefit most from carotid endarterectomy?

   A. Stenosis of 70% to 99% (not near occlusion)
   B. Stenosis of 50% to 69%
   C. String sign (tight stenosis with distal vessel collapse)
   D. Stenosis of 30% to 50%
   E. Stenosis less than 30%

Answer: A

90. Stroke associated with migraine most commonly involves which of the following arterial territories?

   A. Anterior choroidal
   B. Anterior cerebral artery
   C. Posterior cerebral artery
   D. Middle cerebral artery
   E. Ophthalmic artery

Answer: C

91. Which of the following is the most common cause of iatrogenic accessory nerve palsy?

   A. Posterior cervical lymph node dissection
   B. Catheter cerebral angiography through a brachial approach
   C. Tracheostomy
   D. Reduction of shoulder subluxation
   E. Lumbar puncture

Answer: A

92. Which of the following is a potential risk of ventriculostomy in the treatment of patients presenting with hydrocephalus and cerebellar infarction?

A. Central herniation
B. Uncal herniation
C. Upward herniation
D. Transfalcine herniation
E. Kernohan notch syndrome

Answer: C

93. Following carotid endarterectomy for treatment of symptomatic 90% stenosis of the right internal carotid artery, a 70-year-old hypertensive man experienced atypical migrainous phenomena, transient focal seizure activity, and a right hemispheric hematoma. Which of the following conditions most likely explains this postoperative complication?

A. Carotid dissection
B. Perioperative hypotension
C. Rupture of undiagnosed intacranial aneurysm
D. Hyperperfusion syndrome
E. Cerebral amyloid angiopathy

Answer: D

94. Which of the following is the most common cause of ischemic stroke?

A. Atherothrombosis
B. Cervicocephalic arterial dissection
C. Vasculitis
D. Prothrombotic state
E. Cervicocephalic fibromuscular dysplasia

Answer: A

95. Most deaths after first-ever stroke are due to which of the following conditions?

A. Pneumonia
B. Urosepsis
C. Renal failure
D. Cardiovascular event and recurrent stroke
E. SIADH

Answer: D

96. Which of the following anatomical structures is mostly responsible for CSF formation?

A. Pineal gland
B. Lamina terminalis
C. Arachnoid granulations
D. Choroid plexus
E. Obex

Answer: D

97. Which of the following anatomical structures is mostly responsible for CSF resorption?

A. Pineal gland
B. Lamina terminalis
C. Arachnoid granulations
D. Choroid plexus
E. Obex

Answer: C

98. Febrile status epilepticus is the major cause of status epilepticus in which of the following age groups?

A. Less than 6 months
B. 1 to 2 years
C. 3 to 5 years
D. 6 to 8 years
E. 9 to 12 years

Answer: B

99. In the acute management of seizures, which of the following drugs has the most favorable absorption after intramuscular administration?

A. Lorazepam
B. Diazepam
C. Clonazepam
D. Midazolam
E. Paraldehyde

Answer: D

100. After intravenous administration, which of the following drugs has the shortest time to peak brain concentration?

    A. Lorazepam   **D.** Phenytoin
    B. Diazepam   **E.** Phenobarbital
    C. Clonazepam

Answer: B

101. When administered as an intravenous loading dose, which of the following drugs has the lowest potential for respiratory depression?

    A. Lorazepam   **D.** Phenytoin
    B. Diazepam   **E.** Phenobarbital
    C. Clonazepam

Answer: D

102. A 65-year-old woman is brought to the emergency room following a fall down the stairs. On examination, she opens her eyes to voice. She does not follow commands but localizes to noxious stimulus and cannot carry on a conversation with one-word appropriate answers. Her Glasgow Coma Scale (GCS) score is

    A. 5   **D.** 14
    B. <8   **E.** 15
    C. 11

Answer: C

103. Which of the following is *not* a paraclinical test used in the diagnosis of brain death?

    A. Cerebral angiography   **D.** Transcranial Doppler ultrasound
    B. Nuclear medicine blood flow study   **E.** MRI and/or MRA of the brain
    C. EEG

Answer: E

104. Which of these clinical features is *not* a significant determinant in determining the prognosis of a patient with an intracerebral hemorrhage?

    A. Etiology of the hemorrhage   **D.** Glasgow Coma Scale
    B. Patient age   **E.** Intraventricular extension
    C. Hematoma volume

Answer: A

105. In a 40-year-old patient with status epilepticus who continues to seize after receiving the maximum dose of intravenous lorazepam and a maximal loading dose of phenytoin (or the equivalent in fosphenytoin), the current preferred next step would be

    A. Give more lorazepam.
    B. Treat with a loading dose of carbamazepine.
    C. Give an additional 20 mg/kg loading dose of phenytoin.
    D. Treat with a propofol or midazolam drip.
    E. Confirm diagnosis by EEG.

Answer: D

106. Which of the following agents is *not* an inhibitor of acetylcholinesterase (AChE)?

    A. Tacrine   **D.** Galantamine
    B. Donepezil   **E.** Selegiline
    C. Rivastigmine

Answer: E

107. Early parkinsonian features, visual hallucinations, and fluctuations in cognitive function are most characteristic of which of the following dementias?

    A. Pick disease   **D.** Hydrocephalic dementia
    B. Alzheimer disease   **E.** Vascular cognitive impairment
    C. Dementia with Lewy bodies

Answer: C

108. Which of the following agents has been associated with an increased risk of stroke?

A. Quetiapine (Seroquel)   D. Risperidone (Risperdal)
B. Olanzapine (Zyprexa)   E. Buspirone (BuSpar)
C. Haloperidol (Haldol)

Answer: B

109. Which of the following brain regions is most severely affected by the presence of neurofibrillary tangles in patients with Alzheimer dementia?

A. Primary motor cortex   D. Entorhinal cortex and hippocampus
B. Visual cortex   E. Anterior nuclei of the thalamus
C. Primary sensory cortex

Answer: D

110. Diagnosis of Alzheimer disease is made by which of the following?

A. Tau protein in CSF
B. Genotyping for apolipoprotein
C. EEG
D. Single photon emission computerized tomography (SPECT) of the brain
E. Clinical criteria

Answer: E

111. Which of the following is the most common clinical form of multiple sclerosis?

A. Relapsing–remitting   D. Baló concentric sclerosis
B. Primary progressive   E. Acute fulminant form (Marburg variant)
C. Devic disease (neuromyelitis optica)

Answer: A

112. A 30-year-old woman has a 3-day history of right orbital pain associated with eye movements and loss of vision of the right eye. On examination, visual acuity is 20/50 on the OD and 20/20 on the OS. There is red desaturation on the right eye, a right cecocentral scotoma, and a right relative afferent pupillary defect. Which of the following is the most likely diagnosis?

A. Central retinal artery occlusion
B. Anterior ischemic optic neuropathy
C. Optic neuritis
D. Posterior ischemic optic neuropathy
E. Cilioretinal artery occlusion

Answer: C

113. Which of the following is the site of origin of the sympathetic pathway to the pupil?

A. Hypothalamus
B. Edinger-Westphal nucleus in the midbrain
C. Pontine paramedian reticular formation
D. Medial longitudinal fasciculus
E. Nucleus accumbens

Answer: A

114. Which of the following is the site of origin of the parasympathetic pathway to the pupil?

A. Hypothalamus
B. Edinger-Westphal nucleus in the midbrain
C. Paramedian pontine reticular formation
D. Medial longitudinal fasciculus
E. Nucleus accumbens

Answer: B

115. Which of the following is the location of the anatomical structures regulating oxygenation and acid–base balance?

    A. Fronto-orbital   **D.** Lower brainstem

    B. Mesial temporal   **E.** Midbrain tectum

    C. Insula of Reil

Answer: D

116. Which of the following is the basic substance for cerebral metabolism?

    A. Phosphorus   **D.** Magnesium

    B. Calcium   **E.** Sodium

    C. Glucose

Answer: C

117. Which of the following interventions should be *avoided* in the early (<4 hours) management of a comatose patient?

    A. 5% dextrose in water intravenous infusion   **D.** Vasoactive substances

    B. Placement of large-bore intravenous catheter   **E.** Gastric lavage

    C. Oropharyngeal airway

Answer: A

118. Flexion of the upper arms against the chest, pronation and flexion of the wrists, and extension of the lower extremities is an indication of which of the following conditions?

    A. Decorticate posturing   **D.** Tetanus

    B. Decerebrate posturing   **E.** Strychnine poisoning

    C. Catatonia

Answer: A

119. Extension of the elbows, pronation and extension of the wrists, and extension of the lower extremities is an indication of which of the following conditions?

    A. Decortication   **D.** Tetanus

    B. Decerebration   **E.** Strychnine poisoning

    C. Catatonia

Answer: B

120. In a comatose patient, extension of the elbows, pronation and extension of the wrists, and extension of the lower extremities is most likely an indication of a lesion at which of the following anatomical locations?

    A. Bilateral orbitofrontal   **D.** Cerebellum

    B. Bilateral thalamic   **E.** Bilateral mesial temporal

    C. Midbrain/upper pons

Answer: C

121. In a comatose patient, flexion of the arms against the chest, pronation and flexion of the wrists, and extension of the lower extremities is most likely an indication of a lesion at which of the following anatomical locations?

    A. Cerebellum   **D.** Medulla oblongata

    B. Midbrain/upper pons   **E.** Cervicomedullary junction

    C. Cerebral hemispheres and diencephalon

Answer: C

122. Which of the following reflexes is tested with the doll's eyes maneuver?

    A. Oculovestibular   **D.** Oculocephalic

    B. Ciliospinal   **E.** Corneomandibular

    C. Cochleopalpebral

Answer: D

123. Which of the following tests is done to evaluate the oculovestibular reflex?

A. Apnea
B. Caloric (ice water)
C. Dix-Hallpike
D. Brainstem auditory evoked potential
E. Electrooculography

Answer: B

124. A 60-year-old woman complains of nocturnal leg paresthesias with an irresistible urge to move the legs. There is partial relief by activity. Which of the following disorders is most commonly associated with her condition?

A. Hyperthyroidism
B. Hypoglycemia
C. Zinc deficiency
D. Iron deficiency anemia
E. Hypocalcemia

Answer: D

125. Which of the following agents used in the treatment of Parkinson disease can precipitate sleepiness with sudden sleep episodes?

A. Amantadine
B. Dopamine receptor agonists
C. Selegiline
D. L-dopa
E. Artane

Answer: B

126. Which of the following is the drug of first choice in the management of restless legs syndrome?

A. Dopamine agonists
B. Benzodiazepines
C. Levodopa
D. Gabapentin
E. Quetiapine

Answer: A

127. Which of the following neurologic disorders can be improved by liver transplantation?

A. Acute intermittent porphyria
B. Fabry disease
C. Wilson disease
D. Chorea–acanthocytosis
E. Menkes disease

Answer: C

128. Which of the following transplant patients are at greater risk of developing central pontine myelinolysis (CPM) perioperatively?

A. Kidney
B. Heart
C. Lung
D. Liver
E. Pancreas

Answer: D

129. Cortical blindness in allograft transplant patients is most commonly the result of toxicity by which of the following agents?

A. Corticosteroids
B. Cyclosporine
C. Azathioprine
D. Imipenem
E. Mycophenolate

Answer: B

130. A 50-year-old obese man complains of morning headaches, mild memory difficulties, and excessive daytime sleepiness. His bed partner reports loud nocturnal snoring. Which of the following is the most likely diagnosis?

A. Narcolepsy
B. Parasomnia
C. Restless legs syndrome
D. Obstructive sleep apnea
E. REM sleep behavior disorder

Answer: D

131. A 55-year-old executive complains of creeping, crawling sensations of the legs associated with irresistible movements of the extremities most severe at bedtime. Symptoms are present at rest and are occasionally relieved by stretching or rubbing. Which of the following is the most likely diagnosis?

A. Narcolepsy
B. Delayed sleep phase syndrome
C. Restless legs syndrome
D. Obstructive sleep apnea
E. REM sleep behavior disorder

Answer: C

132. An 18-year-old college student complains of excessive daytime sleepiness and irresistible episodes of falling asleep during classes and while driving. Which of the following is the most appropriate ancillary diagnostic test?

A. CSF levels of orexin (hypocretin)
B. Nocturnal polysomnography and multiple sleep latency
C. Apnea–hypopnea index
D. HLA typing
E. Neuropsychological testing

Answer: B

133. Which of the following short-lasting headache types responds to indomethacin?

A. Trigeminal neuralgia
B. Cluster headaches
C. Paroxysmal hemicrania
D. Short-lasting unilateral neuralgiform headache attacks with conjunctival injection and tearing (SUNCT)
E. Hypnic headaches

Answer: C

134. Retroperitoneal fibrosis is a potential complication of which of the following drugs used for the treatment of headaches?

A. Topiramate
B. Methysergide
C. Divalproex sodium
D. Diltiazem
E. Sumatriptan

Answer: B

135. Which of the following is *not* a characteristic clinical feature of cluster headaches?

A. Lacrimation
B. Nasal congestion
C. Rhinorrhea
D. Mydriasis
E. Sense of restlessness during headache

Answer: D

136. Diffuse meningeal enhancement on gadolinium-enhanced MRI is most characteristic of which of the following headache types?

A. Cluster
B. Paroxysmal hemicrania
C. Short-lasting unilateral neuralgiform headache attacks with conjunctival injection and tearing (SUNCT)
D. Chronic daily headache
E. Intracranial hypotension and low-pressure headache

Answer: E

137. Which of the following interventions reduces the risk of postdural puncture headache?

A. Use of large-gauge needles
B. Use of cutting-tip needles
C. Warning about postdural puncture headache
D. Replacing stylet
E. Lying supine for 4 hours after procedure

Answer: D

138. Which of the following is the most common cause of nontraumatic coma?

A. Hypoxia–ischemia
B. Cerebral infarction
C. Hepatic encephalopathy
D. Hyponatremia
E. Brain mass lesions

Answer: A

139. Which of the following clinical/paraclinical features is **not** a poor prognostic indicator in patients with nontraumatic coma?

A. Glasgow Coma Scale (GCS) motor score of 6 at day 3
B. Absent pupillary response to light at day 3
C. Isoelectric EEG after 1 week
D. Bilateral absence of N20 after median nerve stimulation after 1 week
E. Burst-suppression EEG after 1 week

Answer: A

140. Which of the following clinical manifestations is among the earliest clinical findings in children with neurofibromatosis type 1?

A. Café au lait spots
B. Axillary and inguinal freckles
C. Lisch nodules
D. Plexiform neurofibromas
E. Scoliosis

Answer: A

141. Which of the following conditions may cause irreversible spinal cord damage in patients with Down syndrome?

A. Dural ectasias
B. Atlantoaxial instability
C. Spinal cord schwannomas
D. Spinal cord meningiomas
E. Subacute combined degeneration

Answer: A

142. Which of the following tumors is most commonly seen in patients with tuberous sclerosis complex?

A. Meningioma
B. Optic nerve glioma
C. Subependymal giant cell astrocytoma
D. Plexiform neurofibroma
E. Hemangioblastoma

Answer: C

143. CNS hemangioblastomas in patients with von Hippel-Lindau disease are typically located in which of the following anatomical regions?

A. Thalamus
B. Optic chiasm
C. Midbrain
D. Occipital lobes
E. Cerebellum

Answer: E

144. Which of the following features best characterizes cluster headaches?

A. Headaches lasting 1 or 2 days and recurring every 1 to 2 weeks in a 20-year-old woman
B. Bilateral moderately severe headaches in a 60-year-old man
C. Unilateral and severe headaches lasting minutes to a few hours, associated with rhinorrhea, ipsilateral miosis, and eyelid ptosis
D. Sudden onset of severe headaches with neck stiffness
E. Lingering orthostatic headaches

Answer: C

145. Intracranial pain-sensitive structures include all of the following *except*

A. Dura mater
D. Brain parenchyma

B. Large cerebral vessels
C. Pial vessels

E. Large venous sinuses

Answer: D

146. Pain-producing intracranial structures are innervated by which of the following cranial nerves?

A. III
B. V
C. VII
D. IX
E. X

Answer: B

147. Which of the following features best characterizes the mechanism of action of triptans?

A. Selective 5-HT1 agonists
B. Cyclooxygenase (COX) 1 inhibitors
C. Serotonin antagonists
D. Reversible monoamine oxidase inhibitors (MAOI)
E. Endothelin antagonists

Answer: A

148. Which of the following is the most common emotional response after stroke?

A. Mania
B. Agitation
C. Emotional lability
D. Depression
E. Anxiety

Answer: D

149. Of the following, which is the major cause of death for American women?

A. Multiple sclerosis
B. Stroke
C. Myasthenia gravis
D. Epilepsy
E. Parkinson disease

Answer: B

150. Which of the following is the most common adverse effect at the onset of therapy with IFN-β-1A for treatment of multiple sclerosis?

A. Headaches
B. Flulike symptoms
C. Seizures
D. Vomiting
E. Myositis

Answer: B

151. Which of the following clinical features increases the risk of dying in patients with acute bacterial meningitis?

A. Fever
B. Arterial hypotension
C. Altered mental state
D. Community-acquired meningitis
E. Lack of neck stiffness

Answer: B

152. A 40-year-old man developed burning right-sided otalgia, followed by periauricular paresthesias, vertigo, and rapidly developing right-sided peripheral facial weakness associated with vesicles in the ipsilateral ear. Which of the following ganglia is involved?

A. Superior cervical
B. Sphenopalatine
C. Geniculate
D. Gasserian
E. Nodose

Answer: C

153. Which of the following cranial nerves is most commonly involved in patients with Lyme disease?

A. II
D. VII

B. III   **E.** XII
C. V

Answer: D

154. Which of the following organisms is the most common etiologic agent of acute bacterial meningitis in adults (18 to 50 years of age) in the United States?
   A. *Haemophilus influenzae*
   B. *Listeria monocytogenes*
   C. *N. meningitidis*
   D. *Streptococcus agalactiae* (group B *streptococcus*)
   E. *S. pneumoniae*

Answer: E

155. Which of the following is the major cause of the aseptic meningitis syndrome?
   A. Nonsteroidal antiinflammatory drugs (NSAIDs)   **D.** Viruses
   B. Antibiotics   **E.** Parasites
   C. IVIG

Answer: D

156. Which of the following is responsible for tetanus?
   A. Tetanospasmin   **D.** Exotoxin of *Clostridium botulinum*
   B. Tetanolysin   **E.** Toxin-producing dinoflagellates
   C. Tetrodotoxin

Answer: A

157. Which of the following dermatomes is most commonly affected by herpes zoster?
   A. Trigeminal nerve   **D.** Lumbar
   B. Cervical   **E.** Sacral
   C. Thoracic

Answer: C

158. Herpetic vesicles on the tip or side of the nose (Hutchinson sign) indicate involvement of which the following nerves?
   A. Frontal nerve   **D.** Maxillary division of the trigeminal nerve
   B. Nasociliary nerve   **E.** Mandibular division of the trigeminal nerve
   C. Lacrimal nerve

Answer: B

159. Capsaicin is a chemical that depletes which of the following transmitters?
   A. Serotonin   **D.** Substance P
   B. Dopamine   **E.** Glutamate
   C. Norepinephrine

Answer: D

160. Which of the following is *not* a typical feature of normal pressure hydrocephalus (NPH)?
   A. Urinary incontinence   **D.** Slowness of thought
   B. Memory impairment   **E.** Short-stepped and broad-based gait
   C. Papilledema

Answer: C

161. Which of the following clinical features is usually the first symptom in patients with normal pressure hydrocephalus (NPH)?
   A. Gait disturbance   **D.** Seizures
   B. Dementia   **E.** Fecal incontinence
   C. Urinary incontinence

Answer: A

162. Which of the following drugs decreases CSF production by the choroid plexus?

A. Hydrochlorothiazide
B. Indapamide
C. Triamterene
D. Acetazolamide
E. Nimodipine

Answer: D

163. Which of the following organisms is most likely to cause meningitis as a complication of a neurosurgical procedure?

A. *L. monocytogenes*
B. *Staphylococcus aureus* and coagulase-negative staphylococci
C. *S. pneumoniae*
D. *N. meningitides*
E. *H. influenzae* type b

Answer: B

164. Which of the following organisms is the most common cause of acute sporadic encephalitis?

A. La Crosse virus
B. Epstein-Barr virus (EBV)
C. Varicella-zoster virus
D. HSV-1
E. Enteroviruses

Answer: D

165. Which of the following organisms is the most common cause of viral meningitis?

A. La Crosse virus
B. Epstein-Barr virus (EBV)
C. Varicella-zoster virus
D. HSV-1
E. Enterovirus

Answer: E

166. Which of the following viral infections in the first 12 weeks of pregnancy is a cause of intracranial calcifications, microcephaly, cataracts, sensorineural hearing loss, cardiac defects, and hepatosplenomegaly?

A. Rubella
B. Measles
C. Lymphocytic choriomeningitis
D. HSV-1
E. Hepatitis C

Answer: A

167. Which of the following ischemic cerebrovascular disorders is *less commonly* associated with headaches?

A. Basilar artery occlusion
B. Stem of middle cerebral artery occlusion
C. Lacunar infarct
D. Internal carotid artery occlusion
E. Posterior cerebral artery occlusion

Answer: C

168. Central nervous system myelin is produced by which of the following cells?

A. Microglia
B. Oligodendrocyte
C. Astrocyte
D. Purkinje
E. Schwann

Answer: B

169. Which of the following disorders is the most common cause of rest tremor?

A. Parkinson disease
B. Essential tremor
C. Alcohol intoxication
D. Wilson disease
E. Peripheral neuropathy

Answer: A

170. Which of the following inclusions in the substantia nigra is characteristic of Parkinson disease?

A. Negri bodies   **D.** Lewy bodies
B. Hirano bodies   **E.** Bunina bodies
C. Lyssa bodies

Answer: D

171. A 55-year-old man is found at autopsy to have focal hemorrhagic lesions of the inferior part of the corpus callosum and dorsolateral quadrants of the rostral brainstem adjacent to the superior cerebellar peduncle, associated with diffuse axonal damage. Which of the following disorders is the most likely diagnosis?

A. Anoxic encephalopathy   **D.** Fat embolism
B. Carbon monoxide intoxication   **E.** Hemorrhagic leukoencephalitis
C. Diffuse axonal injury

Answer: C

172. Which of the following features is **not** characteristic of cytomegalovirus polyradiculopathy in HIV disease?

A. Subacute lower back pain   **D.** Urinary difficulties
B. Areflexic paraparesis   **E.** Normal CSF
C. Distal sensory loss

Answer: E

173. Which of the following is the most common peripheral nerve manifestation in seroconversion-related neuropathies in HIV disease?

A. Facial nerve palsy
B. Syphilitic polyradiculopathy
C. Hepatitis C infection–related neuropathy
D. Cytomegalovirus-related polyradiculopathy
E. Motor neuron disease syndrome

Answer: A

174. Which of the following aphasias is most commonly seen in the early stages of Alzheimer disease?

A. Broca
B. Wernicke
C. Anomic
D. Conduction
E. Transcortical sensory

Answer: C

175. Which of the following organisms is most commonly associated with subdural effusions in infants?

A. S. pneumoniae   **D.** H. influenzae type b
B. N. meningitides   **E.** S. agalactiae
C. L. monocytogenes

Answer: D

176. Which of the following intracranial tumors is most commonly associated with neurofibromatosis type 2?

A. Acoustic neuromas (vestibular schwannomas)
B. Cerebellar hemangioblastomas
C. Subependymal giant cell astrocytomas
D. Colloid cysts of the third ventricle
E. Medulloblastomas

Answer: A

177. Which of the following drugs is most effective in the treatment of trigeminal neuralgia associated with multiple sclerosis?

A. Topiramate
B. Misoprostol
C. Cannabis
D. Levetiracetam
E. Primidone

Answer: B

178. Which of the following clinical features of patients with aneurysmal subarachnoid hemorrhage (SAH) increases the risk of misdiagnosis?

A. Right-sided aneurysms
B. Hunt-Hess grade I or II
C. Left-sided aneurysms
D. Aneurysm size 7 to 10 mm
E. Lack of prior history of headaches

Answer: B

179. For any given duration of ischemia following cardiac arrest, which of the following CNS regions is most vulnerable?

A. Thalamus
B. Midbrain
C. Pons
D. Cerebral cortex
E. Spinal cord

Answer: D

180. Which of the following disorders is associated with elevation of myelin basic protein in the CSF?

A. Stroke
B. Multiple sclerosis
C. Head injury
D. Intracranial tumors
E. All of the above

Answer: E

181. What percentage of the population harbors an unruptured intracranial aneurysm?

A. 3
B. 15
C. 20
D. 25
E. 30

Answer: A

182. Which of the following unruptured intracranial aneurysms has the lowest annualized risk of subarachnoid hemorrhage (SAH)?

A. Anterior circulation aneurysms < 7 mm
B. Basilar artery aneurysms
C. Giant aneurysms
D. Aneurysms < 10 mm with associated SAH from another aneurysm
E. MCA aneurysms

Answer: A

183. Which of the following best characterizes cerebral edema due to stroke?

A. Response to corticosteroid therapy
B. Response to barbiturates
C. Peak occurrence 3 to 5 days after stroke
D. Less severe among younger patients with MCA stem occlusion
E. Response to NMDA receptor antagonists

Answer: C

184. What is the 30-day mortality rate for aneurysmal subarachnoid hemorrhage (SAH)?

A. 2%
B. 5%
C. 10%
D. 15%
E. 45%

Answer: E

185. Which of the following is the most powerful predictor of 30-day mortality following aneurysmal subarachnoid hemorrhage (SAH)?

A. Anterior circulation aneurysms
B. Cerebral vasospasm
C. Volume of initial SAH
D. Hunt-Hess grade I or II
E. Family history of aneurysmal SAH

Answer: C

186. Which of the following electrolyte/metabolic abnormality causes a depression of the muscle stretch reflexes?

A. Hypoglycemia
B. Hypermagnesemia
C. Hyperkalemia
D. Hyponatremia
E. Hypocalcemia

Answer: B

187. Which of the following is best avoided in the management of aneurysmal SAH in the ICU?

A. Induced hypertension
B. Hypothermia
C. Nimodipine
D. Hypovolemia
E. Hyperventilation

Answer: D

188. Which of the following best predicts the occurrence of cerebral vasospasm in patients with aneurysmal SAH?

A. Male gender
B. Hunt-Hess grade I or II
C. Hyperglycemia
D. Volume of SAH on initial CT
E. Lack of intraventricular hemorrhage

Answer: D

189. Which of the following movement disorders is most commonly associated with the chronic administration of opioids?

A. Tics
B. Chorea
C. Parkinsonism
D. Myoclonus
E. Athetosis

Answer: D

190. Which of the following is the most commonly affected cranial nerve in sarcoidosis?

A. II
B. III
C. V
D. VII
E. VIII

Answer: D

191. Which of the following is a major side effect of mitoxantrone?

A. Depression
B. Flulike symptoms
C. Cardiomyopathy
D. Neuropathy
E. Injection-site reactions

Answer: C

192. Which of the following arthropathies may cause a cauda equina syndrome?

A. Osteoarthritis
B. Rheumatoid arthritis
C. Gout
D. Ankylosing spondylitis
E. Pseudogout

Answer: D

193. Which of the following electrophysiologic testing is especially helpful in detecting clinically silent lesions in patients with multiple sclerosis?

   A. Visual evoked potentials
   B. Brainstem auditory evoked potentials
   C. Electronystagmogram
   D. Electroretinogram
   E. EEG

   Answer: A

194. Among all brain tumors, which of the following is the most common?

   A. Oligodendroglioma
   B. Glioblastoma multiforme
   C. Ependymoma
   D. Meningioma
   E. Metastases

   Answer: E

195. Which of the following is the most common primary brain tumor?

   A. Oligodendroglioma
   B. Glioblastoma multiforme
   C. Ependymoma
   D. Meningioma
   E. Primary CNS lymphoma

   Answer: B

196. A 50-year-old woman has an intracranial meningioma. Examination shows anosmia, ipsilateral optic atrophy, and contralateral papilledema. Which of the following is the location of the tumor?

   A. Cavernous sinus
   B. Cerebellopontine angle
   C. Olfactory groove
   D. Sphenoid wing
   E. Subfrontal

   Answer: C

197. Which of the following is the most common complication of medulloblastoma?

   A. Deafness
   B. Facial nerve palsy
   C. Hydrocephalus
   D. Third cranial nerve palsy
   E. Seizures

   Answer: C

198. In patients with childhood epileptic encephalopathy (Lennox-Gastaut syndrome), corpus callosotomy is effective in reducing which of the following type of seizures?

   A. Axial tonic
   B. Drop attacks
   C. Atypical absences
   D. Complex partial
   E. Generalized tonic–clonic

   Answer: B

199. Which of the following is a major complication of rapid correction of hyperglycemia and hyperosmolality in a patient with type II diabetes and nonketotic hyperosmolar state (NKHS)?

   A. Central pontine myelinolysis
   B. Marchiafava-Bignami disease
   C. Cerebral edema
   D. Orthostatic hypotension
   E. Hypothermia

   Answer: C

200. Which of the following choreatic disorders is associated with an axonal sensorimotor polyneuropathy with amyotrophy?

   A. Sydenham
   B. Huntington
   C. Wilson
   D. Neuroacanthocytosis
   E. Paroxysmal kinesigenic dyskinesia

   Answer: D

201. Which of the following cardiac disorders is a complication of the vein of Galen malformation?

    A. Complete heart block
    B. Prolonged QT interval
    C. High-output cardiac failure
    D. Restrictive cardiomyopathy
    E. Torsades de pointes

    Answer: C

202. A 15-year-old adolescent boy has progressive muscle wasting and weakness in a scapulohumeroperoneal distribution, elbow, neck contractures, and cardiac conduction defects. Which of the following is the most likely diagnosis?

    A. Duchenne muscular dystrophy
    B. Becker muscular dystrophy
    C. Myotonic dystrophy
    D. Emery-Dreifuss muscular dystrophy
    E. Limb–girdle muscular dystrophy

    Answer: D

203. Which of the following syndromes causing intellectual disability is associated with a trinucleotide repeat expansion?

    A. Down
    B. Fragile X
    C. Cri-du-chat
    D. Prader-Willi
    E. Angelman

    Answer: B

204. Dystonia with diurnal variation (worse later in the day) in a 10-year-old girl is best treated with which of the following drugs?

    A. Carbamazepine
    B. Valproate
    C. Lamotrigine
    D. Levodopa
    E. Mestinon

    Answer: D

205. Which of the following peroxisomal disorders is associated with a typical posterior white matter involvement on MRI?

    A. Adrenoleukodystrophy
    B. Zellweger syndrome
    C. Refsum disease
    D. Hyperoxaluria type 1
    E. Glutaryl CoA oxidase deficiency

    Answer: A

206. Which of the following autonomic disturbances in alcoholic neuropathy is due to sympathetic dysfunction?

    A. Dysphagia
    B. Dysphonia
    C. Sleep apnea
    D. Orthostatic hypotension
    E. Depressed reflex heart response

    Answer: D

207. Central pontine myelinolysis (CPM) may result from rapid correction of which of the following electrolyte disorders?

    A. Hypomagnesemia
    B. Hypophosphatemia
    C. Hyponatremia
    D. Hypocalcemia
    E. Hypokalemia

    Answer: C

208. Which of the following is the most common cause of sudden worsening of spasticity in multiple sclerosis?

    A. Cold showers
    B. Sleep deprivation
    C. Aerobic exercise
    D. Urinary tract infection
    E. Pain

    Answer: D

209. Which of the following is the most sensitive test for the diagnosis of multiple sclerosis?

A. MRI of brain
B. CT scan of brain
C. Visual evoked potentials
D. CSF analysis
E. Electronystagmogram

Answer: A

210. Which of the following is the most common cause of vitamin B_{12} (cobalamin) deficiency?

A. Tropical sprue
B. Pernicious anemia
C. Blind loop syndrome
D. Methylmalonic aciduria
E. Whipple disease

Answer: B

211. Which of the following CNS areas is mostly affected by gross atrophy in Huntington disease?

A. Cerebellar vermis
B. Pontine tegmentum
C. Caudate nucleus
D. Superficial layers of cerebral cortex
E. Thalamus

Answer: C

212. Which of the following sensory modalities is interrupted by a syrinx?

A. Light touch
B. Vibration
C. Joint position sense
D. Pain and temperature
E. None of the above

Answer: D

213. Which of the following sensory modalities is affected early in the course of subacute combined degeneration due to cobalamin (B_{12}) deficiency?

A. Light touch
B. Joint position and vibration
C. Pain
D. Temperature
E. None of the above

Answer: B

214. A 10-year-old boy with mild kyphoscoliosis has progressive limb and gait ataxia. Examination shows distal weakness of the legs and feet and loss of position and vibration sense. Muscle stretch reflexes are absent in the legs. Plantar responses are extensor bilaterally. Which of the following is the most likely diagnosis?

A. Homocystinuria
B. Neuroacanthocytosis
C. Friedreich ataxia
D. Chronic inflammatory demyelinating polyneuropathy
E. Refsum disease

Answer: C

215. Which of the following is the most common form of diabetic neuropathy?

A. Cranial neuropathy
B. Lumbosacral polyradiculopathy
C. Autonomic neuropathy
D. Distal sensorimotor polyneuropathy
E. Trunk mononeuropathy

Answer: D

216. Which of the following is the most common location of a hypertensive intraparenchymal hemorrhage?

A. Cerebellum
B. Lobar
C. Pons
D. Putamen
E. Thalamus

Answer: D

217. Which of the following is a major cause of lobar hemorrhage in an elderly normotensive person?

A. Bleeding diathesis
B. Aspirin therapy
C. Ruptured cavernous malformations
D. Telangiectasias
E. Cerebral amyloid angiopathy

Answer: E

218. Which of the following is the most common focal opportunistic brain infection in patients with AIDS?

A. Cryptococcoma
B. Tuberculoma
C. Syphilitic gumma
D. Cerebral toxoplasmosis
E. *Nocardia* brain abscess

Answer: D

219. Which of the following is the treatment of choice in patients with AIDS and single or multiple focal brain lesions?

A. Radiation therapy
B. Empiric trial of pyrimethamine, sulfadiazine, and folinic acid
C. Intravenous amphotericin B and fluconazole
D. High-dose intravenous dexamethasone
E. Intravenous ceftriaxone or penicillin

Answer: B

220. Which of the following vessels is most commonly involved in patients with acute epidural hematoma?

A. Anterior ethmoidal artery
B. Middle meningeal artery
C. Transverse sinus
D. Sigmoid sinus
E. Superior sagittal sinus

Answer: B

221. Chronic subdural hematoma is most commonly the result of rupture of which of the following vessels?

A. Anterior ethmoidal artery
B. Middle meningeal artery
C. Transverse sinus
D. Cortical bridging veins
E. Superior sagittal sinus

Answer: D

222. Which of the following antiepileptic drugs (AEDs) may increase the risk of myoclonic seizures in patients with juvenile myoclonic epilepsy?

A. Valproic acid (Depakene)
B. Lamotrigine (Lamictal)
C. Topiramate (Topamax)
D. Carbamazepine (Tegretol)
E. Divalproex sodium (Depakote)

Answer: D

223. Which of the following visual field deficits is most characteristic of chiasmal compression?

A. Bitemporal superior quadrantanopia
B. Bilateral central scotomas
C. Bilateral superior altitudinal defects
E. Bilateral enlargement of the blind spots

Answer: A

224. Which of the following is the characteristic interictal EEG pattern in patients with infantile spasms (West syndrome)?

A. Burst suppression
B. Hypsarrhythmia
C. Unifocal or multifocal delta activity
D. Multifocal sharp waves
E. Positive rolandic sharp waves

Answer: B

225. Which of the following is the treatment of choice for HSV-1 encephalitis?

    A. Vidarabine
    B. Acyclovir
    C. Famciclovir
    D. Didanosine
    E. Zalcitabine

Answer: B

226. Which of the following vitamins reduces the risk of neural tube defects in the general population?

    A. Vitamin E
    B. Cobalamin
    C. Thiamine
    D. Folic acid
    E. Vitamin D

Answer: D

227. Which of the following antiepileptic drugs (AEDs) may result in oral contraceptive failure?

    A. Gabapentin
    B. Carbamazepine
    C. Valproic acid
    D. Lamotrigine
    E. Felbamate

Answer: B

228. Which of the following paraneoplastic disorders is associated with anti–calcium channel antibodies (N and P/Q types)?

    A. Sensory neuronopathy
    B. Cerebellar degeneration
    C. Lambert-Eaton myasthenic syndrome (LEMS)
    D. Opsoclonus–myoclonus
    E. Limbic encephalitis

Answer: C

229. Which of the following primary brain tumors is more common in women with breast cancer?

    A. Low-grade astrocytoma
    B. Oligodendroglioma
    C. Ependymoma
    D. Primary CNS lymphoma
    E. Meningioma

Answer: E

230. Which of the following vitamin excess states results in sensory ataxia?

    A. Vitamin A
    B. Vitamin K
    C. Cobalamin
    D. Pyridoxine
    E. Thiamine

Answer: D

231. Which of the following drugs can cause a toxic myopathy with abnormal mitochondria resembling ragged red fibers?

    A. Pentazocine
    B. Glucocorticoids
    C. Zidovudine (AZT)
    D. Penicillamine
    E. Lovastatin

Answer: C

232. Which of the following microorganisms has been associated with the axonal form of Guillain-Barré syndrome?

    A. *Karwinskia humboldtiana*
    B. *Campylobacter jejuni*
    C. *Citrobacter diversus*
    D. *Pseudallescheria*
    E. *Cladosporium*

Answer: B

233. Which of the following is an exclusion for the use of intravenous tPA in acute ischemic stroke?

A. Lacunar stroke
B. NIH stroke scale < 8
C. Systolic blood pressure > 200 mm Hg
D. Platelet count < 150,000
E. CT scan evidence of leukoaraiosis

Answer: C

234. Which of the following is the most common involuntary movement disorder in metabolic encephalopathy?

A. Tremor
B. Chorea
C. Hemiballismus
D. Dystonia
E. Myoclonus

Answer: E

235. Which of the following cranial nerves may be injured as a result of carotid endarterectomy?

A. III
B. V
C. VI
D. VII
E. XII

Answer: E

For each disorder, select the most appropriate diagnosis/answer.

236. Abrupt onset, abrupt ending

A. Complex partial seizures
B. Absence seizures
C. Both
D. Neither

Answer: B

237. Unawareness

A. Complex partial seizures
B. Absence seizures
C. Both
D. Neither

Answer: C

238. Increased risk of neural tube defects

A. Valproate
B. Carbamazepine
C. Both
D. Neither

Answer: C

239. Cerebral edema of metastatic brain disease

A. Cytotoxic
B. Vasogenic
C. Interstitial
D. Ischemic
E. Pyogenic

Answer: B

240. Diabetes insipidus

A. Craniopharyngioma
B. Neurosarcoidosis
C. Both
D. Neither

Answer: C

241. Paraneoplastic cerebellar degeneration

A. Anti-Yo antibodies
B. Anti-Hu antibodies
C. Both
D. Neither

Answer: C

242. Hyperprolactinemia

A. Antipsychotics
B. Primary hypothyroidism
C. Both
D. Neither

Answer: C

243. Pheochromocytoma

    A. Neurofibromatosis   **C.** Both

    B. von Hippel-Lindau disease   **D.** Neither

Answer: C

244. Mees lines

    A. Arsenic toxicity   **C.** Both

    B. Thallium toxicity   **D.** Neither

Answer: C

245. Spasticity in multiple sclerosis

    A. Baclofen   **C.** Both

    B. Tizanidine   **D.** Neither

Answer: C

246. Medulloblastoma

    A. Turcot syndrome (glioma polyposis syndrome)   **C.** Both

    B. von Hippel-Lindau disease   **D.** Neither

Answer: A

247. Autosomal dominant

    A. Huntington disease   **C.** Both

    B. Friedreich ataxia   **D.** Neither

Answer: A

248. Autosomal recessive

    A. Huntington disease   **C.** Both

    B. Friedreich ataxia   **D.** Neither

Answer: B

249. Trinucleotide repeat expansion

    A. Huntington disease   **C.** Both

    B. Friedreich ataxia   **D.** Neither

Answer: C

250. Higher risk of Bell palsy

    A. Diabetes mellitus   **C.** Both

    B. Pregnancy   **D.** Neither

Answer: C

251. Tendon xanthomata

    A. Familial hypercholesterolemia   **C.** Both

    B. Cerebrotendinous xanthomatosis   **D.** Neither

Answer: C

252. Physical complaints seen as intentional, voluntary, and consciously produced

    A. Malingering   **C.** Both

    B. Conversion disorder   **D.** Neither

Answer: A

253. Alien limb phenomenon

    A. Corticobasal degeneration   **C.** Both

    B. Callosal infarction   **D.** Neither

Answer: C

254. The first and second most common adult-onset focal dystonias are
   A. Cervical dystonia and oromandibular dystonia
   B. Cervical dystonia and writer's cramp
   C. Cervical dystonia and blepharospasm
   D. Cervical dystonia and brachial dystonia
   E. Blepharospasm and oromandibular dystonia (Meige syndrome)
   Answer: C

255. This disorder is responsive to low doses of L-dopa
   A. Myoclonic dystonia (DYT 11)   C. Both
   B. Paroxysmal kinesigenic dyskinesia (DTY 10)   D. Neither
   Answer: D

256. Retinal hemorrhages
   A. Optic neuritis   C. Both
   B. Anterior ischemic optic neuropathy   D. Neither
   Answer: B

257. Compared to adults with optic neuritis, optic neuritis in children is more often
   A. Bilateral   C. Both
   B. Parainfectious demyelinating   D. Neither
   Answer: C

258. Idiopathic intracranial hypertension (pseudotumor cerebri)
   A. Elevated CSF opening pressure above 180 mm water measured in lateral decubitus position
   B. Elevated CSF opening pressure above 250 mm of water measured in lateral decubitus position
   C. Both
   D. Neither
   Answer: B

259. Conjunctival injection
   A. Cluster headache   C. Both
   B. Trigeminal neuralgia   D. Neither
   Answer: A

260. More common in women
   A. Migraine headache   C. Both
   B. Chronic paroxysmal hemicrania   D. Neither
   Answer: C

261. A 42-year-old woman with elbow injury has difficulty making a pinching grasp between the fingertips of her thumb and index finger. Which is the syndromic term, and to what nerve does the problem localize?
   A. Kiloh-Nevin syndrome, ulnar nerve
   B. Froment prehensile thumb sign, median nerve
   C. Reverse Kiloh-Nevin syndrome, ulnar nerve
   D. Froment prehensile thumb sign, ulnar nerve
   E. Wartenberg sign, median nerve
   Answer: C

262. In a case of suspected ulnar neuropathy affecting abduction of the fifth (abductor digiti minimi) and index finger (first dorsal interosseous), which finding is most helpful in localizing the lesion to below the elbow?
   A. Hypesthesia in the medial dorsal and palmar hand
   B. Preserved flexion of the distal phalanges of the fourth and fifth fingers

    C. Preserved flexion of the proximal phalanges of the fourth and fifth fingers
    D. Preserved adduction of the fifth finger
    E. Preserved radial flexion of the wrist
    Answer: B

263. Which of the following is the most frequent cause of femoral neuropathy after femoral arterial or venous catheterizations?

    A. Prolonged digital pressure
    B. Retroperitoneal hemorrhage
    C. Local hematoma or pseudoaneurysm
    D. Intraneural injection
    E. Ilioinguinal blockade
    Answer: C

264. In a case of foot drop, weakness in which muscle and hypesthesia in which area would support L5 radiculopathy over peroneal neuropathy?

    A. Weakness in flexor digitorum longus and hypesthesia in dorsomedial foot/big toe
    B. Weakness in flexor digitorum longus and hypesthesia in lateral leg and dorsum of the foot
    C. Weakness in flexor hallucis longus and hypesthesia in dorsomedial foot/big toe
    D. Weakness in extensor digitorum longus and hypesthesia in skin between first and second toes
    E. Weakness in extensor hallucis longus and hypesthesia in skin between first and second toes
    Answer: A

265. A 54-year-old man with wasting of the hand, areflexia, and a dissociated sensory loss with hypesthesia to pain and temperature but preservation of proprioception in a half-cape distribution could have any of the following, *except*

    A. Syringomyelia
    B. Meningioma
    C. Intramedullary ependymoma
    D. Intramedullary hemangioblastoma
    E. Cavernous malformation
    Answer: B

266. Which of the following abnormalities would be least likely in a patient with Chiari II malformation?

    A. Myelomeningocele
    B. Spina bifida occulta
    C. "Kinking" of the cervicomedullary junction
    D. Hydrocephalus
    E. Idiopathic syringomyelia
    Answer: E

267. Anti–glutamic acid decarboxylase (GAD) antibodies can lead to any of the following phenotypes, *except*

    A. Adult-onset epilepsy
    B. Stiff person syndrome
    C. Diabetes mellitus type 1
    D. Diabetes mellitus type 2
    E. Cerebellar ataxia
    Answer: D

268. Besides stiff person syndrome, which disorder is associated with high rather than low concentration of antibodies against GAD?

    A. Adult-onset epilepsy
    B. Cerebellar ataxia
    C. Pernicious anemia
    D. Vitiligo
    E. Hyperthyroidism
    Answer: B

269. The spasms in hyperekplexia can be distinguished from those of stiff person syndrome by which of the following?

    A. Slow onset, slow offset, short duration
    B. Slow onset, rapid offset, short duration

    C. Rapid onset, rapid offset, short duration
    D. Rapid onset, slow offset, short duration
    E. Rapid onset, slow offset, long duration
    Answer: C

270. A 43-year-old woman developed posterior cord sensory deficits and sensory ataxia after a surgical procedure involving nitrous oxide anesthesia. Her vitamin B_{12} levels are normal. Which test is most sensitive to support the diagnostic suspicion of subacute combined degeneration of the spinal cord when cobalamin in serum is normal?

    A. Complete blood count (pancytopenia)
    B. Mean corpuscular volume (high, macrocytosis)
    C. Methylmalonic acid and homocysteine (both high)
    D. Blood smear (hypersegmentation of neutrophils)
    E. Lactate dehydrogenase and indirect bilirubin (high, ineffective erythropoiesis)
    Answer: C

271. A 64-year-old man with history of coronary artery disease and left internal carotid artery stenosis developed nonfluent aphasia with impaired comprehension after several syncopal episodes due to severe hypotension. Further assessment revealed normal repetition and echolalia. This phenomenon is reported as

    A. Transcortical sensory aphasia   **D.** Broca aphasia
    B. Mixed transcortical aphasia   **E.** Wernicke aphasia
    C. Transcortical motor aphasia
    Answer: B

272. The nondominant hemisphere lesion equivalent of Broca aphasia (e.g., right MCA, superior division) is

    A. "Expressive" aprosodia   **D.** Alien hand syndrome
    B. Akinetic mutism   **E.** Transcortical motor aphasia
    C. "Acquired sociopathy"
    Answer: A

273. The nondominant hemisphere lesion equivalent of Wernicke aphasia (e.g., right MCA, inferior division) is

    A. Neglect   **D.** Ideomotor apraxia
    B. Anosodiaphoria   **E.** Anosodiaphoria
    C. Acquired amusia (musical deafness)
    Answer: C

274. Name the Wernicke-type aphasia with preserved repetition and the most common aphasia type into which Wernicke aphasia may evolve.

    A. Mixed transcortical aphasia/transcortical sensory aphasia
    B. Transcortical sensory aphasia/conduction aphasia
    C. Transcortical sensory aphasia/mixed transcortical aphasia
    D. Transcortical motor aphasia/conduction aphasia
    E. Transcortical motor aphasia/anomic aphasia
    Answer: B

275. The nondominant hemisphere lesion equivalent of the semantic dementia variant of primary progressive aphasia (e.g., right temporal lobe atrophy) is

    A. Neglect   **D.** Progressive prosopagnosia
    B. Tactile agnosia   **E.** Apperceptive visual agnosia
    C. Constructional apraxia
    Answer: D

276. Appearance of weakness (suggestive of motor neuron disease) in a suspected case of frontotemporal dementia raises the odds for which underlying pathology?

A. Ubiquitinopathy due to a *C9ORF72* mutation
B. Ubiquitinopathy due to a *progranulin* mutation
C. Ubiquitinopathy due to a *FUS* mutation
D. Ubiquitinopathy due to a *TDP-43* mutation
E. Tauopathy due to a *MAPT* mutation

Answer: A

277. Frontotemporal lobar degeneration can arise within the following phenotypes, *except*

A. Progressive supranuclear palsy syndrome
B. Corticobasal syndrome
C. Primary progressive aphasia
D. Dementia of Alzheimer type
E. Dementia with Lewy bodies

Answer: E

278. The most common genetic mutation in frontotemporal dementia associated with parkinsonism is

A. *MAPT*   D. *CHMP2B*
B. *FUS*   E. *C9orf72*
C. *PGRN*

Answer: C

279. The most common genetic mutation in frontotemporal dementia associated with parkinsonism and motor neuron disease

A. *MAPT*   D. *CHMP2B*
B. *FUS*   E. *C9orf72*
C. *PGRN*

Answer: E

280. A 64-year-old man developed hand dystonia, ideomotor apraxia, and levitation. Which additional feature is most predictive of corticobasal degeneration pathology?

A. Hyperreflexia   D. High-frequency tremor
B. Stimulus-sensitive myoclonus   E. Cortical sensory loss
C. Spontaneous myoclonus

Answer: C

281. Which syndrome is expected to develop in a patient with a prior frontal alien hand syndrome with new right ACA stroke?

A. Amnesia   D. Akinetic mutism
B. Confabulation   E. Pseudopsychopathic disorder
C. Executive dysfunction

Answer: D

282. Which syndrome is expected to develop in a patient with prior alexia without agraphia with a new right PCA stroke?

A. Balint syndrome   D. Hemiachromatopsia
B. Prosopagnosia   E. Optic aphasia
C. Astereopsis

Answer: B

283. The most typical manifestation of mesial temporal lobe injury from herpes simplex virus (HSV) encephalitis or posterior cerebral artery (PCA) stroke, affecting the hippocampi, amygdalae, and entorhinal and parahippocampal cortices is

A. Anterograde amnesia   D. Impaired retrieval of proper names

B. Retrograde amnesia   E. Semantic memory impairment
C. Surface dyslexia

Answer: A

284. The earliest neuropsychological features in patients suspected of having dementia with Lewy bodies are

A. Visuospatial disorientation and encoding-impaired short-term memory loss
B. Visuospatial disorientation and retrieval-impaired short-term memory loss
C. Phonemic verbal fluency and semantic memory
D. Semantic verbal fluency and working memory
E. Attention impairment and poor episodic memory

Answer: B

285. The most specific psychiatric feature of dementia with Lewy bodies is

A. Delusions of persecution   D. Capgras syndrome
B. False sense of presence   E. Auditory hallucinations
C. Visual hallucinations

Answer: D

286. Recurrent visual hallucinations in dementia with Lewy bodies are best described as

A. They occur spontaneously or after treatment with dopaminergic drugs.
B. They rarely complicate treatment with anticholinergic drugs.
C. They do not worsen by infectious or metabolic derangements.
D. They are always associated with impaired insight.
E. They are always preceded by illusions.

Answer: A

287. The clinical finding most helpful to distinguish essential tremor from dystonic tremor is

A. Response to alcohol   D. Combined head, arms, and voice tremor
B. Family history of tremor   E. Isolated hand tremor
C. Isolated head tremor

Answer: D

288. Reliable clinical descriptors for dystonia are all of the following, *except*

A. Action-induced   D. Sensory trick–responsive
B. Position-dependent   E. Alcohol-responsive
C. Task-specific

Answer: E

289. Positive family history and alcohol responsiveness are

A. Core historic findings of patients with essential tremor
B. Core historic findings of patients with dystonic tremor
C. Helpful findings present about equally in patients with essential and dystonic tremor
D. Helpful findings more common in essential tremor than dystonic tremor
E. Helpful findings more common in dystonic tremor than essential tremor

Answer: C

290. Isolated head tremor is a finding most suggestive of

A. Essential tremor   D. Holmes tremor
B. Dystonic tremor   E. Parkinsonian tremor
C. Cerebellar tremor

Answer: B

291. A high-frequency tremor (>8 Hz) is seen in the following disorders, *except*

A. Holmes tremor   D. Drug-induced tremor

B. Enhanced physiologic tremor   **E.** Essential tremor
C. Orthostatic tremor

Answer: A

292. Patients with multiple system atrophy can be best distinguished from PD by the documentation of the following feature

A. Absent or poor levodopa response
B. No dyskinetic complications of levodopa therapy
C. Presence of dysautonomia
D. Presence of myoclonus
E. Presence of cognitive impairment

Answer: D

293. The most supportive neuroimaging feature for the clinical diagnosis of multiple system atrophy is

A. Caudate-predominant atrophy   **D.** Frontal lobe–predominant atrophy
B. Midbrain-predominant atrophy   **E.** Thalamic T2-weighted hyperintensity
C. Putaminal-predominant atrophy

Answer: C

294. The alien limb variant seen in the corticobasal syndrome consists of

A. Instinctive avoidance and firm grasping
B. Intermanual conflict and manual interference of the nondominant hand
C. Intermanual conflict and manual interference of the dominant hand
D. Exploratory reaching, grasping reflex, and manual groping
E. Severe grasping and intermanual conflict

Answer: A

295. All of the following signs localize to the parietal lobe and support the clinical diagnosis of corticobasal syndrome, *except*

A. Arm levitation   **D.** Exploratory reaching
B. Inability to release an object from grasp   **E.** Agraphesthesia
C. Hemihypesthesia

Answer: D

296. Progressive supranuclear palsy (PSP) pathology can arise within each of the following phenotypes, *except*

A. Primary progressive freezing of gait
B. Balint syndrome
C. Pure akinesia
D. Asymmetric parkinsonism with resting tremor
E. Corticobasal syndrome

Answer: B

297. The earliest oculomotor abnormality in progressive supranuclear palsy (PSP) is

A. Impairment of upgaze   **D.** Impaired optokinetic response
B. Impairment of downgaze   **E.** Saccadic pursuit
C. Square-wave jerks

Answer: C

298. Progressive supranuclear palsy (PSP) and corticobasal syndrome may be presenting phenotypes of frontotemporal lobar degeneration when the following additional features are present, *except*

A. Early dysexecutive dementia   **D.** Visual impairment
B. Motor neuron disease   **E.** Personality disorders
C. Language impairment

Answer: D

299. Isolated head tremor is most likely an expression of
   A. Essential tremor
   B. Dystonic tremor
   C. Cerebellar tremor
   D. Parkinson disease
   E. Psychogenic tremor
   Answer: B

300. Cervical dystonia with prominent anterocollis or laterocollis appearing in the context of parkinsonism is often indicative of
   A. Parkinson disease
   B. Progressive supranuclear palsy
   C. Multiple system atrophy
   D. Corticobasal degeneration
   E. Frontotemporal dementia with parkinsonism
   Answer: C

301. Cervical dystonia with prominent retrocollis appearing in the context of parkinsonism is often indicative of
   A. Parkinson disease
   B. Progressive supranuclear palsy
   C. Multiple system atrophy
   D. Corticobasal degeneration
   E. Frontotemporal dementia with parkinsonism
   Answer: B

302. Paroxysmal retrocollis is a clinical hallmark of
   A. Tardive dystonia   D. Rapid-onset dystonia parkinsonism
   B. Tardive dyskinesia   E. Lubag disease (sex-linked dystonia parkinsonism)
   C. Acute dystonic reaction
   Answer: A

303. In a 26-year-old man who has had hypotonia at birth, dystonia in childhood, and macrocephaly and whose neuroimaging studies show relative frontotemporal atrophy with increased subarachnoid spaces, you suspect that his diagnosis of cerebral palsy should be revised to
   A. Lesch-Nyhan syndrome   D. Argininemia
   B. Pyruvate dehydrogenase deficiency   E. Cytochrome oxidase deficiency
   C. Glutaric aciduria type 1
   Answer: C

304. In a 14-year-old boy with athetoid "cerebral palsy," you identified marked abnormalities in the brain MRI, including agenesis of the corpus callosum agenesis and cystic lesions in the basal ganglia, cerebellum, and brainstem. You suspect the correct diagnosis is
   A. Lesch-Nyhan syndrome   D. Argininemia
   B. Pyruvate dehydrogenase deficiency   E. Cytochrome oxidase deficiency
   C. Glutaric aciduria type 1
   Answer: B

305. The discovery of retinitis pigmentosa in a 24-year-old woman with sensory ataxia and areflexia, previously suspected of having Friedreich ataxia, most likely indicate
   A. Vitamin E deficiency   D. Refsum disease
   B. Abetalipoproteinemia   E. Kearns-Sayre syndrome
   C. Aceruloplasminemia
   Answer: A

306. The most important cause of disability and death in Friedreich ataxia is

A. Progressive scoliosis
B. Diabetes mellitus
C. Cardiomyopathy
D. Dysphagia
E. Postural impairment and falls

Answer: C

307. Proprioceptive loss and Romberg sign is a feature of the following ataxic syndromes, *except*

A. Copper deficiency
B. Nitrous oxide myeloneuropathy
C. HIV myelopathy
D. Ataxia–telangiectasia
E. Miller Fisher syndrome

Answer: D

308. A 49-year-old wheelchair-bound man developed sudden-onset left hemiparesis, dysarthria, and diplopia. Several months later he developed a progressively disabling left arm tremor. Examination showed skew deviation, left hemiparesis, left hemianesthesia, truncal ataxia, palatal tremor, worse on the left distal soft palate, and a postural and action proximal left arm tremor. The lesion is most likely located in

A. Left superior cerebellar peduncle with right olivary pseudohypertrophy
B. Left pons or upper medulla with left olivary pseudohypertrophy
C. Right superior cerebellar peduncle with left olivary pseudohypertrophy
D. Right pons or upper medulla with right olivary pseudohypertrophy
E. Left dentate nucleus with right olivary pseudohypertrophy

Answer: D

309. A palatal tremor is suspected to be essential rather than symptomatic when

A. It is present in the distal rather than proximal soft palate
B. Tremor may extend into the vocal cords and ocular muscles
C. It remains active during sleep
D. It is of sudden onset
E. Ear clicks are reported

Answer: E

310. All of the following disorders can be associated with increased T1-weighted hyperintensity in the basal ganglia, *except*

A. Wilson disease
B. Chorea–acanthocytosis
C. Acquired hepatolenticular degeneration
D. Manganese transporter deficiency
E. Ephedronic encephalopathy due to methcathinone toxicity

Answer: B

311. Chorea may be associated with the following paraneoplastic/autoimmune antibodies, *except*

A. Anti-CRMP5 antibodies
B. Anti–N-methyl-D-aspartate receptor antibodies
C. Anti-Ma antibodies
D. Anti-Hu antibodies
E. Antiphosphatidylserine antibodies

Answer: C

312. A 59-year-old man was evaluated for a 6-month history of left eye blinking followed by upper face twitching and continuous facial discomfort without pain. On examination, the movements, which were present during sleep, had tonic and myoclonic components that partially attenuated but not disappeared during volitional tasks. The myoclonic component between the perioral and periocular region was not synchronous. The rest of the neurological examination was normal. The best next step is to

A. Proceed with chemodenervation of involved facial muscles
B. Obtain a brain MRI
C. Obtain a nerve conduction study of the facial nerve
D. Obtain an electromyographic study of the facial nerve
E. Obtain an EEG

Answer: E

313. The most important screening test for a 54-year-old man with a 6-year history of progressive motor tics, chorea, tongue thrusting when chewing, cognitive impairment, peripheral neuropathy, and areflexia is

A. Blood count and smear
B. Serum uric acid
C. Serum copper and ceruloplasmin
D. Slitlike lamp examination
E. EMG and NCV

Answer: A

314. A 60-year-old homeless man, with prior history of schizophrenia and cocaine abuse, is taken to the ER within 7 days of a prior evaluation for psychotic bout. He had retrocollis, jaw-opening dystonia, and right arm dystonia, with internal rotation and wrist flexion. Of the drugs given 7 days previously, which one may have backfired?

A. Dextrose administration followed by thiamine
B. Meperidine administration in the setting of ongoing treatment with bupropion
C. Oxycodone in the setting of prior cocaine exposure
D. Haloperidol in the setting of prior cocaine exposure
E. Lorazepam in the setting of prior cocaine exposure

Answer: D

315. Which is the only opioid that can be given safely in an acute setting for someone at risk for serotonin syndrome?

A. Oxycodone
B. Meperidine
C. Morphine
D. Hydrocodone
E. Fentanyl

Answer: C

316. A 43-year-old man complains of hearing loss and constriction of the visual fields. On examination, he had cerebellar ataxia, postural and action tremor, and stocking–glove hypesthesia, developing over several years. These deficits point in the direction of a/an

A. Autoimmune etiology: anti-GAD antibodies
B. Chronic toxic etiology: mercury poisoning
C. Iatrogenic etiology: chronic phenytoin treatment
D. Paraneoplastic etiology: anti-Hu antibodies
E. Metabolic etiology: vitamin E deficiency

Answer: B

317. A 24-year-old woman with sensory ataxia, areflexia, and mild scoliosis is suspected of having Friedreich ataxia. However, her fundi showed abnormally pigmented retina. The clinician should suspect which Friedreich ataxia–like disorder?

A. Neurologic celiac disease
B. Vitamin B_{12} deficiency
C. Refsum disease
D. Abetalipoproteinemia
E. Biotinidase deficiency

Answer: D

318. In North America, the most common "pure" form of autosomal dominant spinocerebellar ataxia (SCA) is

A. SCA 1
D. SCA 6

B. SCA 2
C. SCA 3

E. SCA 8

Answer: D

319. Spinocerebellar ataxia type 3 (SCA 3) can present with any of the following, *except*

A. Parkinsonism
B. Dystonia
C. Chorea

D. Myoclonus
E. Spasticity

Answer: D

320. Familial ataxias that can mimic Parkinson disease at some stage include all of the following, *except*

A. SCA 1
B. SCA 2
C. SCA 3

D. SCA 12
E. SCA 18

Answer: E

321. The following oculomotor findings may be documented in a patient with SCA 3, *except*

A. Square-wave jerks
B. Downbeat nystagmus
C. Gaze-evoked nystagmus

D. Slow saccades
E. Supranuclear gaze palsy

Answer: B

322. Besides ataxia, the following feature would greatly support the diagnosis of MSA if present

A. Inspiratory stridor
B. Brachial dystonia
C. High-amplitude tremor

D. Cognitive impairment
E. Cortical sensory loss

Answer: A

323. The diagnostic suspicion of MSA-C in a 63-year-old man with ataxia and early dysautonomia may instead need revision into fragile X tremor–ataxia syndrome (FXTAS) if any of the following features are present, *except*

A. Postural and action tremor
B. Cognitive impairment
C. Downgaze nystagmus

D. Hyperintensity in the middle cerebellar peduncle
E. Generalized cerebral atrophy

Answer: C

324. Supranuclear gaze palsy associated with ataxia should suggest any of the following, *except*

A. Tay-Sachs disease
B. Niemann-Pick type C
C. Gaucher disease

D. Spinocerebellar ataxia type 3
E. Spinocerebellar ataxia type 6

Answer: E

325. A 16-year-old boy with ataxia and supranuclear gaze palsy is suspected of having Niemann-Pick type C. Which feature would strongly favor a diagnostic switch from this disorder to cerebrotendinous xanthomatosis?

A. Peripheral neuropathy
B. Seizures
C. Cataracts

D. Upper motor neuron pattern of weakness
E. Chorea

Answer: C

326. Ataxia–telangiectasia can be suspected in a patient with neither ataxia nor telangiectasia if

A. Chorea is associated with increased CK
B. Chorea is associated with abnormal liver function tests

    C. Dystonia is associated with hypoalbuminemia
    D. Dystonia is associated with IgA deficiency
    E. Myoclonus is associated with increased BUN and creatinine

    Answer: D

327. A patient with alexia without agraphia may have any of the following associated findings, *except*

    A. Impaired visual confrontation naming of concrete entities, colors, and actions
    B. Impaired acquisition of declarative verbal material
    C. Visual object agnosia
    D. Prosopagnosia
    E. Color agnosia

    Answer: D

328. Hyperintensity in any or all of the following regions suggest Wernicke encephalopathy, *except*

    A. Superior cerebellar vermis   **D.** Middle cerebellar peduncles
    B. Dorsomedial thalamus   **E.** Brainstem tegmentum
    C. Mamillary bodies

    Answer: D

329. Which of the following regions affected by Wernicke encephalopathy is always spared in Wernicke-like presentation of Leigh syndrome?

    A. Superior cerebellar vermis   **D.** Middle cerebellar peduncles
    B. Dorsomedial thalamus   **E.** Brainstem tegmentum
    C. Mamillary bodies

    Answer: C

330. Which extraneurological manifestations may develop in individuals with B_1 deficiency?

    A. Glucose intolerance   **D.** Liver insufficiency
    B. Congestive heart failure   **E.** Pancreatic insufficiency
    C. Gastroparesis

    Answer: B

331. Chronic alcoholism has been associated with all of the following, *except*

    A. Wernicke encephalopathy   **D.** Central pontine myelinolysis
    B. Foix-Chavany-Marie syndrome   **E.** Cerebellar degeneration
    C. Marchiafava-Bignami disease

    Answer: B

332. A case of postencephalitic parkinsonism is strengthened when any of the following are present, *except*

    A. Oculogyric crisis   **D.** Thalamic hyperintensities on brain MRI
    B. Obsessive–compulsive behaviors   **E.** Sleep–wake inversion
    C. Hiccups

    Answer: D

333. Response to levodopa in patients with postencephalitic parkinsonism is most favorable when the brain MRI demonstrates lesions in

    A. Substantia nigra only   **D.** Putamen and caudate nucleus
    B. Substantia nigra and putamen   **E.** Putamen and pallidum
    C. Putamen only

    Answer: A

334. Which of the following is the most common arthropod-borne human encephalitis worldwide is also the most common cause of postencephalitic parkinsonism.

    A. Epstein-Barr virus   **D.** Japanese B encephalitis

B. ECHO virus 25   **E.** Coxsackie B3 and B4

C. St. Louis encephalitis

Answer: D

335. Cortical or cerebral blindness may be caused by any of the following, *except*

  A. Heidenhain variant of Creutzfeldt-Jakob disease

  B. Adrenoleukodystrophy

  C. Chronic methyl mercury poisoning

  D. Bismuth-induced encephalopathy

  E. Eclampsia

Answer: D

336. A form of corticobasal syndrome, presenting with a sensory or parietal form of alien limb syndrome (withdrawal or avoidance of the nondominant hand) is most often the result of

  A. Corticobasal degeneration   **D.** Frontotemporal dementia

  B. Alzheimer disease   **E.** Paraneoplastic encephalopathy

  C. Creutzfeldt-Jakob disease

Answer: C

337. Development of hemichorea or hemiballism in a patient with HIV is most often indicative of which of the following complications?

  A. Primary CNS lymphoma   **D.** Histoplasmosis

  B. Toxoplasmosis   **E.** Progressive multifocal leukoencephalopathy

  C. Cryptococcal meningitis

Answer: B

338. The following features are typical of a patient affected with benign positional paroxysmal vertigo, *except*

  A. Torsional nystagmus

  B. Latency of seconds between position change and nystagmus

  C. Fatigability of the vertigo after repeating the triggering position

  D. Nystagmus is suppressible with fixation.

  E. Fast phase of the nystagmus follows direction of gaze.

Answer: E

339. The following features are typical of a patient with Ménière disease, *except*

  A. Torsional nystagmus

  B. Loud noises may induce transient vertigo.

  C. The fast phase of the nystagmus is toward the abnormal ear.

  D. Nystagmus is suppressible with fixation.

  E. Direction of nystagmus changes on eccentric gaze.

Answer: E

340. If the rhythmic contractions of the face and palate shown in the case of epilepsia partialis continua were to be slightly slower (~1 Hz), a lesion in which of the following structures could be suspected?

  A. Contralateral superior cerebellar peduncle

  B. Contralateral central tegmental tract

  C. Contralateral dentate nucleus

  D. Ispilateral dentate nucleus

  E. Ipsilateral red nucleus

Answer: A

341. A 67-year-old man is evaluated for bizarre nocturnal movement reminiscent of dream enactment behaviors, with repetitive kicking and shouting, about which he is amnestic.

Routine EEG is normal. Polysomnographic evidence shows that these episodes occur more frequently in stage 2 of sleep. The most likely diagnosis is

A. Psychogenic movement disorder
B. REM sleep behavior disorder
C. Sleep terror
D. Confusional arousals
E. Frontal lobe epilepsy

Answer: E

342. Which of the following behaviors would **not** support the diagnosis of nocturnal frontal lobe seizures?

A. Ambulation
B. Pelvic thrusting
C. Genital manipulation
D. Paroxysmal arousals
E. Repetitive vocalization

Answer: D

343. Which of the following events **never** lead to a neurally mediated syncope?

A. Cough
B. Swallowing
C. Chiropractic manipulation
D. Light therapy
E. Urination

Answer: D

344. A 56-year-old man with hypertension and diabetes has developed fainting episodes following prolonged coughing spells. The intervention most likely to benefit is

A. Chest X-ray to evaluate for respiratory problems
B. EKG to evaluate for cardiac conduction abnormalities
C. Replace lisinopril with another antihypertensive drug
D. Replace Glucophage with another hypoglycemic drug
E. Treat cough symptomatically with guaifenesin

Answer: C

345. A 65-year-old man with progressive gait impairment may not have Parkinson disease if his gait examination shows

A. Festination
B. Wide base
C. Freezing of gait
D. Trembling in place
E. Dystonic foot

Answer: B

346. The most likely underlying neuropathology in the brain of a 67-year-old woman with a 4-year history of progressive gait impairment leading to frequent episodes of gait freezing but without rigidity, tremor, bradykinesia, or any other impairment (including a normal oculomotor exam) is

A. Parkinson disease
B. Corticobasal degeneration
C. Progressive supranuclear palsy
D. Multiple system atrophy
E. Vascular parkinsonism

Answer: C

347. The following disorder is not typically associated with a lower-body parkinsonism

A. Binswanger disease
B. Posterior reversible encephalopathy syndrome
C. Cerebral autosomal dominant arteriopathy with subcortical infarcts and leukoencephalopathy (CADASIL)
D. Enlarged Virchow-Robin perivascular spaces
E. Frontal lobe meningioma

Answer: B

348. One of the most important clinical findings predicting lack of response to cerebrospinal fluid (CSF) diversion is

A. Impaired postural reflexes
B. Hyperreflexia
C. Wide-based gait
D. Dysexecutive cognitive impairment
E. Early neurogenic bladder

Answer: A

349. The onset of motor complications in Parkinson disease is driven primarily by

A. Duration of levodopa exposure
B. Cumulative exposure to levodopa
C. Amount of levodopa per dose
D. Disease duration
E. Prior use of dopamine agonists

Answer: D

350. The "fear" of development of levodopa-induced dyskinesias in patients with Parkinson disease should not prevent efforts to titrate the dose to optimize motor function because

A. Levodopa-induced dyskinesias are a rare occurrence.
B. Levodopa-induced dyskinesias are predominantly nontroublesome.
C. Levodopa-induced dyskinesias contribute less to impairing quality of life than rigidity and bradykinesia.
D. A and B
E. B and C

Answer: E

351. Which of the following disorders is a true cause of focal dystonia (rather than pseudo-dystonia) in adults?

A. Carpopedal spasm
B. Reflex sympathetic dystrophy
C. Stiff person syndrome
D. Parkinson disease
E. Cramp–fasciculation syndrome

Answer: D

352. A reliable feature of dystonic gait is the improvement in gait with

A. Botulinum toxin injections
B. Backward walking
C. Double tasking
D. Anticholinergic drugs
E. Prosthetic apparatuses

Answer: B

353. The most common pattern of isolated psychogenic gait impairment is

A. Astasia–abasia
B. Excessive slowness of gait
C. Knee buckling
D. Dystonic gait
E. Bizarre gait

Answer: C

354. The diagnosis of psychogenic movement disorders can be based with accuracy only with

A. Applying established clinical criteria
B. After ruling out potential organic disorders
C. After ruling out psychiatric comorbidities
D. After serially evaluating the patient
E. After confirming the disorder normalizes when the patient is unobserved

Answer: A

355. Increased T2-weighted and FLAIR signal in the mesial temporal lobes is most often due to which paraneoplastic disorder?

A. Anti–CRMP-5
B. Anti-Hu
C. Anti-Ri
D. Anti-Ma
E. Anti-Yo

Answer: B

356. Increased T2-weighted and FLAIR signal in the striatum is most often due to which paraneoplastic disorder?

A. Anti–CRMP-5
B. Anti-Hu
C. Anti-Ri
D. Anti-Ma
E. Anti-Yo

Answer: A

357. Paraneoplastic cerebellar degeneration associated with adenocarcinomas of the breast is most common due to which paraneoplastic disorder?

A. Anti–CRMP-5
B. Anti-Hu
C. Anti-Ri
D. Anti-Ma
E. Anti-Yo

Answer: C

358. A 63-year-old homeless man with history of schizophrenia was given haloperidol during his most recent emergency room evaluation. His risk of returning to the emergency room with an acute dystonic reaction within a week is increased 40-fold because he

A. Was not given prophylactic treatment with benztropine
B. Did not comply with haloperidol treatment as outpatient
C. Used metoclopramide as antiemetic
D. Had prior history of cocaine abuse
E. Had family history of parkinsonism

Answer: D

359. A 67-year-old woman was noted to have difficulties with driving, misjudging the distance from other cars and getting lost in previously familiar routes. During an episode of urinary tract infection, she developed paranoia and hallucinations, which was worsened after the administration of quetiapine. This patient's most likely diagnosis is

A. Delirium
B. Vascular dementia
C. Dementia with Lewy bodies
D. Frontotemporal dementia
E. Alzheimer disease

Answer: C

360. Which of the following drugs can acutely worsen restless leg syndrome?

A. Clonazepam
B. Methadone
C. Gabapentin
D. Propoxyphene
E. Diphenhydramine

Answer: E

361. In a patient with restless leg syndrome and comorbid renal insufficiency, the best first-line drug for his symptomatic treatment is

A. Pramipexole
B. Ropinirole
C. Clonazepam
D. Oxycodone
E. Propoxyphene

Answer: B

362. Loss or alteration of motor or sensory function, not intentionally produced to resolve an unacceptable but obvious conflict (external gain) is most likely due to which of the following disorders?

A. Malingering
B. Conversion disorder
C. Factitious disorder
D. Somatization disorder
E. Hypochondriasis

Answer: B

363. Excessive preoccupation with the fear of having a serious disease based on misinterpretation of symptoms and despite negative investigations and reassurances to the contrary, without obvious external gain or voluntary production of symptoms is most likely due to which of the following disorders?

A. Malingering
B. Conversion disorder
C. Factitious disorder
D. Somatization disorder
E. Hypochondriasis

Answer: E

364. Excessive and persistent concern about multiple somatic complaints for which there is neither secondary gain nor intentional production of symptoms but deep conviction of illness is indicative of which of the following disorders?

A. Malingering
B. Conversion disorder
C. Factitious disorder
D. Somatization disorder
E. Hypochondriasis

Answer: D

365. The diagnosis of psychogenic tremor can be made with clinically definite diagnostic certainty if

A. It disappears when patients are unobserved
B. Laboratory and imaging evaluations are normal
C. Clinical criteria are applied
D. Clear stressor is identified at or before the onset of the tremor
E. Psychiatric comorbidity is present

Answer: C

366. Which of the following clinical features does not assist in the diagnosis of psychogenic tremor?

A. Disappearance with distracting maneuvers
B. Persistence during walking
C. Cocontraction sign
D. Entrainment of tremor rate
E. Variability of tremor amplitude

Answer: B

367. The classic anterograde amnesia of anoxic encephalopathy after cardiac arrest results from which of the following?

A. Systemic inflammatory response
B. Watershed cortical infarcts
C. Postischemic neurodegeneration
D. Loss of pyramidal cells in the CA1 region of the hippocampi
E. Gliosis of the mammillary bodies

Answer: D

368. A neurologist should be mindful that Chvostek and Trousseau signs can appear within the context of treatment with phenobarbital, phenytoin, carbamazepine, foscarnet, and cimetidine by virtue of their development of iatrogenic

A. Hyperphosphatemia
B. Hypophosphatemia
C. Hypocalcemia
D. Hypercalcemia
E. Hypermagnesemia

Answer: C

369. Carpopedal spasm or tetany in the setting of high PTH and phosphorus may result from any of the following disorders, *except*

A. Pseudohypoparathyroidism
B. Rhabdomyolysis
C. Tumor lysis syndrome
D. Liver insufficiency
E. Renal insufficiency

Answer: D

370. The range of pathology associated with antibodies to voltage-gated potassium channels (VGKC) includes the following, *except*

A. Acquired neuromyotonia

B. Lambert-Eaton myasthenic syndrome

C. Morvan syndrome

D. Limbic encephalitis

E. Faciobrachial dystonic seizures

Answer: B

371. The same voltage-gated potassium channels (VGKC) functionally blocked by antibodies in neuromyotonia can also be blocked by which toxin?

A. Dendrotoxin

B. Conotoxin

C. Tetrodotoxin

D. Saxitoxin

E. Ziconotide

Answer: A

372. The vascular supply of the putamen arises from which of the following vessels?

A. Lenticulostriate arteries

B. Artery of Percheron

C. Posterior choroidal artery

D. Anterior choroidal artery

E. Basilar artery bifurcation

Answer. A

373. A 52-year-old woman with "Parkinson disease" demonstrates, within 3 years from symptom onset, reddish, mottled hands; anterocollis; and inspiratory stridor. Her most likely diagnosis is

A. Progressive supranuclear palsy

B. Corticobasal degeneration

C. Multiple system atrophy

D. Vascular parkinsonism

E. Perry syndrome

Answer: C

INDEX

A

Abducens nerve palsy, 168–169
Abetalipoproteinemia, 314
Absence seizures, 275, 304
Accessory nerve palsy, 285
Acetazolamide, cerebrospinal fluid suppression, 295
Acetylcholinesterase inhibitor, Alzheimer disease
    management, 64, 65
Acquired amusia, 308
Acute dystonic reaction, 133–135
Acyclovir, 178, 303
Adie tonic pupil, 161–162
Adrenoleukodystrophy, 300
Adult-onset focal dystonias, 306
AICA. *See* Anterior inferior cerebellar artery
AION. *See* Anterior ischemic optic neuropathy
Akinetic mutism, 309
Alcoholic neuropathy, 300
Alexia, 55–56, 96–98, 316
Alien hand syndrome, 54–55
Alien limb phenomenon, 305
ALS. *See* Amyotrophic lateral sclerosis
Alzheimer disease
    aphasia, 296
    diagnosis, 288
    early disease, 62–64
    late disease, 64–66
    neurofibrillary tangle localization, 288
    positron emission tomography, 285
Amantadine, progressive supranuclear palsy
    management, 117
Amitriptyline
    progressive supranuclear palsy management, 117
    sensory neuronopathy management, 14
Amnesia, 60–61
Amyotrophic lateral sclerosis, 22, 274, 275
Angiitis, 260–261
Anosognosia, 277
Anoxic encephalopathy, 321
Anterior cerebral artery, watershed infarcts, 85
Anterior inferior cerebellar artery, 137
Anterior interosseous neuropathy, 2, 284
Anterior ischemic optic neuropathy, 163–164, 306
Anterior opercular syndrome, 58–59
Anterograde amnesia, 61, 309–310
Anticholinergics, acute dystonic reaction
    management, 135
Antiepileptic drugs
    epilepsia partialis continua management, 216
    partial complex seizure management,
        211–213
Anti-glutamic acid decarboxylase antibodies, 307

Antiphospholipid antibody syndrome
    arterial thrombosis, 83
    cerebral infarctions, 82–83
    ischemic myelopathy, 36–38
    posterior cerebral artery occlusion, 172–174
APAS. *See* Antiphospholipid antibody syndrome
Aphasia
    Alzheimer disease, 296
    evaluation test, 47
    left frontal infarction, 41–44
    left internal carotid artery occlusion, 44–45
    left middle cerebral artery infarction, 48–49
    left posterior temporal infarction, 46–47
    primary progressive aphasia, 50–51
Arsenic toxicity, 305
Arterial thrombosis, 83
Arthropod-borne human encephalitis, 316–317
Aseptic meningitis, 178–180, 294
Aspirin, stroke risk reduction, 76
Asymptomatic carotid artery stenosis, 70–71
Ataxia
    cerebellar ataxia, 141–142
    Friedreich ataxia, 138–140
    hereditary ataxia, 143–144
    lipid storage ataxia, 149–150
    multiple sclerosis, 153–155
    posterior inferior cerebellar artery infarction,
        136–137
    sensory ataxia, 303
Ataxia–telangiectasia, 315–316
Ataxic hemiparesis, 77–78
Atrial fibrillation, stroke risks, 76
Atypical facial pain, 206–207
Autoantibodies
    antiphospholipid antibody syndrome (*See*
        Antiphospholipid antibody syndrome)
    calcium voltage channel antibodies in Lambert-
        Eaton myasthenic syndrome, 303
    myasthenia gravis, 24
    paraneoplastic cerebellar degeneration, 304
Autoimmune myelopathy, 33–35
Autosomal dominant primary dystonia, 119
Autosomal recessive and X-linked dystonias, 119
Azathioprine, myositis management, 265
AZT. *See* Zidovudine

B

Baclofen, spasticity management, 231
Bacterial meningitis, 293, 294
Basilar artery
    aneurysm, 281
    stenosis, 72–73, 279

Behavioral variant of frontotemporal dementia, 52–53
Bell's palsy, 7–8, 305
Benign paroxysmal positional vertigo, 186
  classical presentation, 191
  clinical features, 281–282, 317
  Dix–Hallpike maneuver, 191
  Epley maneuver, 191–193
  management, 190
  nystagmus, 193
  vertigo, 186
Benzodiazepines, spasticity management, 231
Benztropine, neuroleptic-induced acute dystonic
      reaction management, 134
Bilateral carpal tunnel, 1–2
Bilateral internuclear ophthalmoplegia, 151–153
Bilateral parietooccipital infarcts, 280
Blepharospasm, 306
Botulinum toxin
  cervical dystonia management, 120, 122
  essential tremor management, 105
  progressive supranuclear palsy management, 117
  spasticity management, 285
  tic disorder management, 131
BPPV. See Benign paroxysmal positional vertigo
Brachial plexus, 10–11. See also Parsonage-Turner
      syndrome
  anatomy, 269–270
  magnetic resonance imaging, 269
  neoplastic brachial plexopathy, 269–270
Brain death, 287
Brainstem, 289
Breast cancer
  neoplastic brachial plexopathy, 269–270
  paraneoplastic cerebellar degeneration, 320
  primary brain tumors, 303
Broca's aphasia, 41–45, 47, 49, 308

C

CAA. See Cerebral amyloid angiopathy
CABG. See Coronary artery bypass graft
CADASIL. See Cerebral Autosomal Dominant Arteri-
      opathy Subcortical Infarcts and Leukoen-
      cephalopathy
Callosal alien hand syndrome, 55
Callosal infarction, 305
Capgras syndrome, 310
Capsaicin, 294
Capsular lacunar infarction, 76–77
Carbamazepine
  juvenile myoclonic epilepsy management, 302
  neuropathic pain management, 14
  oral contraceptive interactions, 303
  trigeminal neuralgia management, 206
Cardiac arrest, 253–255
Cardiac tamponade, thrombolytic therapy risks, 282
Cardiac transplantation, aspergillosis, 277
Cardiomyopathy
  Friedreich's ataxia, 140, 313
  mitoxantrone toxicity, 298
Carotid artery angioplasty and stenting, 71
Carotid artery stenosis, 70–71, 285, 304
Carpal spasm, 256–257
Carpal tunnel syndrome, 1–2, 272, 280
Carpopedal spasm, 321
Cataplexy, 222
Catheter arteriography, 98, 261

Cauda equina syndrome, 298
Cavernous sinus lesion
  differential diagnosis, 166
  progressive oculomotor nerve palsy, 167–168
  third nerve palsy, 165–166
CBD. See Corticobasal degeneration
CBS. See Corticobasal syndrome
Central artery of Percheron, 279
Central pontine myelinolysis, 290
Cerebellar ataxia, 141–142, 307
Cerebellar infarction
  arterial occlusions, 137
  posterior inferior cerebellar artery, 243–244
  ventriculostomy risk, 286
Cerebellopontine angle syndrome, 187–188
Cerebral amyloid angiopathy, 91–92, 302
Cerebral angiography
  dysphagia, 75
  intracerebral hemorrhage, 91
  primary CNS angiitis, 96
  varicella-zoster virus infection, 89
Cerebral angiopathy, 57–58, 89, 91–92
Cerebral Autosomal Dominant Arteriopathy with
      Subcortical Infarcts and Leukoencepha-
      lopathy, 284
Cerebral blindness, 317
Cerebral edema, 297, 299, 304
Cerebral infarction, 89–90
Cerebral palsy, 121–122, 312
Cerebral Performance Categories Scale, 254
Cerebral vasospasm, 298
Cerebral venous thrombosis, 100
Cerebrospinal fluid
  acetazolamide suppression, 295
  aseptic meningitis, 179
  formation, 286
  leptomeningeal malignancy, 239
  lymphoma detection, 239
  multiple sclerosis diagnosis, 152, 156
  myelin basic protein elevation, 297
  primary central nervous system angiitis, 260
  resorption, 286
  sarcoidosis evaluation, 32
Cerebrotendinous xanthomatosis, 196–197, 262–263, 305
Cervical dystonia, 118–120, 306, 312
Cervical myelopathy, 31–33
Cervical syringomyelia, 27–29
Cervicocephalic arterial dissection, 79–80
Chenodeoxycholic acid, cerebrotendinous
      xanthomatosis management, 263
Chiari II malformation, 307
Chiasmal compression, 302
Chorea, 127–128, 313
Choroid plexus, 286
Chronic alcoholism, 316
Chronic hand weakness, 6
Chronic progressive external ophthalmoplegia, 170–172
Chvostek sign, 321
CJD. See Creutzfeldt–Jakob disease
Claw hand deformity, 3, 4
Clonazepam
  stiff person syndrome management, 34
  tic disorder management, 131
Clonidine, tic disorder management, 131
Clozapine, dementia with Lewy bodies management, 69
Cluster headache, 199–201, 291, 292, 306
Cobalamin deficiency, 39–40

Coma, nontraumatic, 292
Combined median and ulnar neuropathy, 5–7
Complex partial seizures, 209–211
Compound muscle action potential, 24
Computed tomography
    brachial plexus, 270
    cervicocephalic arterial dissection, 80
    cough syncope, 219
    posterior fossa ischemic stroke, 244
    spine, 38
    syringomyelia, 29
    Takayasu's arteritis, 88
Conduction aphasia, 42, 45, 47, 49, 308
Congenital myotonic dystrophy, 26
Conjunctival injection, 306
Conversion disorder, 320
    gait effects, 247–248
    speech effects, 248–250
Coronary artery bypass graft, stroke risks,
    277, 280
Corpus callosotomy, 299
Corticobasal degeneration, 110, 309
Corticobasal syndrome
    alien limb variant, 311
    clinical features, 113–114
    Creutzfeldt–Jakob disease, 317
    diagnosis, 311
    magnetic resonance imaging, 114
    Parkinson disease, 110
    phenotypes, 311
Corticosteroids
    cerebral amyloid angiopathy, 92
    epilepsia partialis continua management, 216
    Ménière disease treatment, 190
    myositis management, 265
Cough syncope, 219–220
CPEO. See Chronic progressive external
    ophthalmoplegia
CPM. See Central pontine myelinolysis
Cranial nerve palsies
    facial nerve palsy, 7–8
    hypoglossal nerve palsy, 9
    sixth nerve palsy, 168–169
    third cranial nerve
Cranial nerve palsies
    cavernous sinus mass and progressive palsy,
        167–168
    postoperative acute palsy, 164–166
Creutzfeldt–Jakob disease, 182–184, 317
CSF. See Cerebrospinal fluid
CT. See Computed tomography
CTX. See Cerebrotendinous xanthomatosis
Cyclophosphamide
    leptomeningeal malignancy management, 239
    primary CNS angiitis management, 261
Cyclosporine
    cortical blindness induction, 290
    myositis management, 265
Cytomegalovirus polyradiculopathy, 296

D

Dandy–Walker malformation, 285
Deafness, 187–188
Decerebrate posturing, 289
Decorticate posturing, 289
Dementia

early Alzheimer disease, 62–64
    hydrocephalic dementia, 287
    late Alzheimer disease, 65–66
Dementia with Lewy bodies, 110, 320
    versus Alzheimer disease, 67–68
    versus dementia, 67
    management, 68–69
    neuropsychological features, 310
    psychiatric feature, 310
    recurrent visual hallucinations, 310
Dendrotoxin, 322
Deprenyl, tic disorder management, 131
Dermatomyositis, 265
Diabetes insipidus, 304
Diabetic ketoacidosis, 124–126
Diabetic neuropathy, 301
Diazepam
    acute attacks treatment, 190
    pharmacokinetics, 287
Diffuse axonal injury, 296
Diphenhydramine
    neuroleptic-induced acute dystonic reaction
        management, 134
    Parkinson disease management, 246
    restless leg syndrome, 320
Disc herniation, 14–16, 274
Dizziness, 189–190, 275
DLB. See Dementia with Lewy bodies
Doll's eyes maneuver, 289
Donepezil, Alzheimer disease management, 64, 65
Dopamine agonists, restless legs syndrome
    management, 290
Down syndrome
    moyamoya syndrome, 86–87
    spinal cord damage and dural ectasia, 292
Dysarthria, primary progressive multiple sclerosis,
    157
Dysphagia
    motor neuron disease, 23
    moyamoya syndrome, 211
    vertebrobasilar ischemia, 74–75
Dystonia, 121
    adult-onset, 118
    childhood-onset, 118
    clinical descriptors for, 310
    focal, 118–120
    generalized, 118
    genetic types of, 119
    hemidystonia and sarcoidosis, 132–133
    management, 300
    neuroleptic-induced acute dystonic reactions,
        134–135
    segmental, 118
    treatment, 122
Dystonic gait, 234–236, 319
Dystonic tremor, 312
    clinical features, 106, 310
    versus essential tremor, 106, 108
    etiology, 106
    management of, 107
    versus parkinsonian tremor, 106

E

Edinger–Westphal nucleus, 288
Elbow, ulnar neuropathy, 3–5, 284
Electric myokymia, 257–258

Electromyography
brachial plexus, 269
carpal tunnel syndrome, 2
cobalamin deficiency, 39
disc herniation, 15
femoral neuropathy, 17
myasthenia gravis, 265
myotonic dystrophy, 26
neuromyotonia, 258
peroneal neuropathy, 21
stiff person syndrome, 35
ulnar neuropathy, 4
Emery–Dreifuss muscular dystrophy, 300
EMG. *See* Electromyography
Enhanced lumbar lordosis, 34
EPC. *See* Epilepsia partialis continua
Epidural hematoma, 302
Epilepsia partialis continua, 215–216, 317
Epilepsy, 210
absence seizures, 304
automatisms in generalized tonic-clonic seizures,
275
complex partial seizures, 276, 304
frontal lobe epilepsy, 317–318
juvenile absence epilepsy, 273
juvenile myoclonic epilepsy, 273, 302
management, 273, 275–276
prevalence, 275
Ergotamine, cluster headache management, 201
Erythrocyte sedimentation rate, vasculitis, 261
ESR. *See* Erythrocyte sedimentation rate
Essential tremor, 103
characteristic features, 104, 310
versus dystonic tremor, 310
primidone and propranolol, 105
red flags in, 107
tremorogenic drugs, 105
Ethosuximide, epilepsy management, 275–276
Expressive aprosodia, 308
Extracranial internal carotid artery dissections, 79–80

F

Fabry disease, 279
Facial nerve palsy, 7–8
Facial pain, atypical, 206–207
Famciclovir, postherpetic neuralgia management, 178
Familial ataxias, 315
Familial hypercholesterolemia, 305
Febrile status epilepticus, 286
Femoral nerve, 17
Femoral neuropathy
computed tomography, 17
electromyography, 17
versus L4 radiculopathy, 18–19
local hematoma and pseudoaneurysm, 307
MRI/MRA, 17, 18
FLE. *See* Frontal lobe epilepsy
Floppy baby, 26
Fludrocortisone
multiple system atrophy, cerebellar type
management, 148
multiple system atrophy, parkinsonian type
management, 112
Fluent aphasia, left posterior temporal infarction,
46–47

Fluphenazine, neuroleptic-induced acute dystonic
reactions, 134
Focal dystonia
adult-onset, 306
Parkinson disease, 319
Foix–Chavany–Marie syndrome, 58–59
Folic acid
neural tube defect prevention, 303
supplementation in women on antiepileptics, 212
Foot drop, 19–21, 272, 307
Forced vital capacity, motor neuron disease, 23
Fragile X syndrome, 300
FRDA. *See* Friedreich's ataxia
Friedreich's ataxia, 276, 301, 305
abetalipoproteinemia, 314
cardiomyopathy, 313
clinical presentation, 138
diagnosis, 139
MRI, 140
pathophysiology, 139–140
treatment, 140
Froment's prehensile thumb sign, 3–4
Frontal alien hand syndrome, 54–55, 309
Frontal lobe epilepsy, 217–218, 317–318
Frontotemporal dementia
behavioral variants, 53
clinical presentation, 52
genetic causes, 53
genetic mutation
motor neuron disease, 309
parkinsonism, 309
ubiquitinopathy, C9ORF72 mutation, 309
Frontotemporal lobar degeneration, 116, 309, 311
FTD. *See* Frontotemporal dementia
FVC. *See* Forced vital capacity

G

Gabapentin
atypical facial pain management, 207
neuropathic pain management, 14
Gait. *See also* Spastic gait
adult-onset dystonic, 234–236
apraxia, 224–226
conversion disorder, 247–248
hemiparkinsonian, 232–233
psychogenic, 236–237
Galantamine, Alzheimer disease management,
64, 65
Gerstmann plus syndrome, 57–58
Glasgow coma score, 287
Glatiramer acetate, multiple sclerosis management,
155
Glioblastoma multiforme, 299
Global aphasia, 42, 49
Glutaric aciduria type 1, 312
Guanfacine, tic disorder management, 131
Guillain–Barré syndrome, 273, 281, 303

H

Haloperidol
cocaine exposure, 314
neuroleptic-induced acute dystonic reactions, 134
Heerfordt syndrome, 133
HELLP syndrome, 57

Hemichorea-hemiballism, 123–125
Hemidystonia, 132–133
Hemifacial spasm, 128–129
Hemiparesis
    ataxic hemiparesis, 77–78
    lacunar stroke and pure motor hemiparesis, 76–77
Hemiparkinsonian gait, 232–233
Hemiplegic gait, 230–231
Hemopericardium, thrombolytic therapy risks, 282
Heparin, pregnancy precautions, 101
Hepatic failure *versus* portosystemic encephalopathy,
        281
Hereditary ataxia, 143–144
Herpes simplex virus
    acute sporadic encephalitis, 295
    encephalitis management, 303
    mesial temporal lobe injury, 309–310
Herpes zoster. *See* Varicella-zoster virus
HMG-CoA reductase inhibitor, cerebrotendinous
        xanthomatosis management, 263
Holmes tremor, 310–311
Holmes–Adie syndrome, 161
Horner's syndrome, 159–160, 270, 281
Human immunodeficiency virus, 296, 302, 317
Huntington's disease, 301, 305
Hutchinson sign, 294
Hydrocephalic dementia, 287
Hydrocephalus, 225, 286, 299
Hyperekplexia *versus* stiff person syndrome, 307–308
Hyperemesis gravidarum, 194–195
Hyperkinetic disorders, 133
Hypermagnesemia, 298
Hyperperfusion syndrome, 286
Hyperprolactinemia, 304
Hypertension, stroke risks, 84, 285
Hypnagogic hallucinations, 222
Hypocalcemia, 321
Hypoglossal nerve
    injury in carotid endarterectomy, 304
    palsy, 9
Hyponatremia, 300
Hypothenar atrophy, 6
Hypoxic-ischemic brain injury, 255

I

ICA. *See* Internal carotid artery
Idiopathic intracranial hypertension, 204–205
IIH. *See* Idiopathic intracranial hypertension
Indomethacin, paroxysmal hemicrania management,
        291
INO. *See* Internuclear ophthalmoplegia
Interferons, multiple sclerosis management, 155, 293
Internal carotid artery
    dissection, 79–80
    infraction, 45
    occlusion, 45
Internuclear ophthalmoplegia, 151–153, 279–280
Intracranial hemorrhage, 91
Intracranial hypertension, 282, 306
Intracranial hypotension syndrome, 201–203, 291
Intrinsic spinal cord lesions, 28
Iron deficiency anemia, 290
Isaac syndrome, 258
Ischemic myelopathy, 36–38
Isolated vestibular syndrome, 185–186

J

Japanese B encephalitis, 316–317
Juvenile absence epilepsy, 273
Juvenile myoclonic epilepsy, 273

K

Kearns–Sayre syndrome, 171
Kiloh–Nevin syndrome, 2
Knee buckling, 319
Korsakoff's syndrome, 195
KSS. *See* Kearns–Sayre syndrome

L

L5 radiculopathy, 14–16
Lacunar hemichoreoathetosis, 94–95
Lacunar infarcts, 77–78
Lacunar stroke. *See* Stroke
Lambert–Eaton myasthenic syndrome, 24, 303
Late Alzheimer disease, 65–66
Lateral medullary syndrome, 81, 159–160
Left internal carotid artery dissection, 79–80
Left posterior temporal infarction, 46–47
Leigh syndrome, 316
LEMS. *See* Lambert–Eaton myasthenic syndrome
Lennox–Gastaut syndrome, 299
Leptomeningeal malignancy, 238–239
Levodopa
    dystonia management, 300
    hemichorea-hemiballism management, 126
    hemiparkinsonian gait management, 233
    Parkinson disease management, 278
    parkinsonian variant of multiple system atrophy
            management, 112
    Parkinson's disease management, 110
Lewy bodies, 296
Lipid storage ataxia, 149–150
Liver insufficiency, 321
Liver transplantation, 290
Locked-in syndrome, 279
Lower brachial plexopathies, 7
Lower limb dystonia, 235
Lower motor neuron, 22
Lower-body parkinsonism, 224–226, 318
Lumbar myelomeningocele, 29–30
Lumbar puncture, headache, 291
Lumbar radiculopathy. *See* Disc herniation
Lymphoma, leptomeningeal, 238–239

M

Machado–Joseph disease, 145–146
Magnetic resonance angiography
    anterior opercular syndrome, 59
    Gerstmann plus syndrome, 57
Magnetic resonance imaging
    abducens nerve palsy, 169
    acute cerebellar infarction, 244
    adrenoleukodystrophy, 300
    adult-onset dystonic gait, 235
    amnesia, 60, 61
    anterior opercular syndrome, 59
    brachial plexus, 11, 269
    cavernous sinus mass lesions, 167

Magnetic resonance imaging (*Continued*)
  cerebellar atrophy, 266, 267, 268
  cerebrotendinous xanthomatosis, 263
  cervicocephalic arterial dissection, 80
  cobalamin deficiency, 39
  corticobasal syndrome, 113, 114
  Creutzfeldt–Jakob disease, 183
  dementia with Lewy bodies, 68
  disc herniation, 15
  femoral neuropathy, 17, 18
  Friedreich ataxia, 140
  Gerstmann plus syndrome, 57
  headache, 291
  hemichorea-hemiballism, 125, 126
  hemifacial spasm, 129
  lower-body parkinsonism, 224–225
  multiple sclerosis, 154–155, 301
  multiple system atrophy, parkinsonian type,
    111, 112
  Niemann-Pick type C, 150
  palatal tremor, 122, 123
  paraneoplastic chorea, 241
  peroneal neuropathy, 21
  post-cardiac arrest encephalopathy, 254
  postencephalitic parkinsonism, 181
  posterior cerebral artery infarction, 60, 61
  posterior fossa ischemic stroke, 244
  primary CNS angiitis, 97
  progressive supranuclear palsy, 116, 117
  regional atrophy, 268
  sarcoidosis, 32
  semantic dementia, 51
  spinal cord, 38
  syringomyelia, 28, 29
  Takayasu's arteritis, 88
  temporal lobe epilepsy, 211
  third nerve palsy, 167–168
  tuberous sclerosis complex, 215
  vascular parkinsonism, 227
  vertebrobasilar circulation TIA, 73
  Wernicke encephalopathy, 175
Malingering, 305
Mamillary bodies, 316
Mannitol, intracranial hypertension management,
  282
MCA. *See* Middle cerebral artery
Medial longitudinal fasciculus, 153
Medial medullary syndrome, 124
Median nerve entrapment, 1–2, 5
Medulloblastoma, 299, 305
Mees lines, 305
Memantine, Alzheimer disease management, 64
Ménière disease, 190, 281–282, 317
Meningioma, 168, 303
Meningitis
  bacterial, 294, 295
  recurrent aseptic meningitis, 178–180, 294
  viral, 196, 295
Mercury poisoning, 314
Mesial temporal lobe injury, 309–310, 319
Metabolic encephalopathy, 304
Metastasis, brain, 299
Methotrexate, myositis management, 265
Methysergide
  cluster headache management
  toxicity, 291

Mexiletine, neuropathic pain management, 14
MG. *See* Myasthenia gravis
Midazolam, acute seizure management, 286
Middle cerebral artery
  ischemic stroke, 44
  watershed infarcts, 85
  Wernicke's aphasia and infarction, 48–49
Midodrine, multiple system atrophy, parkinsonian
    type management, 112
Migraine
  pregnancy, 198–199
  stroke association, 172–174, 285
  women, 306
Migrainous infarction, 174
Mini-Mental State Examination, 64, 65
Minnesota Multiphasic Personality Inventory, 249
Misoprostol
  atypical facial pain management
  trigeminal neuralgia management in multiple
    sclerosis, 297
Mitochondrial encephalomyopathies, 171
Mitoxantrone
  multiple sclerosis management, 155
  toxicity, 298
Mixed transcortical aphasia, 308
MMSE. *See* Mini-Mental State Examination
Mobile dystonia, 132
Mollaret's meningitis, 180
Morphine, serotonin syndrome management, 314
Motor neuron disease, 22–23, 283
Moyamoya syndrome, 86–87, 276
MSA. *See* Multiple system atrophy
MSA-C. *See* Multiple system atrophy, cerebellar type
Multifocal motor neuropathy, 22
Multiple lobar hemorrhage, 91–92
Multiple sclerosis
  bilateral internuclear ophthalmoplegia, 151–153
  diagnosis, 299, 301
  forms, 288
  management, 155, 293
  nystagmus and ataxia, 153–155
  pontine lesion, 155–156
  primary progressive, 157
  primary progressive disease, 157
  spasticity
    treatment, 305
    urinary tract infection, 300
  trigeminal neuralgia management, 297
Multiple strokes, 84
Multiple system atrophy, 110
  cervical dystonia with anterocollis, 312
  diagnosis, 311
  inspiratory stridor, 315
  versus PD, 311
Multiple system atrophy, cerebellar type, 147–148,
  266–268, 315
Multiple system atrophy, parkinsonian type,
  111–112
Myasthenia gravis
  chronic progressive external ophthalmoplegia
    differential diagnosis, 171
  diagnosis and management, 265, 274
  management, 24
  mimicking disorders, 25
  myositis differential diagnosis, 264–265
  neurophysiologic studies, 24

ocular symptoms, 272, 274
serologic studies, 24
Mycophenolate, myositis management, 265
Myelin basic protein, 297
Myelodysplasia, 30
Myelominingocele, 29–30
Myelopathy, cervical sarcoid myelopathy, 31–33
Myoclonus, 298, 304
Myositis, 264–265
Myotonic dystrophy, 25–26, 272, 283–284

N

NA-AION. *See* Nonarteritic anterior ischemic optic
neuropathy
Narcolepsy, 222
Nasociliary nerve, 294
Neoplastic brachial plexopathy, 269–270
Neurally mediated syncope, 318
Neuroacanthocytosis, 299
Neurofibromtosis
pheochromocytoma, 305
type 1, 292
type 2, 296
Neuroleptic-induced acute dystonic reactions,
134–135
Neuromyotonia, 257–258
Neuropathic pain, management, 14
Neurosarcoidosis, 33
Nicotine, tic disorder management, 131
Niemann-Pick C, 149–150
Nimodipine, subarachnoid hemorrhage manage-
ment, 282
Nitrous oxide, paraparesis after anesthesia, 39–40
NKHS. *See* Nonketotic hyperosmolar state
N-methyl-D-aspartate receptor antagonist, Alzheimer
disease management, 64
Nocturnal frontal lobe seizures, 318
Nocturnal polysomnography and multiple sleep
latency, 291
Nonantipsychotic neuroleptic drugs, 134
Nonarteritic anterior ischemic optic neuropathy,
163–164
Nonfluent aphasia
left frontal infarction, 41–44
LICA occlusion, 44–45
Nonketotic hyperosmolar state, 299
Nonperisylvian aphasias, 45
Normal pressure hydrocephalus, 225–229, 294
Nortriptyline, neuropathic pain management, 14
NPC. *See* Niemann-Pick C
NPH. *See* Normal pressure hydrocephalus
Nystagmus
central *versus* peripheral, 193
multiple sclerosis, 153–155

O

Obstructive sleep apnea, 221–223, 290
Oculocephalic reflex, 289
Oculomotor brainstem syndromes, 152
Oculomotor nerve palsy
cavernous sinus mass and progressive palsy,
167–168
postoperative acute palsy, 164–166
Oculovestibular reflex, 290

Olanzapine, stroke risks, 288
Olfactory groove tumor, 299
Oligoclonal bands, 152
Oligodendrocyte, myelin synthesis, 295
Opioids
myoclonus induction, 298
serotonin syndrome, 298
Optic aphasia, 56
Optic neuritis, 288, 306
Optic neuropathy, 278
Orthostatic hypotension, 148, 268, 300
OSA. *See* Obstructive sleep apnea

P

PAGF. *See* Pure akinesia gait freezing
Palatal myoclonus, 122–124
Palatal tremor, 122–124, 313
Paraneoplastic syndrome
autoantibodies, 304
breast cancer, 320
chorea, 240–242
chorea and sensory neuronopathy, 127–128
T2-weighted and FLAIR signal, 319–320
Paraparesis, 39–40
Paresthesia, carpal tunnel syndrome, 1–2, 272
Parkinson's disease, 245–246
cardinal features, 102, 109
clinical features, 296
corticobasal syndrome, 110
dementia, 68
dementia with Lewy bodies, 110
diagnosis, 322
focal dystonia, 319
levodopa-induced dyskinesia, 319
Lewy bodies, 296
motor complications, 319
multiple system atrophy, 110
nonmotor manifestations, 109
versus NPH and vascular parkinsonism, 225
parkinsonian tremor, 102–103
progressive supranuclear palsy, 109
therapeutic options for, 110
treatment, 278, 290
Paroxysmal hemicrania, 291
Paroxysmal retrocollis, 312
Pars caudalis, 277
Parsonage–Turner syndrome, 10–11
Partial proximal median nerve injury, 7
Partial seizures
complex, 209–211
with elementary symptomatology, 211–213
PCA. *See* Posterior cerebral artery
PDD. *See* Parkinson disease dementia
PEG. *See* Percutaneous endoscopic gastrostomy
PEP. *See* Postencephalitic parkinsonism
Percutaneous endoscopic gastrostomy, motor neuron
disease patients, 23
Pergolide, tic disorder management, 131
Peripheral facial nerve palsy, 7–8
Pernicious anemia, 39–40
Peroneal neuropathy, 19–21, 272, 284
Phencyclidine, acute dystonic reaction management,
135
Phenobarbital, epilepsia partialis continua
management, 216

Phenytoin
  epilepsia partialis continua management, 216
  respiratory effects, 287
Pheochromocytoma, 305
PICA. *See* Posterior inferior cerebellar artery
PMD. *See* Psychogenic movement disorder
PME. *See* Progressive myoclonic encephalopathy
PMH. *See* Pure motor hemiparesis
Polymyositis, 264–265, 273–274
Polyneuropathy, 12–14
Pontine lesion, 155–156
Positron emission tomography, Alzheimer disease, 285
Post-cardiac arrest syndrome, 253–255
Postencephalitic parkinsonism
  arthropod-borne human encephalitis, 316–317
  cerebrospinal fluid analysis, 182
  levodopa, MRI, 316
  magnetic resonance imaging, 181, 182
Posterior alien limb syndrome, 114
Posterior cerebral artery
  alexia following stroke, 55–56, 96
  amnesia following stroke, 60–61
  anatomy, 279
  antiphospholipid antibody syndrome and
      occlusion, 172–174
  cardioembolism and exclusion, 280
  hemaniopa with macular sparing in occlusion, 280
  infarction, 45
  right homonymous hemianopsia, 172–174
  watershed infarcts, 85
Posterior cervical lymph node dissection, 285
Posterior inferior cerebellar artery
  acute infarction with early hydrocephalus,
      243–244
  infarction and ataxia, 136–137
Posterior interosseus neuropathy, 272
Posterior-variant alien hand syndrome, 55
Posttraumatic cervical syringomyelia, 27–29
PPA. *See* Primary progressive aphasia
PPFG. *See* Primary progressive freezing of gait
Prednisolone, myositis management, 265
Prednisone, postherpetic neuralgia management, 178
Preeclampsia, 2
Pregnancy
  carpal tunnel syndrome, 1–2
  heparin precautions, 101
  migraine headaches, 198–199
  neural tube defects, 303, 304
  stroke, 56–58
  warfarin precautions, 101
Primary angiitis, 97–98
Primary central nervous system angiitis, 260–261
Primary progressive aphasia, 50–51, 308
Primary progressive freezing of gait, 226
Primidone, essential tremor management, 105
Progressive gait impairment, 318
Progressive myoclonic encephalopathy, 215–216
Progressive supranuclear palsy, 278
  cervical dystonia with retrocollis, 312
  clinical presentation, 116
  magnetic resonance imaging, 116, 117
  oculomotor abnormality in, 311
  parkinsonism, 109–110
  phenotypes, 311
  treatment, 117
Propranolol, essential tremor management, 105

Proprioceptive loss, 313
Prosopagnosia, 309
Proximal myotonic myopathy, 26
Pseudobulbar palsy, 84
Pseudotumor cerebri, 306
PSP. *See* Progressive supranuclear palsy
Psychogenic gait, 236–237, 247–248, 319
Psychogenic movement disorder, 237, 319
Psychogenic stuttering, 248–250
Psychogenic tremor, 250–251, 321
Pupil, sympathetic and parasympathetic pathways,
      288
Pure akinesia gait freezing, 226
Pure motor hemiparesis, 76–77
Pure sensory stroke, 93
Putamen, 301, 322
Putaminal-predominant atrophy, 311
Pyramidal tract, 277
Pyridoxine excess, 303
Pyruvate dehydrogenase deficiency, 312

Q

Quetiapine, dementia with Lewy bodies management,
      68–69

R

Ramsay Hunt syndrome, 89–90
Relapsing-remitting multiple sclerosis, 153–155
Rendu–Osler–Weber syndrome, 276
Reserpine, tic disorder management, 131
Resting tremor, 102–103
Restless legs syndrome, 290, 291, 320
Retinal hemorrhages, 306
Retinal ischemia, 279
Retinitis pigmentosa, 312
Retrograde amnesia, 61
Retrohumeral radial neuropathy, 272
Retroperitoneal fibrosis, 291
Reverse Kiloh–Nevin syndrome, ulnar nerve, 306
Rheumatologic disease, acquired neuromyotonia,
      257–258
Richardson syndrome. *See* Progressive supranuclear
      palsy
Rivastigmine
  Alzheimer disease management, 64, 65
  dementia with Lewy bodies management, 69
Romberg sign, 313
Ropinirole
  comorbid renal insufficiency treatment, 320
  restless leg syndrome treatment, 320
Ross syndrome, 161–162
Rubella, 295

S

Sagittal sinus thrombosis, 99–101
SAH. *See* Subarachnoid hemorrhage
Sarcoidosis
  cervical myelopathy, 31–33
  hemidystonia, 132–133
  vestibulocochlear nerve involvement, 298
SCA. *See* Spinocerebellar ataxia; Superior cerebellar
      artery
Sciatica, lumbar disc disease management, 15

Sensory dissociation syndrome, 28
Sensory neuronopathy
  causes of, 12–13
  differential diagnosis, 13–14
  management, 14
  paraneoplastic syndrome, 127–128
Sildenafil, optic neuropathy risks, 279
Sixth nerve palsy, 168–169
Sleep apnea. *See* Obstructive sleep apnea
Sleep attacks, 222
Sleep paralysis, 222
Slow chorea, 132
Somatization disorder, 321
Somatoform disorders, 247–250. *See also* Conversion
  disorder
Spastic gait
  management, 231
  primary progressive multiple sclerosis, 157
  stroke, 177–178
Spasticity, 230–231
Spina bifida, 29–30
Spinal accessory nerve, 284–285
Spinal cord degeneration, 308
Spinal cord infarction, 36–38, 274, 280–281
Spinal cord injury, cervical syringomyelia, 27–29
Spinal dysraphism, 30
Spinocerebellar ataxia, 314–315
Spinocerebellar ataxia type 3, 145–146
SPS. *See* Stiff person syndrome
Statins, cerebrotendinous xanthomatosis management, 263
Steele–Richardson–Olszewski syndrome, 53
Stiff person syndrome, 33–35, 266–268
Stroke
  alexia, 96–98
  alien hand syndrome, 54–55
  amnesia, 60
  antiphospholipid antibody syndrome and cerebral
    infarctions, 82–83
  asymptomatic carotid artery stenosis, 70–71
  atherothrombosis, 286
  carotid artery stenosis, 70–71
  cerebral edema, 297
  children, 276
  coronary artery bypass grafting risks, 45,
    277, 280
  depression, 293
  Gerstmann plus syndrome, 57
  hypertension as risk factor, 84, 285
  intracerebral hemorrhage
    aneurysms and rupture, 282
    diagnosis, 297
    lobar hemorrhage and cerebral amyloid
      angiopathy, 90–92
    mortality of subarachnoid hemorrhage, 298
    thalamic hemorrhage and pure sensory stroke,
      92–93
  intracranial hypertension, 282
  lacunar stroke
    ataxic hemiparesis, 77–78
    hemichorea and hemiballismus, 95
    pure motor hemiparesis, 76–77
  migraine association, 172–174, 285
  palatal tremor due to medullary infarction,
    122–124
  posterior fossa ischemic stroke, 243–244

posterior inferior cerebellar artery infarction and
  ataxia, 136–137
pregnancy, 56–58
prognosis, 288
pseudobulbar palsy, 83–84
risk after TIA, 73
superior sagittal sinus thrombosis, 101
thalamic hemorrhage and pure sensory stroke, 93
watershed infarcts, 85
Subarachnoid hemorrhage
  aneurysms risk, 297
  cerebral vasospasm, 298
  management, 298
  misdiagnosis risk, 297
  mortality rate, 297, 298
Subdural hematoma, 302
Substance P, 294
Sumatriptan, cluster headache management, 201
Superior cerebellar artery, 137
Superior sagittal sinus thrombosis, 99–101
Supranuclear gaze palsy, 116, 315
Symptomatic palatal tremor, 123–124
Syncope, 219–220
Syringomyelia, 28–29

T

Takayasu's arteritis, 87–88
Tardive dystonia, 312
Tendon xanthoma, 263, 305
Tetanus, 294
Tetany, 256–257
Tetrabenazine, tic disorder management, 131
Thalamic hemorrhage, 93
Thallium toxicity, 305
Thenar atrophy, 6
Therapeutic hypothermia, 255
Third cranial nerve palsy, 164–166
Thrombolytic therapy
  cardiac tamponade risks, 282
  contraindications, 304
Thymectomy, myasthenia gravis management, 24
TIA. *See* Transient ischemic attack
Tic disorder, 130–131
Tinnitus, 187–188
Tissue plasminogen activator, cervicocephalic arterial
  dissection, 80
Tizanidine, spasticity management, 231
Topiramate
  cluster headache management, 201
  epilepsy management, 273
Torticollis, 118–120
Tourette syndrome, 130–131
Toxoplasmosis, 302, 317
Transcortical sensory aphasia, 308
Transient ischemic attack, 71. *See also* Stroke
  basilar artery stenosis, 72–74
  stroke risks, 73
Transtentorial herniation, 209–210
Transverse myelitis, 274
Trigeminal neuralgia, 205–206, 281, 293, 297
Trousseau signs, 321
TS. *See* Tourette syndrome
TSC. *See* Tuberous sclerosis complex
Tuberous sclerosis complex, 213–215, 292
Turcot syndrome, 305

U

Ubiquitinopathy, 309
Ulnar neuropathy, 3–5, 284, 306–307
Unruptured intracranial aneurysm, 297
Upbeat nystagmus, 174–176
Upper trunk brachial plexopathy, 10–11
Upward herniation, 286
Urinary tract infection, multiple sclerosis, 300

V

Vagus nerve stimulation, 273
Valacyclovir, postherpetic neuralgia management,
    178
Van Bogaert's disease. *See* Cerebrotendinous
    xanthomatosis
Varicella-zoster virus infection
    herpes zoster oticus, 89–90
    postherpetic neuralgia, 177–178
Vascular dementia, 62–65
Vascular parkinsonism, 225–229
Vasculitides, 88, 260–261
Vasculopathic sixth nerve palsy, 169
Vein of Galen malformation, 300
Verapamil
    cluster headache treatment, 201
    tic disorder management, 131
Vertebral artery
    dissection, 81
    stenosis, 74–75, 279
Vertebrobasilar artery dissection, 81
Vertebrobasilar circulation transient ischemic attack,
    72–74
Vertiginous dizziness, 189–190
Vertigo
    acute vestibular syndrome, 185–187
    cerebellar infarction, 275
    dizziness, 189–190
Vestibular neuritis, 188
Vestibular schwannoma, 187–188

Vestibular syndrome, 185–186
Vestibulocochlear nerve, 293–294, 298
Viral meningitis, 295
Visual evoked potentials, 299
Visuospatial disorientation and retrieval-impaired
    short-term memory loss, 310
Vitamin B$_1$ deficiency, 316
Vitamin B$_{12}$ deficiency
    causes, 301
    paraparesis after nitrous oxide anesthesia, 39–40
    sensory defect, 301
Vitamin E deficiency, 312
Voltage-gated potassium channels, 322
Von Hippel-Lindau disease, 292, 305
VZV. *See* Varicella-zoster virus

W

Wallenberg syndrome
    corneal reflex, 277
    Horner syndrome, 159–160
    vertebral artery dissection, 81
Warfarin
    antiphospholipid antibody syndrome
        management, 83
    pregnancy precautions, 101
    stroke risk reduction, 76
Watershed infarcts, 85
Wernicke aphasia, 308
Wernicke encephalopathy, 316
    hyperemesis gravidarum, 194–195
    Leigh syndrome, 316
    upbeat nystagmus, 174–176
Wernicke's aphasia, 42–44, 48–49
West syndrome, 302
Wilson disease, 290
Wrist flexion weakness, 6

Z

Zidovudine, toxicity, 303